Eosinophilic Esophagitis

Editor

IKUO HIRANO

GASTROENTEROLOGY CLINICS OF NORTH AMERICA

www.gastro.theclinics.com

Consulting Editor
GARY W. FALK

June 2014 • Volume 43 • Number 2

ELSEVIER

1600 John F. Kennedy Boulevard ● Suite 1800 ● Philadelphia, Pennsylvania, 19103-2899
http://www.theclinics.com

GASTROENTEROLOGY CLINICS OF NORTH AMERICA Volume 43, Number 2
June 2014 ISSN 0889-8553, ISBN-13: 978-0-323-29921-3

Editor: Kerry Holland
Developmental Editor: Susan Showalter

Gastroenterology Clinics of North America (ISSN 0889-8553) is published quarterly by Elsevier Inc., 360 Park Avenue South, New York, NY 10010-1710. Months of issue are March, June, September, and December. Business and Editorial Offices: 1600 John F. Kennedy Blvd., Suite 1800, Philadelphia, PA 19103-2899. Customer Service Office: 6277 Sea Harbor Drive, Orlando, FL 32887-4800. Periodicals postage paid at New York, NY and additional mailing offices. Subscription prices are $320.00 per year (US individuals), $160.00 per year (US students), $530.00 per year (US institutions), $350.00 per year (Canadian individuals), $651.00 per year (Canadian institutions), $445.00 per year (international individuals), $220.00 per year (international students), and $651.00 per year (international institutions). Foreign air speed delivery is included in all *Clinics* subscription prices. All prices are subject to change without notice. **POSTMASTER:** Send address changes to *Gastroenterology Clinics of North America*, Elsevier Health Sciences Division, Subscription Customer Service, 3251 Riverport Lane, Maryland Heights, MO 63043. Telephone: 1-800-654-2452 (U.S. and Canada); 314-447-8871 (outside U.S. and Canada). Fax: 314-447-8029. E-mail: journalscustomerservice-usa@elsevier.com (for print support); journalsonlinesupport-usa@elsevier.com (for online support).

Reprints. For copies of 100 or more, of articles in this publication, please contact the Commercial Reprints Department, Elsevier Inc., 360 Part Avenue South, New York, New York 10010-1710. Tel. 212-633-3874, Fax: 212-633-3820, E-mail: reprints@elsevier.com.

Gastroenterology Clinics of North America is also published in Italian by Il Pensiero Scientifico Editore, Rome, Italy; and in Portuguese by Interlivros Edicoes Ltda., Rua Commandante Coelho 1085, 21250 Cordovil, Rio de Janeiro, Brazil.

Gastroenterology Clinics of North America is covered in *MEDLINE/PubMed (Index Medicus)*, *Excerpta Medica*, *Current Contents/Clinical Medicine*, *Science Citation Index*, *ISI/BIOMED*, and *BIOSIS*.

Contributors

CONSULTING EDITOR

GARY W. FALK, MD, MS
Professor of Medicine, Division of Gastroenterology, Hospital of the University of Pennsylvania, University of Pennsylvania Perelman School of Medicine, Philadelphia, Pennsylvania

EDITOR

IKUO HIRANO, MD
Director, Esophageal Center; Professor of Medicine, Division of Gastroenterology, Northwestern University Feinberg School of Medicine, Chicago, Illinois

AUTHORS

SEEMA S. ACEVES, MD, PhD
Associate Professor, Division of Allergy and Immunology, Departments of Pediatrics and Medicine, University of California, San Diego, Rady Children's Hospital, San Diego, La Jolla, California

JEFFREY A. ALEXANDER, MD, FACP
Associate Professor of Medicine, Division of Gastroenterology and Hepatology, Mayo Clinic School of Medicine, Mayo Clinic, Rochester, Minnesota

STEPHEN E. ATTWOOD, FRCS
North Tyneside Hospital, North Shields, United Kingdom

PAUL J. BRYCE, PhD
Associate Professor, Division of Allergy-Immunology, Department of Medicine, Feinberg School of Medicine, Northwestern University, Chicago, Illinois

EDAIRE CHENG, MD
Assistant Professor, Departments of Pediatrics and Internal Medicine, Esophageal Diseases Center, Children's Medical Center, VA North Texas Health Care System, University of Texas Southwestern Medical Center, Dallas, Texas

MARGARET H. COLLINS, MD
Professor of Pathology, Division of Pathology and Laboratory Medicine, Cincinnati Children's Hospital Medical Center, Cincinnati, Ohio

EMILY M. CONTRERAS, MD
Assistant Professor of Clinical Pediatrics, Division of Pediatric Gastroenterology, Hepatology, and Nutrition, Department of Pediatrics, Riley Hospital for Children, Indiana University School of Medicine, Indianapolis, Indiana

EVAN S. DELLON, MD, MPH
Division of Gastroenterology and Hepatology, Department of Medicine, Center for Esophageal Diseases and Swallowing, Center for Gastrointestinal Biology and Disease, University of North Carolina School of Medicine, Chapel Hill, North Carolina

GARY W. FALK, MD, MS
Professor of Medicine, Division of Gastroenterology, Hospital of the University of Pennsylvania, University of Pennsylvania Perelman School of Medicine, Philadelphia, Pennsylvania

GLENN T. FURUTA, MD
Director, Gastrointestinal Eosinophilic Diseases Program, Children's Hospital Colorado; Professor of Pediatrics, University of Colorado School of Medicine, Aurora, Colorado

LAURA M. GOBER, MD
Division of Allergy, Immunology, and Infectious Diseases; Attending Physician, Center for Pediatric Eosinophilic Disorders, The Children's Hospital of Philadelphia, Philadelphia, Pennsylvania

NIRMALA GONSALVES, MD
Associate Professor of Medicine, Division of Gastroenterology & Hepatology, Northwestern University-Feinberg School of Medicine, Chicago, Illinois

SANDEEP K. GUPTA, MD
Professor of Clinical Pediatrics and Clinical Medicine, Division of Pediatric Gastroenterology, Hepatology, and Nutrition, Department of Pediatrics, Riley Hospital for Children, Indiana University School of Medicine, Indianapolis, Indiana

IKUO HIRANO, MD
Director, Esophageal Center; Professor of Medicine, Division of Gastroenterology, Northwestern University Feinberg School of Medicine, Chicago, Illinois

AMIR F. KAGALWALLA, MD
Associate Professor of Pediatrics, Division of Gastroenterology, Hepatology & Nutrition, Ann & Robert H. Lurie Children's Hospital of Chicago, Northwestern University-Feinberg School of Medicine, Chicago, Illinois

DAVID A. KATZKA, MD
Professor of Medicine, Division of Gastroenterology and Hepatology, Mayo Clinic, Rochester, Minnesota

CHRIS A. LIACOURAS, MD
Co-Director of the Center for Pediatric Eosinophilic Disorders; Division of Gastroenterology, Hepatology and Nutrition, The Children's Hospital of Philadelphia; Professor of Pediatrics, Perelman School of Medicine, University of Pennsylvania, Philadelphia, Pennsylvania

CALMAN PRUSSIN, MD
Senior Clinical Investigator, Laboratory of Allergic Diseases, National Institute of Allergy and Infectious Diseases, National Institutes of Health, Bethesda, Maryland

MARC E. ROTHENBERG, MD, PhD
Professor, Division of Allergy and Immunology, Department of Pediatrics, Cincinnati Children's Hospital Medical Center, University of Cincinnati College of Medicine, Cincinnati, Ohio

ALAIN M. SCHOEPFER, MD
Division of Gastroenterology and Hepatology, Centre Hospitalier Universitaire Vaudois/CHUV, Lausanne, Switzerland

JOSEPH D. SHERRILL, PhD
Instructor, Division of Allergy and Immunology, Department of Pediatrics, Cincinnati Children's Hospital Medical Center, University of Cincinnati College of Medicine, Cincinnati, Ohio

RHONDA F. SOUZA, MD
Professor, Department of Internal Medicine, Esophageal Diseases Center, Children's Medical Center, VA North Texas Health Care System, Harold C. Simmons Comprehensive Cancer Center, University of Texas Southwestern Medical Center, Dallas, Texas

STUART JON SPECHLER, MD
Professor, Department of Internal Medicine, Esophageal Diseases Center, Children's Medical Center, VA North Texas Health Care System, Harold C. Simmons Comprehensive Cancer Center, University of Texas Southwestern Medical Center, Dallas, Texas

JONATHAN SPERGEL, MD
Co-Director of the Center for Pediatric Eosinophilic Disorders; Division of Allergy, Immunology, and Infectious Diseases, The Children's Hospital of Philadelphia; Professor of Pediatrics, Perelman School of Medicine, University of Pennsylvania, Philadelphia, Pennsylvania

ALEX STRAUMANN, MD
Chairman, Swiss EoE Clinic and Swiss EoE Research Network, Olten, Switzerland

JOSHUA B. WECHSLER, MD
Instructor, Division of Gastroenterology, Hepatology and Nutrition, Department of Pediatrics, Ann & Robert H. Lurie Children's Hospital of Chicago, Chicago, Illinois

Contents

Initial case series describing children and adults with symptoms related to esophageal dysfunction and dense esophageal eosinophilia lead to recognition of a "new" disease, eosinophilic esophagitis (EoE). Clinical, basic, and translational studies have provided a deeper understanding of this somewhat enigmatic disease that mechanistically is defined as an antigen-driven condition limited to the esophagus. This article summarizes many of the key historical features of EoE and provides a glimpse of potential future developments.

In this article, the epidemiology of eosinophilic esophagitis (EoE) is reviewed. Demographic features and natural history are described, the prevalence and incidence of EoE are highlighted, and risk factors for EoE are discussed. EoE can occur at any age, there is a male predominance, it is more common in whites, and there is a strong association with atopic diseases. EoE is chronic, relapses are frequent, and persistent inflammation increases the risk of fibrostenotic complications. The prevalence is currently estimated at 0.5–1 in 1000, and EoE is now the most common cause of food impaction. The incidence of EoE is approximately 1/10,000 new cases per year, and the increase in incidence is outpacing increases in recognition and endoscopy volume, but the reasons for this evolving epidemiology are not yet fully delineated.

Eosinophilic esophagitis (EoE) is increasing in western nations. Symptoms in infants and young children include feeding difficulties, failure to thrive, and gastroesophageal reflux. School-aged children may present with vomiting, abdominal pain, and regurgitation; adolescents and adults with dysphagia and food impaction. Delayed diagnosis increases risk of stricture formation. Children with untreated EoE have tissue changes resembling airway remodeling. Endoscopy does not always correlate. Management centers on food elimination. Approaches include skin prick and patch testing, removal of foods, or an amino acid formula diet.

has been made in an effort to rectify this lack and to improve understanding of the factors that cause EoE. This article highlights key advances in elucidating the genetic (and epigenetic) components involved in EoE.

Eosinophilic esophagitis is rapidly increasing in incidence. It is associated with food antigen–triggered, eosinophil-predominant inflammation, and the pathogenic mechanisms have many similarities to other chronic atopic diseases. Studies in animal models and from patients have suggested that allergic sensitization leads to food-specific IgE and T-helper lymphocyte type 2 cells, both of which seem to contribute to the pathogenesis along with basophils, mast cells, and antigen-presenting cells. In this review our current understandings of the allergic mechanisms that drive eosinophilic esophagitis are outlined, drawing from clinical and translational studies in humans as well as experimental animal models.

In eosinophilic esophagitis (EoE), remodeling changes are manifest histologically in the epithelium and subepithelium where lamina propria fibrosis, expansion of the muscularis propria, and increased vascularity occur. The clinical symptoms and complications of EoE are largely consequences of esophageal remodeling. Available therapies have demonstrated variable ability to reverse existing remodeling changes of the esophagus. Systemic therapies have the potential of addressing subepithelial remodeling. Esophageal dilation remains a useful, adjunctive therapeutic maneuver in symptomatic adults with esophageal stricture. As novel treatments emerge, it is essential that therapeutic end points account for the fundamental contributions of esophageal remodeling to overall disease activity.

Eosinophilic gastroenteritis (EGE) represents one member within the spectrum of diseases collectively referred to as eosinophilic gastrointestinal disorders, which includes eosinophilic esophagitis (EoE), gastritis, enteritis, and colitis. EGE is less common than EoE and involves a different site of disease but otherwise shares many common features with EoE. The clinical manifestations of EGE are protean and can vary from nausea and vomiting to protein-losing enteropathy or even bowel obstruction requiring surgery. Although systemic corticosteroids are an effective treatment for EGE, their use results in substantial corticosteroid toxicity. Accordingly, there is a great need for improved therapies for these patients.

A validated disease-specific symptom-assessment tool for eosinophilic esophagitis (EoE) has yet to be approved by regulatory authorities for use in clinical trials. Relevant end points for daily practice include EoE-related symptoms and esophageal eosinophilic inflammation. Endoscopic features should also be taken into account when establishing a therapy plan. A reasonable clinical goal is to achieve a reduction in EoE-related symptoms and esophageal eosinophilic inflammation. Evidence is increasing to support an anti-inflammatory maintenance therapy, as this can reduce esophageal remodeling. In EoE patients in clinical remission, annual disease monitoring with symptom, endoscopic, and histologic assessments of sustained treatment response is recommended.

Swallowed fluticasone and oral viscous budesonide are effective first-line therapies for eosinophilic esophagitis in children. Side effects are minimal without evidence of Cushing syndrome, as seen in treatment with systemic corticosteroids. New studies on alternative delivery systems and different corticosteroids (eg, ciclesonide) are encouraging. As knowledge of corticosteroids in eosinophilic esophagitis expands, newer questions continue to arise concerning dose, delivery, and choice of corticosteroids; long-term adverse effects; and maintenance therapies.

Topical steroid therapy has been used to treat eosinophilic esophagitis (EoE) for more than 15 years. We review the treatment trials of topical steroid therapy in adult patients with EoE. Currently, there is no commercially available preparation designed to deliver the steroid to the esophagus. Current regimens consist of swallowing steroid preparations designed for inhalation treatment for asthma. In the short term, steroids are associated with an approximately 15% to 25% incidence of asymptomatic esophageal candidiasis, but otherwise appear to be well tolerated.

Emerging evidence supports impaired epithelial barrier function as the key initial event in the development of eosinophilic esophagitis (EoE) and other allergic diseases. Symptom resolution, histologic remission, and prevention of both disease and treatment-related complications are the goals of treatment. Successful dietary treatments include elemental, empirical elimination and allergy test directed diets. Dietary therapy with exclusive elemental diet offers the best response. Cow's milk, wheat, egg, soy, peanut/tree nut, and fish/shellfish are the 6 food antigens most likely to induce esophageal inflammation.

Twenty years have passed since eosinophilic esophagitis was first recognized as a new and distinct entity. Current treatment modalities for eosinophilic esophagitis include the "3 Ds": drugs, allergen avoidance with diet, and esophageal dilation. Drugs entail the limitation that only corticosteroids have a proven efficacy; most other compounds evoke only a minimal effect. Diets must be maintained continuously and they interfere markedly with the quality of life, possibly even involving some risk of malnutrition. A greater understanding of the immunopathogenesis, natural history, and disease spectrum will inevitably lead to improved therapeutic outcomes for this emerging entity.

GASTROENTEROLOGY
CLINICS OF NORTH AMERICA

Foreword

Eosinophilic Esophagitis

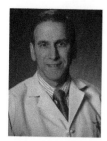

Gary W. Falk, MD, MS
Editor

Eosinophilic esophagitis (EoE) is a disease that was virtually unheard of 20 years ago. Yet, in recent years, there has been an explosive increase in the number of children and adults afflicted with the disease along with our understanding of the fundamental pathogenesis and clinical management of this fascinating disorder. The pace of change continues to be rapid as can be attested to by the publication of three sets of EoE clinical guidelines since 2007. Furthermore, recent studies suggest that delay in diagnosis leads to an increase in dysphagia symptoms and the findings of fibrostenotic disease at the time of endoscopy. This observation has important implications for disease recognition and management.

Given our rapidly evolving understanding of EoE, now is a good time to get a good "lay of the land" of this disease. Ikuo Hirano, an international leader and pioneer in EoE, has assembled well-recognized experts in the field to provide you with a state-of-the-art, practical understanding of EoE for both children and adults in 2014. Topics you will find in this issue of *Gastroenterology Clinics of North America* include the epidemiology, clinical presentation, diagnosis, and management of EoE as well as a glimpse into what the future holds. In addition, articles dedicated to mechanisms of disease pathogenesis and complications complete this comprehensive assessment of the field at present.

I know that this issue of the *Gastroenterology Clinics of North America* will enhance your understanding of EoE and I hope you enjoy it.

Gary W. Falk, MD, MS
Division of Gastroenterology
Hospital of the University of Pennsylvania
University of Pennsylvania Perelman School of Medicine
9 Penn Tower
One Convention Avenue
Philadelphia, PA 19104, USA

E-mail address:
gary.falk@uphs.upenn.edu

Gastroenterol Clin N Am 43 (2014) xiii
http://dx.doi.org/10.1016/j.gtc.2014.03.002
0889-8553/14/$ – see front matter © 2014 Elsevier Inc. All rights reserved.

gastro.theclinics.com

Preface

Eosinophilic Esophagitis

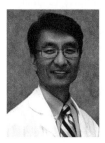

Ikuo Hirano, MD
Editor

Eosinophilic esophagitis (EoE) has emerged over the past two decades as an important cause of upper gastrointestinal symptoms in both adults and children. Defined as a chronic, immune/antigen-mediated esophageal disease, EoE presents in children with manifestations of nausea, vomiting, abdominal pain, and feeding difficulty; in adults, it presents as a leading cause of dysphagia. Food impaction requiring emergent endoscopic extraction is a common, untoward consequence of unrecognized and untreated EoE. Once considered rare, the prevalence of EoE is currently estimated at 0.5 to 1 case per 1000, approaching the prevalence of inflammatory bowel disease. Furthermore, the prevalence continues to steadily rise, paralleling the rise of atopic diseases.

This issue of *Gastroenterology Clinics of North America* includes perspectives and reviews by clinicians and investigators dedicated to the advancement of our knowledge of EoE. Although eosinophilic gastrointestinal disorders are now recognized worldwide, there are many areas of controversy and uncertainty. Insights into the rising prevalence, diagnostic criteria, genetic predisposition, allergic mechanisms, interactions with gastroesophageal reflux disease, and measurement of disease activity have generated as many questions as answers. Therapeutic options of medications, endoscopically directed esophageal dilation, and diet therapy by eliminating food triggers are utilized in practice but no pharmaceutical treatments are currently approved by the US Food and Drug Administration. Indeed, the definition, appropriate assessment, and optimal management of EoE continue to evolve.

This issue begins and ends with unique perspectives from three of the individuals credited with the initial recognition and advancement of EoE. The intervening articles are authored by international experts from pediatric and adult gastroenterology, immunology, allergy, pathology, and basic science research, emphasizing the important and fundamental collaborative efforts inspired by this new and interdisciplinary entity. Central contributions from dieticians and health care psychologists are evident in the discussions on the primary role of diet therapy and disease impact on quality of life,

Gastroenterol Clin N Am 43 (2014) xv–xvi
http://dx.doi.org/10.1016/j.gtc.2014.03.001
0889-8553/14/$ – see front matter © 2014 Elsevier Inc. All rights reserved.

respectively. The topic of "extraesophageal" eosinophilic gastrointestinal disorders is addressed in a specific article as well as in the review on histopathology. Finally, I would like to acknowledge that many of the articles in this issue were authored by members of The International Gastrointestinal Eosinophil Researchers (TIGERS). Over the past decade, TIGERS has led educational and research efforts to define eosinophilic gastrointestinal disorders. The consensus recommendations authored by the TIGERS group in 2007 and 2011 have fundamentally shaped the current concepts and identification of unmet needs in eosinophilic gastrointestinal disorders.

I thank my distinguished colleagues for contributing to this issue of *Gastroenterology Clinics of North America*. I hope you will find the information useful for current clinical practice and future investigations into this important disease.

Ikuo Hirano, MD
Division of Gastroenterology
Northwestern University Feinberg School of Medicine
676 North Saint Clair, Suite 1400
Chicago, IL 60611, USA

E-mail address:
i-hirano@northwestern.edu

Eosinophilic Esophagitis
Historical Perspective on an Evolving Disease

Stephen E. Attwood, FRCS[a], Glenn T. Furuta, MD[b],*

KEYWORDS

- Eosinophilic esophagitis • Eosinophilic oesophagitis • Dysphagia
- Food bolus obstruction

KEY POINTS

- Mild-to-severe dysphagia and food impaction are the most common symptoms of eosinophilic esophagitis (EoE) in adults and teenagers.
- Vomiting, feeding difficulties, and abdominal pain are the most common symptoms of EoE in children.
- EoE is diagnosed by clinical features and esophageal biopsy.

INTRODUCTION

During the last two decades, a new disease, eosinophilic esophagitis (EoE) emerged as one of the leading causes of food impaction and dysphagia in adults and vague reflux-like symptoms in children. Early case series describing adult patients indicated that this disease possessed distinct features that differentiated it from gastroesophageal reflux disease (GERD). Following these early descriptions, a tide of reports provided a clearer symptom complex in children and adults that ultimately helped to define EoE as a clinicopathological condition characterized by symptoms of esophageal dysfunction and dense esophageal epithelial eosinophilia (>15 eosinophils per high-power field [eos/HPF]). Clinical, basic, and translational studies have provided a deeper understanding of this somewhat enigmatic disease that mechanistically is defined as an antigen-driven condition limited to the esophagus. This article summarizes many of the key historical features of EoE and provides a glimpse of potential future developments.

This work was supported by NIH Grant K24 DK100303 (G.T. Furuta).
a North Tyneside Hospital, Rake Lane, North Shields NE29 8NH, UK; b Gastrointestinal Eosinophilic Diseases Program, Children's Hospital Colorado, 13123 East 16th Avenue, B290, Aurora, CO 80045, USA
* Corresponding author.
E-mail address: glenn.furuta@childrenscolorado.org

INITIAL DESCRIPTIONS OF ESOPHAGEAL EOSINOPHILIA

Although eosinophils reside in most the gastrointestinal mucosae, they are not present in the normal esophageal epithelia. Initial reports of esophageal eosinophilia associated this histologic finding with GERD.[1,2] How and why acid affected the esophageal epithelium in some but not all patients still escapes our understanding; however, the association of GERD with esophageal eosinophilia held firm for several years. Interestingly, these early reports characterized eosinophilia as more than 1 eos/HPF and the size of the HPF was not standardized. In 1985, Lee[3] reported eosinophilic infiltration in esophageal mucosal biopsy in 11 patients with average age of 14.6 years; these patients had reflux symptoms and their eosinophil density was low. In retrospect, these were probably patients with GERD.

GERD IS NOT THE ONLY DISEASE ASSOCIATED WITH ESOPHAGEAL EOSINOPHILIA

Although GERD-associated eosinophilia was thought to be the predominant cause of esophagitis for years, several case series began to report clinical features that were somewhat different from those associated with classic GERD. In 1978, Landres and colleagues[4] reported an isolated case of vigorous achalasia in a patient with marked smooth muscle hypertrophy and eosinophilic infiltration of esophagus. He concluded that this patient likely represented a variant of eosinophilic gastroenteritis, which predisposed to esophageal motor disorder. This case is unusual in that large numbers of eosinophils are not commonly found in esophageal tissues affected by achalasia or other defined motor disorders. In 1981, Picus and Frank[5] reported a case of 16-year-old boy with progressive dysphagia for 1.5 years and dense esophageal eosinophilia. Endoscopic findings revealed multiple 1 mm nodular filling defects near a stricture and proximal dilation. Radiological studies showed luminal narrowing and wall rigidity; peripheral blood showed high circulating eosinophil count. Again, the investigators assumed it was a variant of eosinophilic gastroenteritis. Following this, a series of case reports provided more details of patients who presented with dysphagia and esophageal eosinophilia, some of who developed esophageal strictures.[6–8]

CRITICAL OBSERVATIONS OF NEW CLINICAL DISORDER: EoE

In 1989, Attwood and colleagues[9] published an abstract in *Gut*, describing "Oesophageal Asthma—an episodic dysphagia with eosinophilic infiltrates." These investigators compared a group of 15 adults who presented with dysphagia without esophageal obstruction and normal pH monitoring with a group of 100 adults with GERD as defined by increased acid exposure in the distal esophagus. Differences between the two groups were that the group without increased acid exposure was found to have significantly greater number of eosinophils than the group with GERD. The key finding of this case series was that it identified patients with dysphagia, with severity up to complete bolus obstruction, who presented with dense esophageal eosinophilia. In 1993, they published these key findings that described adults with dysphagia, normal pH monitoring, and dense esophageal eosinophilia (>20 eos/HPF) and termed this esophageal eosinophilia with dysphagia, a distinct clinicopathological syndrome.[10] Importantly, control patients with proven GERD had a mean of 3.3 eos/HPF in the esophageal epithelium. Endoscopic appearances using fiberoptic technology likely limited descriptions of the full details now observed in this disease and may partially explain why no endoscopic abnormalities were visualized in this series. Seven patients had food hypersensitivity and all required advanced intervention (dilatation and/or steroids in one case) for resolution of symptoms.

In 1994, Straumann and colleagues[11] described a series of 10 patients with acute recurrent dysphagia seen over a 4-year period, who showed discrete endoscopic changes and high concentrations of epithelial esophageal eosinophils, who improved following systemic steroid and antihistamine treatment. From this series, it was clear that the endoscopic findings, including rings, white exudates, and furrows, were variably expressed because some patients' esophageal mucosae appeared relatively normal. The investigators termed this idiopathic EoE.

Taken together, these two reports from two different investigators, described key clinical findings observed in adults with dysphagia who had dense mucosal eosinophilia that was limited to the esophagus who did not have GERD. Importantly, endoscopic findings were variable, leading to the necessity of procuring endoscopic pinch biopsy to make the diagnosis. Because this practice was not widespread and because of the lack of diagnostic usefulness, larger recognition of this newfound disease remained somewhat limited.

These two series, published by a gastroenterologist in private practice, Straumann, and a surgeon, Attwood, formed the beginnings of their quest to define key clinical features and therapeutic approaches during the next 20 years.

INCREASING AWARENESS OF EoE IN THE PEDIATRIC GASTROENTEROLOGY COMMUNITY

With the emergence of improved sedation practices in the early 1990s, pediatric gastroenterologists began to perform fiberoptic endoscopy with increased frequency. Coincident with this increased practice, was the recognition that histologic evidence of inflammation could be present despite an endoscopically normal appearing mucosa.[12] This observation lead to the practice of procuring mucosal samples as a standard of care for children undergoing endoscopic assessment of symptoms, a key difference from adult practice.

During this time, an increasing number of children were observed to have symptoms that persisted despite antacid blockade. Children ranging from toddlers to teenagers presented with a wide range of symptoms, including vomiting, regurgitation, feeding problems, and abdominal pain, that were unresponsive to H2 receptor antagonists or proton pump inhibitors (PPIs) and who, at the time of endoscopy, were found to have dense mucosal eosinophilia limited to the esophagus.[13–20] Associated clinical features observed in these patients included a male predominance, radiologic evidence of strictures, and endoscopic findings of white exudates, edema, and rings. Consistent with the initial reports in adults, some children seemed to experience a high degree of concomitant atopic diseases, including food allergy, eczema, and asthma.

EoE MAY BE A FOOD ALLERGY DISEASE

With the increasing clinical descriptions, lack of therapeutic approaches, and potential allergic mechanism underlying this disease, Kelly and colleagues[13] took a novel approach in 1995. They provided a detailed description of 10 children who experienced vomiting and abdominal pain, dense esophageal eosinophilia (>20/HPF), and lack of response to either acid blockade or fundoplication (n = 2), who responded clinically and histologically to an amino acid–based formula. Strict use of the formula lead to normalization of the esophagus and, when allergenic food was added back into the diet, symptoms and esophageal eosinophilia returned. This study set the stage for several future studies that have examined the allergic diathesis and mechanisms of EoE. Development of therapeutic regimens included removing the six most common food allergens and instituting a diet based on the removal of foods based on food allergy testing.[21,22] In addition, the global concept of EoE being a chronic disease was initiated because patients relapsed once foods were added back into the diet.

ALTERNATIVE APPROACHES TO TREAT EoE

Because of difficulties adhering to diet restriction and the impact of steroids in other eosinophilic diseases, investigators took two different approaches. In 1998, Liacouras and colleagues[16] demonstrated that subjects with EoE responded clinically and histologically to prednisone but that symptoms recurred when the medication was stopped. In the same year, Faubion and colleagues[15] adapted a novel approach to provide topical steroids to the esophageal mucosa. They hypothesized that steroid sprayed from the metered dose inhaler used for asthma could be delivered by the saliva to the esophageal mucosa, leading to an antiinflammatory response. In their series of four patients, they found that this delivery mechanism was effective in relieving symptoms and, when examined, diminished esophageal eosinophilia. Subsequent studies using a variety of different preparations in adults and children have shown this approach to significantly decrease symptoms and mucosal eosinophilia.[23–40] Other approaches toward modulating the immune system to treat EoE include leukotriene antagonist as described by Attwood and colleagues,[41] antibody-based approaches to block interleukin (IL)-5, and a chemoattractant receptor-homologous molecule on Th2 cells (CRTH2) antagonist.[42–46]

With the increasing identification of fixed narrowings in patients with EoE, dilatation has been very helpful in EoE management. Some early reports of perforation risk were perhaps overstated, which may be accounted for by the use of rigid esophagoscopy and bougie dilatation.[47] However, the increased use of flexible endoscopic approaches with either balloon or bougie have shown to provide safe outcomes with a risk of perforation less than 1% per procedure, a risk similar to dilatation of peptic stricture.[48–50]

More clinical experiences and prospective research studies continue to emphasize the chronic nature of EoE in that when treatments are stopped symptoms and inflammation return.

WIDER ACCEPTANCE OF EoE AND INCREASING FREQUENCY OF DIAGNOSIS

Following these articles, there was a nearly logarithmic rise in articles focusing on the new entity, EoE. Within these bodies of works, reports surfaced that documented EoE as a disease occurring primarily in white males with an overall incidence of 1 in 10,000.[51] From 2003 to 2007, work began to focus on defining the clinical phenotype of EoE. Symptoms in children included vomiting, abdominal pain, and feeding difficulties; adults were characterized by the stereotypical features of food impaction, dysphagia, and, in some circumstances, chest pain.[22,27,52–68] Endoscopic patterns of linear furrows, circular ridges, and more defined rings (trachealization); the presence of white microabscesses; and the complication of severe strictures in some patients, were all manifestations of EoE.[27,52,63,69–79] Retrospective studies detailing experiences with diet elimination, topical steroids, and other treatments emerged.[21,22,24–26,28,42,47,78,80–84] Overall, a growing acceptance of a "new" disease became manifest and patient diagnoses and treatments ensued.

DEVELOPMENT OF CONSENSUS RECOMMENDATIONS FOR DIAGNOSIS AND TREATMENT

Despite this increased recognition, several problems emerged that stymied not only clinical care but also an emerging research interest in this disease.[85] How many eosinophils were required to make the diagnosis? What is the size of diagnostic HPF? What symptoms are necessary to diagnose a patient with EoE? Most problematic was determining the criteria necessary to make a diagnosis of EoE. To address this, the North American Society of Pediatric Gastroenterology, Hepatology, and Nutrition held the First International Gastrointestinal Eosinophil Research Symposium in Orlando, Florida, in 2006. This meeting represented the culmination of a multidisciplinary team of experts' yearlong work to develop diagnostic recommendations and treatment approaches. The following year, the first consensus recommendations were published founded on expert clinical experience as well as the published literature, works that consisted primarily of case series, and retrospective analyses.[86] This multidisciplinary team of physicians and clinical scientists determined that EoE was a clinicopathological disease that required symptoms characterizing esophageal dysfunction and dense esophageal eosinophilia (>15 eos/HPF) to make the diagnosis. Alternative causes for eosinophilia were ruled out and other parts of the gastrointestinal tract were normal. This publication provided strong support for the efforts of the advocacy organization, the American Partnership for Eosinophilic Disorders (APFED.org) to spearhead efforts in 2008, 15 years after the first case series was published, to obtain approval for the *International Classification of Diseases, Ninth Revision* classification (530.13) for EoE. Since then, three more guidelines have been published, each with new and improved recommendations based on expert opinion and, even more, on prospective studies.[87–89] During that time, the original acronym EE was changed to EoE to avoid confusion with the previous use of EE to describe erosive esophagitis. Taken together, these guidelines provide a basis for both clinical care and research studies.

DEFINING EoE PHENOTYPES

With increased clinical experiences, the clinical diversity of EoE continues to undergo definition. For instance, EoE is likely the most common cause of food impaction in adults and children.[58,90–99] A range of features characterize luminal narrowings associated with EoE, including isolated esophageal strictures and rings, long segment narrowings, and crepe paper esophagus. Although rare, esophageal perforation can occur because of dilation or as a spontaneous event. In fact, EoE is now likely the most common cause of spontaneous perforation of the esophagus, although it is usually a partial perforation and treated differently than the original complete disruption originally described by Boorhaeve.[65,100–102] In addition, clinical phenotypes related to therapeutic responses have been identified. For instance, patients with an FK506-binding protein 5 (FKBP51) genotype are steroid responsive thus pointing to a future role for molecular techniques to define personalized medicine.[32]

HISTOLOGIC CONUNDRUMS: WHAT IS PPI-RESPONSIVE ESOPHAGEAL EOSINOPHILIA?

One of the more confounding clinical problems that has arisen relates to determining whether the primary driver of esophageal eosinophilia is related to peptic or allergic causes. To address this, clinicians either have treated patients with high-dose PPIs or performed pH monitoring of the distal esophagus.[103] These practices have revealed a group of patients with symptoms of esophageal dysfunction, dense esophageal eosinophilia, and normal pH monitoring who respond clinically and histologically to PPIs. For instance, Molina-Infante and colleagues,[104] and Molina-Infante and Zamorano,[105] identified many patients thought to not have GERD who responded to PPI therapy. Cheng and colleagues[106] provide a potential mechanism for this finding in studies in which omeprazole was shown to downregulate EoE-related cytokines, including IL-4, IL-13, and eotaxin-3 signaling in esophageal epithelial cells through a signal transducer and activator of transcription factor 6 (STAT6)-dependent process.[107] Whether this represents undocumented GERD or an alternative action of PPIs related to its potential antiinflammatory effect is not yet certain. Further studies defining the molecular features of EoE may lend insights into this clinical finding.

UNDERSTANDING OF CHRONICITY

Following these initial case series, very little progress was apparent in the literature until the detailed description of the chronic nature and natural history of EoE. Straumann[108] described the longest follow-up of 30 adults with EoE (22 men, mean age, 40.6 years; range, 16–71 years). The presenting symptom was almost exclusively dysphagia with food impaction and diagnosis was delayed an average of 4.6 years (range, 0–17 years). During the follow-up period of 1.4 to 11.5 years, 23% of patients reported increasing dysphagia and 36.7% reported stable symptoms. No change in endoscopic features was identified in six of seven patients in whom a subepithelial component could be analyzed but an increase in fibrosis and thickening was documented. Follow-up studies by the same group demonstrated that delay in diagnosis increased risk for stricture formation.[109]

MOLECULAR TECHNIQUES ADVANCE CARE AND PATHOGENETIC UNDERSTANDING

In 2006, Blanchard reported the seminal finding that EoE was defined by a uniquely conserved gene-expression profile that included overexpression of eotaxin-3.[110] Work from this group and others has defined several gene profiles for children and adults with EoE that have identified novel therapeutic targets. In addition, murine models and ex vivo systems continue to dissect pathogenetic pathways, in particular, those associated with IL-5, IL-13, and thymic stromal lymphopoietin (TSLP).[111–119] Most recently, Wen and colleagues[120] described a novel molecular testing that provides a diagnostic platform for patients with EoE in a rapid and objective manner using mucosal biopsies. These approaches will likely pave the way for future diagnostic and therapeutic approaches leading to a more personalized approach to care.

FUTURE CONCERNS AND DIRECTIONS
Expanding Diagnostic Criteria Beyond a Number

Whereas eosinophil counts remain the gold standard biomarker for diagnosis and primary endpoints, few diseases are characterized by just one cell's number. Problems associated with this approach include lack of standardization of HPF size, location of biopsy, limited size of biopsy sample compared with the total surface area of the esophagus, variability in enumeration techniques, and a broad range of eosinophilia associated with peptic and allergic inflammation.[121–123] In this regard, future studies that determine endoscopic, histologic, or molecular features that further define EoE are critical.

Challenges in Monitoring Disease Activity

Assessment of disease activity is complicated by three factors. First, symptoms do not always reflect esophageal inflammation.[124] Second, measurement of esophageal inflammation requires endoscopy and biopsy. Third, measurement of esophageal function, as it relates to EoE, has not been standardized. Each of these areas is undergoing study and rapid progress has been made during the last few years. Several minimally invasive tools (esophageal string and sponge tests) that would preclude endoscopy and sedation are undergoing development.[125,126] Functional tests, such as the EndoFLIP (Crospon Ireland, Galway, Ireland, and Carlsbad, CA, USA), show great potential in identifying critical features of clinically significant fibrosis and remodeling.[127–129] This last concern is critical because our current understanding of this disease has been developed based on events described within the esophageal epithelia as documented by mucosal pinch biopsies. In fact, this snapshot may only reveal part of the story in that the inflammation, characterized by not only eosinophils but also by T cells, B cells, mast cells, basophils, fibroblasts, and endothelia, may lead to remodeling that affects deeper layers of the esophageal wall.

The clinical impact of this concern relates to the adult symptoms of dysphagia, food bolus obstruction, and chest pain. The term regurgitation is sometimes used but it is usually only of the swallowed fluids above the obstructed esophagus. When taking patient history, it is useful to try to distinguish the type of regurgitation in EoE (swallowed fluids) versus the type of regurgitation seen in GERD (acid reflux from the stomach). In addition, the use of the term vomiting in EoE usually refers to the efforts the patients make to wretch to move the blocked food bolus, often trying to bring it up into the pharynx. This is not vomiting in the normal sense and it is best described as retching. When talking with patients it is useful to distinguish the vomiting they might suffer when the stomach empties itself through the esophagus in contrast to the retching and heaving that occurs from a food bolus obstruction in the esophagus. Several studies are now seeking to provide characterization of symptoms, quality of life, and endoscopic appearances of patients with EoE with the hope of developing patient-reported outcomes and other metrics that can be used in prospective therapeutic trials.[130–135]

Developing New Therapeutic Approaches

EoE treatments that include topical steroids and diet exclusion of antigens induce remission in 50% to 75% of patients, representing excellent therapeutic responses. However, topical steroids can be difficult to administer and carry potential side effects. Diet treatment can be complicated by identifying the specific allergen and maintaining adherence. To date, no cure has been identified for EoE thus emphasizing the urgent need for future studies dedicated to developing treatments approved by the US Food and Drug Administration.[136,137]

SUMMARY

Initial case series describing children and adults with symptoms related to esophageal dysfunction and dense esophageal eosinophilia lead to recognition of a "new" disease, EoE. Clinical experiences and a growing body of research have rapidly lead to diagnostic criteria, therapeutic interventions, and identification of complications. Future works will delineate more refined approaches to diagnosis, new therapeutic targets, and the natural history of this enigmatic disease.[136,137]

REFERENCES

1. Biller JA, Winter HS, Grand RJ, et al. Are endoscopic changes predictive of histologic esophagitis in children? J Pediatr 1983;103:215–8.
2. Brown LF, Goldman H, Antonioli DA. Intraepithelial eosinophils in endoscopic biopsies of adults with reflux esophagitis. Am J Surg Pathol 1984;8:899–905.
3. Lee RG. Marked eosinophilia in esophageal mucosal biopsies. Am J Surg Pathol 1985;9:475–9.

4. Landres RT, Kuster GG, Strum WB. Eosinophilic esophagitis in a patient with vigorous achalasia. Gastroenterology 1978;74:1298–301.
5. Picus D, Frank PH. Eosinophilic esophagitis. AJR Am J Roentgenol 1981;136: 1001–3.
6. Feczko P, Halpert R, Zonca M. Radiographic abnormalities in eosinophilic esophagitis. Gastrointest Radiol 1985;10:321–4.
7. Matzinger MA, Daneman A. Esophageal involvement in eosinophilic gastroenteritis. Pediatr Radiol 1983;13:35–8.
8. Munch R, Kuhlmann U, Makek M, et al. Eosinophilic esophagitis, a rare manifestation of eosinophilic gastroenteritis. Schweiz Med Wochenschr 1982;112:731–4 [in German].
9. Attwood SE, Smyrk TC, Demeester TR. Eosinophilic asthma-episodic dysphagia with eosinophilic infiltrates. Gut 1989;30:A1493.
10. Attwood SE, Smyrk TC, Demeester TC, et al. Esophageal eosinophilia with dysphagia. A distinct clinicopathologic syndrome. Dig Dis Sci 1993;38:109–16.
11. Straumann A, Spichtin HP, Bernoulli R, et al. Idiopathic eosinophilic esophagitis: a frequently overlooked disease with typical clinical aspects and discrete endoscopic findings. Schweiz Med Wochenschr 1994;124:1419–29 [in German].
12. Schmidt-Sommerfeld E, Kirschner BS, Stephens JK. Endoscopic and histologic findings in the upper gastrointestinal tract of children with Crohn's disease. J Pediatr Gastroenterol Nutr 1990;11:448–54.
13. Kelly KJ, Lazenby AJ, Rowe PC, et al. Eosinophilic esophagitis attributed to gastroesophageal reflux: improvement with an amino acid-based formula. Gastroenterology 1995;109:1503–12.
14. Mahajan L, Wyllie R, Petras R, et al. Idiopathic eosinophilic esophagitis with stricture formation in a patient with long-standing eosinophilic gastroenteritis. Gastrointest Endosc 1997;46:557–60.
15. Faubion WA Jr, Perrault J, Burgart LJ, et al. Treatment of eosinophilic esophagitis with inhaled corticosteroids. J Pediatr Gastroenterol Nutr 1998;27:90–3.
16. Liacouras CA, Wenner WJ, Brown K, et al. Primary eosinophilic esophagitis in children: successful treatment with oral corticosteroids. J Pediatr Gastroenterol Nutr 1998;26:380–5.
17. Orenstein SR, Shalaby TM, Di Lorenzo C, et al. The spectrum of pediatric eosinophilic esophagitis beyond infancy: a clinical series of 30 children. Am J Gastroenterol 2000;95:1422–30.
18. Siafakas CG, Ryan CK, Brown MR, et al. Multiple esophageal rings: an association with eosinophilic esophagitis: case report and review of the literature. Am J Gastroenterol 2000;95:1572–5.
19. Fox VL, Nurko S, Teitelbaum JE, et al. High-resolution EUS in children with eosinophilic "allergic" esophagitis. Gastrointest Endosc 2003;57:30–6.
20. Khan S, Orenstein SR, Di Lorenzo C, et al. Eosinophilic esophagitis: strictures, impactions, dysphagia. Dig Dis Sci 2003;48:22–9.
21. Kagalwalla AF, Sentongo TA, Ritz S, et al. Effect of six-food elimination diet on clinical and histologic outcomes in eosinophilic esophagitis. Clin Gastroenterol Hepatol 2006;4:1097–102.
22. Spergel JM, Andrews T, Brown-Whitehorn TF, et al. Treatment of eosinophilic esophagitis with specific food elimination diet directed by a combination of skin prick and patch tests. Ann Allergy Asthma Immunol 2005;95:336–43.
23. Teitelbaum J, Fox V, Twarog F, et al. Eosinophilic esophagitis in children: immunopathological analysis and response to fluticasone propionate. Gastroenterology 2002;122:1216–25.

24. Arora AS, Perrault J, Smyrk TC. Topical corticosteroid treatment of dysphagia due to eosinophilic esophagitis in adults. Mayo Clin Proc 2003;78:830–5.
25. Aceves SS, Dohil R, Newbury RO, et al. Topical viscous budesonide suspension for treatment of eosinophilic esophagitis. J Allergy Clin Immunol 2005;116: 705–6.
26. Konikoff MR, Noel RJ, Blanchard C, et al. A randomized, double-blind, placebo-controlled trial of fluticasone propionate for pediatric eosinophilic esophagitis. Gastroenterology 2006;131:1381–91.
27. Remedios M, Campbell C, Jones DM, et al. Eosinophilic esophagitis in adults: clinical, endoscopic, histologic findings, and response to treatment with fluticasone propionate. Gastrointest Endosc 2006;63:3–12.
28. Aceves SS, Bastian JF, Newbury RO, et al. Oral viscous budesonide: a potential new therapy for eosinophilic esophagitis in children. Am J Gastroenterol 2007; 102(10):2271–9.
29. Lucendo AJ, De Rezende L, Comas C, et al. Treatment with topical steroids downregulates IL-5, eotaxin-1/CCL11, and eotaxin-3/CCL26 gene expression in eosinophilic esophagitis. Am J Gastroenterol 2008;103:2184–93.
30. Schaefer ET, Fitzgerald JF, Molleston JP, et al. Comparison of oral prednisone and topical fluticasone in the treatment of eosinophilic esophagitis: a randomized trial in children. Clin Gastroenterol Hepatol 2008;6:165–73.
31. Aceves SS, Newbury RO, Chen D, et al. Resolution of remodeling in eosinophilic esophagitis correlates with epithelial response to topical corticosteroids. Allergy 2010;65:109–16.
32. Caldwell JM, Blanchard C, Collins MH, et al. Glucocorticoid-regulated genes in eosinophilic esophagitis: a role for FKBP51. J Allergy Clin Immunol 2010;125: 879–88.e8.
33. Dohil R, Newbury R, Fox L, et al. Oral viscous budesonide is effective in children with eosinophilic esophagitis in a randomized, placebo-controlled trial. Gastroenterology 2010;139:418–29.
34. Peterson KA, Thomas KL, Hilden K, et al. Comparison of esomeprazole to aerosolized, swallowed fluticasone for eosinophilic esophagitis. Dig Dis Sci 2010;55: 1313–9.
35. Straumann A, Conus S, Degen L, et al. Budesonide is effective in adolescent and adult patients with active eosinophilic esophagitis. Gastroenterology 2010;139:1526–37, 1537.e1.
36. Abu-Sultaneh SM, Durst P, Maynard V, et al. Fluticasone and food allergen elimination reverse sub-epithelial fibrosis in children with eosinophilic esophagitis. Dig Dis Sci 2011;56:97–102.
37. Straumann A, Conus S, Degen L, et al. Long-term budesonide maintenance treatment is partially effective for patients with eosinophilic esophagitis. Clin Gastroenterol Hepatol 2011;9(5):400–9.e1.
38. Alexander JA, Jung KW, Arora AS, et al. Swallowed fluticasone improves histologic but not symptomatic response of adults with eosinophilic esophagitis. Clin Gastroenterol Hepatol 2012;10:742–9.e1.
39. Dellon ES, Sheikh A, Speck O, et al. Viscous topical is more effective than nebulized steroid therapy for patients with eosinophilic esophagitis. Gastroenterology 2012;143:321–4.e1.
40. Schroeder S, Fleischer DM, Masterson JC, et al. Successful treatment of eosinophilic esophagitis with ciclesonide. J Allergy Clin Immunol 2012;129:1419–21.
41. Attwood SE, Lewis CJ, Bronder CS, et al. Eosinophilic oesophagitis: a novel treatment using Montelukast. Gut 2003;52:181–5.

42. Garrett JK, Jameson SC, Thomson B, et al. Anti-interleukin-5 (mepolizumab) therapy for hypereosinophilic syndromes. J Allergy Clin Immunol 2004;113:115–9.

43. Assa'ad AH, Gupta SK, Collins MH, et al. An antibody against IL-5 reduces numbers of esophageal intraepithelial eosinophils in children with eosinophilic esophagitis. Gastroenterology 2011;141:1593–604.

44. Spergel JM, Rothenberg ME, Collins MH, et al. Reslizumab in children and adolescents with eosinophilic esophagitis: results of a double-blind, randomized, placebo-controlled trial. J Allergy Clin Immunol 2012;129:456–63, 463.e1–3.

45. Otani IM, Anilkumar AA, Newbury RO, et al. Anti-IL-5 therapy reduces mast cell and IL-9 cell numbers in pediatric patients with eosinophilic esophagitis. J Allergy Clin Immunol 2013;131:1576–82.

46. Straumann A, Hoesli S, Bussmann C, et al. Anti-eosinophil activity and clinical efficacy of the CRTH2 antagonist OC000459 in eosinophilic esophagitis. Allergy 2013;68:375–85.

47. Lucendo AJ, De Rezende L. Endoscopic dilation in eosinophilic esophagitis: a treatment strategy associated with a high risk of perforation. Endoscopy 2007;39:376 [author reply: 377].

48. Jacobs JW Jr, Spechler SJ. A systematic review of the risk of perforation during esophageal dilation for patients with eosinophilic esophagitis. Dig Dis Sci 2010;55:1512–5.

49. Riley SA, Attwood SE. Guidelines on the use of oesophageal dilatation in clinical practice. Gut 2004;53(Suppl 1):i1–6.

50. Schoepfer AM, Gonsalves N, Bussmann C, et al. Esophageal dilation in eosinophilic esophagitis: effectiveness, safety, and impact on the underlying inflammation. Am J Gastroenterol 2010;105:1062–70.

51. Noel RJ, Putnam PE, Rothenberg ME. Eosinophilic esophagitis. N Engl J Med 2004;351:940–1.

52. Croese J, Fairley SK, Masson JW, et al. Clinical and endoscopic features of eosinophilic esophagitis in adults. Gastrointest Endosc 2003;58:516–22.

53. Liacouras CA. Eosinophilic esophagitis in children and adults. J Pediatr Gastroenterol Nutr 2003;37(Suppl 1):S23–8.

54. Straumann A, Spichtin HP, Grize L, et al. Natural history of primary eosinophilic esophagitis: a follow-up of 30 adult patients for up to 11.5 years. Gastroenterology 2003;125:1660–9.

55. Lucendo AJ, Carrion G, Navarro M, et al. Eosinophilic esophagitis in adults: an emerging disease. Dig Dis Sci 2004;49:1884–8.

56. Potter JW, Saeian K, Staff D, et al. Eosinophilic esophagitis in adults: an emerging problem with unique esophageal features. Gastrointest Endosc 2004;59:355–61.

57. Sant'Anna AM, Rolland S, Fournet JC, et al. Eosinophilic esophagitis in children: symptoms, histology and pH probe results. J Pediatr Gastroenterol Nutr 2004;39:373–7.

58. Desai TK, Stecevic V, Chang CH, et al. Association of eosinophilic inflammation with esophageal food impaction in adults. Gastrointest Endosc 2005;61:795–801.

59. Liacouras CA, Spergel JM, Ruchelli E, et al. Eosinophilic esophagitis: a 10-year experience in 381 children. Clin Gastroenterol Hepatol 2005;3:1198–206.

60. Cherian S, Smith NM, Forbes DA. Rapidly increasing prevalence of eosinophilic oesophagitis in Western Australia. Arch Dis Child 2006;91:1000–4.

61. Gonsalves N, Policarpio-Nicolas M, Zhang Q, et al. Histopathologic variability and endoscopic correlates in adults with eosinophilic esophagitis. Gastrointest Endosc 2006;64:313–9.
62. Parfitt JR, Gregor JC, Suskin NG, et al. Eosinophilic esophagitis in adults: distinguishing features from gastroesophageal reflux disease: a study of 41 patients. Mod Pathol 2006;19:90–6.
63. Aceves SS, Newbury RO, Dohil R, et al. Distinguishing eosinophilic esophagitis in pediatric patients: clinical, endoscopic, and histologic features of an emerging disorder. J Clin Gastroenterol 2007;41:252–6.
64. Chehade M, Sampson HA, Morotti RA, et al. Esophageal subepithelial fibrosis in children with eosinophilic esophagitis. J Pediatr Gastroenterol Nutr 2007;45: 319–28.
65. Cohen MS, Kaufman A, Dimarino AJ Jr, et al. Eosinophilic esophagitis presenting as spontaneous esophageal rupture (Boerhaave's Syndrome). Clin Gastroenterol Hepatol 2007;5:A24.
66. Kerlin P, Jones D, Remedios M, et al. Prevalence of eosinophilic esophagitis in adults with food bolus obstruction of the esophagus. J Clin Gastroenterol 2007; 41:356–61.
67. Pasha SF, DiBaise JK, Kim HJ, et al. Patient characteristics, clinical, endoscopic, and histologic findings in adult eosinophilic esophagitis: a case series and systematic review of the medical literature. Dis Esophagus 2007;20:311–9.
68. Prasad GA, Talley NJ, Romero Y, et al. Prevalence and predictive factors of eosinophilic esophagitis in patients presenting with dysphagia: a prospective study. Am J Gastroenterol 2007;102(12):2627–32.
69. Sundaram S, Sunku B, Nelson SP, et al. Adherent white plaques: an endoscopic finding in eosinophilic esophagitis. J Pediatr Gastroenterol Nutr 2004;38: 208–12.
70. Kaplan M, Mutlu EA, Jakate S, et al. Endoscopy in eosinophilic esophagitis: "feline" esophagus and perforation risk. Clin Gastroenterol Hepatol 2003;1: 433–7.
71. Straumann A, Rossi L, Simon HU, et al. Fragility of the esophageal mucosa: a pathognomonic endoscopic sign of primary eosinophilic esophagitis? Gastrointest Endosc 2003;57:407–12.
72. Nurko S, Teitelbaum JE, Husain K, et al. Association of Schatzki ring with eosinophilic esophagitis in children. J Pediatr Gastroenterol Nutr 2004;38:436–41.
73. Straumann A, Spichtin HP, Bucher KA, et al. Eosinophilic esophagitis: red on microscopy, white on endoscopy. Digestion 2004;70:109–16.
74. Prasad GA, Arora AS. Spontaneous perforation in the ringed esophagus. Dis Esophagus 2005;18:406–9.
75. Mecklenburg I, Weber C, Folwaczny C. Spontaneous recovery of dysphagia by rupture of an esophageal diverticulum in eosinophilic esophagitis. Dig Dis Sci 2006;51:1241–2.
76. Zuber-Jerger I, Ratiu N, Kullman F. Long-lasting effect of endoscopic dilatation of an esophageal stenosis due to eosinophilic esophagitis. J Gastrointestin Liver Dis 2006;15:167–70.
77. Lee GS, Craig PI, Freiman JS, et al. Intermittent Dysphagia for solids associated with a multiringed esophagus: clinical features and response to dilatation. Dysphagia 2007;22:55–62.
78. Lucendo AJ, Pascual-Turrion JM, Navarro M, et al. Endoscopic, bioptic, and manometric findings in eosinophilic esophagitis before and after steroid therapy: a case series. Endoscopy 2007;39:765–71.

79. Muller S, Puhl S, Vieth M, et al. Analysis of symptoms and endoscopic findings in 117 patients with histological diagnoses of eosinophilic esophagitis. Endoscopy 2007;39:339–44.

80. Zeiter DK, Hyams JS. Gastroesophageal reflux: pathogenesis, diagnosis, and treatment. Allergy Asthma Proc 1999;20:45–9.

81. Markowitz JE, Spergel JM, Ruchelli E, et al. Elemental diet is an effective treatment for eosinophilic esophagitis in children and adolescents. Am J Gastroenterol 2003;98:777–82.

82. Noel RJ, Putnam PE, Collins MH, et al. Clinical and immunopathologic effects of swallowed fluticasone for eosinophilic esophagitis. Clin Gastroenterol Hepatol 2004;2:568–75.

83. Stein ML, Collins MH, Villanueva JM, et al. Anti-IL-5 (mepolizumab) therapy for eosinophilic esophagitis. J Allergy Clin Immunol 2006;118:1312–9.

84. Shah A, Hirano I. Treatment of eosinophilic esophagitis: drugs, diet, or dilation? Curr Gastroenterol Rep 2007;9:181–8.

85. Dellon ES, Aderoju A, Woosley JT, et al. Variability in diagnostic criteria for eosinophilic esophagitis: a systematic review. Am J Gastroenterol 2007;102(10):2300–13.

86. Furuta GT, Liacouras CA, Collins MH, et al. Eosinophilic esophagitis in children and adults: a systematic review and consensus recommendations for diagnosis and treatment. Gastroenterology 2007;133:1342–63.

87. Liacouras CA, Furuta GT, Hirano I, et al. Eosinophilic esophagitis: updated consensus recommendations for children and adults. J Allergy Clin Immunol 2011;128:3–20.e6 [quiz: 21–2].

88. Dellon ES, Gonsalves N, Hirano I, et al. ACG clinical guideline: evidenced based approach to the diagnosis and management of esophageal eosinophilia and eosinophilic esophagitis (EoE). Am J Gastroenterol 2013;108:679–92 [quiz: 693].

89. Papadopoulou A, Koletzko S, Heuschkel R, et al. Management guidelines of eosinophilic esophagitis in childhood. J Pediatr Gastroenterol Nutr 2014;58:107–18.

90. Focht DR, Kaul A. Food impaction and eosinophilic esophagitis. J Pediatr 2005; 147:540.

91. Lucendo Villarin AJ, Carrion Alonso G, Navarro Sanchez M, et al. Eosinophilic esophagitis in adults, an emerging cause of dysphagia. Description of 9 cases. Rev Esp Enferm Dig 2005;97:229–39.

92. Luis AL, Rinon C, Encinas JL, et al. Non stenotic food impaction due to eosinophilic esophagitis: a potential surgical emergency. Eur J Pediatr Surg 2006;16: 399–402.

93. Smith CR, Miranda A, Rudolph CD, et al. Removal of impacted food in children with eosinophilic esophagitis using Saeed banding device. J Pediatr Gastroenterol Nutr 2007;44:521–3.

94. Nonevski IT, Downs-Kelly E, Falk GW. Eosinophilic esophagitis: an increasingly recognized cause of dysphagia, food impaction, and refractory heartburn. Cleve Clin J Med 2008;75:623–6, 629–33.

95. Hurtado CW, Furuta GT, Kramer RE. Etiology of esophageal food impactions in children. J Pediatr Gastroenterol Nutr 2011;52:43–6.

96. Sperry SL, Crockett SD, Miller CB, et al. Esophageal foreign-body impactions: epidemiology, time trends, and the impact of the increasing prevalence of eosinophilic esophagitis. Gastrointest Endosc 2011;74:985–91.

97. El-Matary W, El-Hakim H, Popel J. Eosinophilic esophagitis in children needing emergency endoscopy for foreign body and food bolus impaction. Pediatr Emerg Care 2012;28:611–3.

98. Akyuz U, Akyuz F, Ozdil K, et al. Food impaction in older age: Think about an eosinophilic esophagitis. World J Gastrointest Endosc 2013;5:79–80.
99. Hudson S, Sampson C, Muntz HR, et al. Foreign body impaction as presentation of eosinophilic esophagitis. Otolaryngology 2013;149(5):679–81.
100. Straumann A, Bussmann C, Zuber M, et al. Eosinophilic esophagitis: analysis of food impaction and perforation in 251 adolescent and adult patients. Clin Gastroenterol Hepatol 2008;6:598–600.
101. Lucendo AJ, Friginal-Ruiz AB, Rodriguez B. Boerhaave's syndrome as the primary manifestation of adult eosinophilic esophagitis. Two case reports and a review of the literature. Dis Esophagus 2011;24:E11–5.
102. Fontillon M, Lucendo AJ. Transmural eosinophilic infiltration and fibrosis in a patient with non-traumatic Boerhaave's syndrome due to eosinophilic esophagitis. Am J Gastroenterol 2012;107:1762.
103. Hirano I. Editorial: should patients with suspected eosinophilic esophagitis undergo a therapeutic trial of proton pump inhibition? Am J Gastroenterol 2013;108:373–5.
104. Molina-Infante J, Ferrando-Lamana L, Ripoll C, et al. Esophageal eosinophilic infiltration responds to proton pump inhibition in most adults. Clin Gastroenterol Hepatol 2011;9(2):110–7.
105. Molina-Infante J, Zamorano J. Distinguishing eosinophilic esophagitis from gastroesophageal reflux disease upon PPI refractoriness: what about PPI-responsive esophageal eosinophilia? Digestion 2012;85:210.
106. Cheng E, Zhang X, Huo X, et al. Omeprazole blocks eotaxin-3 expression by oesophageal squamous cells from patients with eosinophilic oesophagitis and GORD. Gut 2013;62:824–32.
107. Zhang X, Cheng E, Huo X, et al. Omeprazole blocks STAT6 binding to the eotaxin-3 promoter in eosinophilic esophagitis cells. PLoS One 2012;7:e50037.
108. Straumann A. The natural history and complications of eosinophilic esophagitis. Thorac Surg Clin 2011;21:575–87.
109. Schoepfer AM, Safroneeva E, Bussmann C, et al. Delay in diagnosis of eosinophilic esophagitis increases risk for stricture formation, in a time-dependent manner. Gastroenterology 2013;145(6):1230–6.e1-2.
110. Blanchard C, Wang N, Stringer KF, et al. Eotaxin-3 and a uniquely conserved gene-expression profile in eosinophilic esophagitis. J Clin Invest 2006;116:536–47.
111. Rothenberg ME, Mishra A, Collins MH, et al. Pathogenesis and clinical features of eosinophilic esophagitis. J Allergy Clin Immunol 2001;108:891–4.
112. Mishra A, Hogan SP, Brandt EB, et al. IL-5 promotes eosinophil trafficking to the esophagus. J Immunol 2002;168:2464–9.
113. Mishra A, Hogan SP, Brandt EB, et al. Enterocyte expression of the eotaxin and interleukin-5 transgenes induces compartmentalized dysregulation of eosinophil trafficking. J Biol Chem 2002;277:4406–12.
114. Mishra A, Rothenberg ME. Intratracheal IL-13 induces eosinophilic esophagitis by an IL-5, eotaxin-1, and STAT6-dependent mechanism. Gastroenterology 2003;125:1419–27.
115. Rothenberg ME, Spergel JM, Sherrill JD, et al. Common variants at 5q22 associate with pediatric eosinophilic esophagitis. Nat Genet 2010;42:289–91.
116. Sherrill JD, Gao PS, Stucke EM, et al. Variants of thymic stromal lymphopoietin and its receptor associate with eosinophilic esophagitis. J Allergy Clin Immunol 2010;126:160–5.e3.

117. Masterson JC, McNamee EN, Hosford L, et al. Local hypersensitivity reaction in transgenic mice with squamous epithelial IL-5 overexpression provides a novel model of eosinophilic oesophagitis. Gut 2014;63(1):43–53.

118. Niranjan R, Rayapudi M, Mishra A, et al. Pathogenesis of allergen-induced eosinophilic esophagitis is independent of interleukin (IL)-13. Immunol Cell Biol 2013;91:408–15.

119. Noti M, Wojno ED, Kim BS, et al. Thymic stromal lymphopoietin-elicited basophil responses promote eosinophilic esophagitis. Nat Med 2013;19:1005–13.

120. Wen T, Stucke EM, Grotjan TM, et al. Molecular diagnosis of eosinophilic esophagitis by gene expression profiling. Gastroenterology 2013;145(6): 1289–99.

121. Ngo P, Furuta G, Antonioli D, et al. Eosinophils in the esophagus—peptic or allergic Eosinophilic Esophagitis? Case series of three patients with esophageal eosinophilia. Am J Gastroenterol 2006;101(7):1666–70.

122. Dohil R, Newbury RO, Aceves S. Transient PPI responsive esophageal eosinophilia may be a clinical sub-phenotype of pediatric eosinophilic esophagitis. Dig Dis Sci 2012;57:1413–9.

123. Schroeder S, Capocelli KE, Masterson JC, et al. Effect of proton pump inhibitor on esophageal eosinophilia. J Pediatr Gastroenterol Nutr 2013;56:166–72.

124. Pentiuk S, Putnam PE, Collins MH, et al. Dissociation between symptoms and histological severity in pediatric eosinophilic esophagitis. J Pediatr Gastroenterol Nutr 2009;48:152–60.

125. Furuta GT, Kagalwalla AF, Lee JJ, et al. The oesophageal string test: a novel, minimally invasive method measures mucosal inflammation in eosinophilic oesophagitis. Gut 2013;62:1395–405.

126. Lao-Sirieix P, Boussioutas A, Kadri SR, et al. Non-endoscopic screening biomarkers for Barrett's oesophagus: from microarray analysis to the clinic. Gut 2009;58:1451–9.

127. Kwiatek MA, Hirano I, Kahrilas PJ, et al. Mechanical properties of the esophagus in eosinophilic esophagitis. Gastroenterology 2011;140:82–90.

128. Lin Z, Kahrilas PJ, Xiao Y, et al. Functional luminal imaging probe topography: an improved method for characterizing esophageal distensibility in eosinophilic esophagitis. Therap Adv Gastroenterol 2013;6:97–107.

129. Nicodeme F, Hirano I, Chen J, et al. Esophageal distensibility as a measure of disease severity in patients with eosinophilic esophagitis. Clin Gastroenterol Hepatol 2013;11(9):1101–7.e1.

130. Dellon ES, Irani AM, Hill MR, et al. Development and field testing of a novel patient-reported outcome measure of dysphagia in patients with eosinophilic esophagitis. Aliment Pharmacol Ther 2013;38(6):634–42.

131. Franciosi JP, Hommel KA, Bendo CB, et al. PedsQL eosinophilic esophagitis module: feasibility, reliability, and validity. J Pediatr Gastroenterol Nutr 2013; 57:57–66.

132. Franciosi JP, Hommel KA, DeBrosse CW, et al. Development of a validated patient-reported symptom metric for pediatric eosinophilic esophagitis: qualitative methods. BMC Gastroenterol 2011;11:126.

133. Franciosi JP, Hommel KA, Greenberg AB, et al. Development of the Pediatric Quality of Life Inventory™ Eosinophilic Esophagitis module items: qualitative methods. BMC Gastroenterol 2012;12:135.

134. Taft TH, Kern E, Kwiatek MA, et al. The adult eosinophilic oesophagitis quality of life questionnaire: a new measure of health-related quality of life. Aliment Pharmacol Ther 2011;34:790–8.

135. Hirano I, Moy N, Heckman MG, et al. Endoscopic assessment of the oesopha-
     geal features of eosinophilic oesophagitis: validation of a novel classification
     and grading system. Gut 2013;62:489–95.
136. Fiorentino R, Liu G, Pariser AR, et al. Cross-sector sponsorship of research in
     eosinophilic esophagitis: a collaborative model for rational drug development
     in rare diseases. J Allergy Clin Immunol 2012;130:613–6.
137. Rothenberg ME, Aceves S, Bonis PA, et al. Working with the US Food and Drug
     Administration: progress and timelines in understanding and treating patients
     with eosinophilic esophagitis. J Allergy Clin Immunol 2012;130:617–9.

Epidemiology of Eosinophilic Esophagitis

Evan S. Dellon, MD, MPH

KEYWORDS

- Eosinophilic esophagitis • Epidemiology • Incidence • Prevalence • Risk factors
- Natural history

KEY POINTS

- Eosinophilic esophagitis (EoE) affects patients of all ages, is more commonly seen in males, and whites, and is strongly associated with atopy.
- EoE is chronic, relapses are frequent after treatment is stopped, and diagnostic delay with persistent inflammation increases the risk of esophageal strictures and fibrostenotic complications.
- The prevalence of EoE is 0.5 to 1 cases/1000 persons.
- The incidence of EoE is approximately 10 cases/10,000 persons per year.
- Elucidating the reasons for the rapid increase in incidence and prevalence of EoE is an active area of research, and possibilities include changes in food allergens and aeroallergens, other environmental factors, the decrease of *Helicobacter pylori*, and early life exposures.

INTRODUCTION

Epidemiology is the study of patterns and causes of diseases in defined populations. It uses observational study designs, such as case control or cohort studies, to make inferences about causes and risk factors for diseases. These results generate hypotheses that can subsequently be tested in experimental study designs, such as clinical trials. Over the past 2 decades, great strides have been made in understanding the epidemiology of eosinophilic esophagitis (EoE). Case reports and case series

This work was supported in part by NIH award number K23 DK090073.

Disclosures: No conflicts of interest pertaining to this article. Dr E.S. Dellon has received research support from AstraZeneca, Meritage Pharma, Olympus, National Institutes of Health, ACG, AGA, and CURED Foundation. Dr E.S. Dellon has been a consultant for Aptalis, Novartis, Receptos, and Regeneron.

Division of Gastroenterology and Hepatology, Department of Medicine, Center for Esophageal Diseases and Swallowing and Center for Gastrointestinal Biology and Disease, University of North Carolina School of Medicine, CB#7080, Bioinformatics Building, 130 Mason Farm Road, UNC-CH, Chapel Hill, NC 27599-7080, USA

E-mail address: edellon@med.unc.edu

Gastroenterol Clin N Am 43 (2014) 201–218
http://dx.doi.org/10.1016/j.gtc.2014.02.002
0889-8553/14/$ – see front matter © 2014 Elsevier Inc. All rights reserved.

provided initial descriptions of clinical characteristics of patients with EoE,[1–4] and then, as larger cohorts were reported and natural history data accumulated,[5–11] formal disease definitions and guidelines were put forth.[12–14] Epidemiologic techniques have been used to estimate the incidence and prevalence of EoE at the single-center, regional, and national levels to provide an understanding of trends in the number of cases as well as the burden of disease attributable to EoE.[15–22] The clear result of these studies is that EoE is rapidly increasing both in incidence and in prevalence. Investigations have also begun to determine potential causes that might explain this evolving epidemiology. In this article, the current knowledge base related to the epidemiology of EoE is reviewed. In particular, demographic features and natural history are described, data summarizing the prevalence and incidence of EoE throughout the world are highlighted, and risk factors for EoE are discussed.

DEMOGRAPHIC FEATURES

EoE has been reported throughout the life span, from infancy to almost 100 years of age.[10,13,23] However, most cases are in children, adolescents, and adults younger than 50 years.[10,13,22–24] There is a consistent gender discrepancy, with males affected 3 to 4 times more commonly than females, and EoE is also more frequently reported in whites compared with other races/ethnicities.[11,13,19,22,24–27] The reason for the male predominance is not known, and as more data accrue from larger centers with more diverse patient populations, increasing numbers of racial minorities have been identified with EoE.[28–31] Although most clinical, endoscopic, and histologic features are shared by patients with EoE of different races, some data suggest that African Americans with EoE may be diagnosed at earlier ages and are less likely to have typical endoscopic findings of EoE.[28,31] EoE is also strongly associated with atopic disease and can run in families; both of these topics, as well as the clinical features and differences in the presentation between adults and children, are addressed in detail in other articles elsewhere in this issue.

NATURAL HISTORY

EoE is considered a chronic disease.[12–14] Data from the placebo arms of randomized clinical trials[32–38] and prospective and retrospective cohort studies[5–7,10,11,39–41] show that EoE does not tend to spontaneously resolve or burn out. Specifically, the endoscopic signs and esophageal eosinophilia persist in the absence of treatment. Moreover, if treatment is stopped, symptoms, endoscopic signs, and esophageal eosinophilia recur in most patients over a period of several months.[8,41–45] There are no published reports of EoE transforming into hypereosinophilic syndrome, extending to involve other areas of the gastrointestinal (GI) tract, or causing a malignancy.[6,7,10,11,40]

Recent data have supported the concept that EoE may progress from an inflammatory-predominant phenotype (primarily seen in children) to a fibrosis-predominant one (seen in adults).[13,46–48] These data help to explain the clinical differences between adults and children,[11,39,49,50] and are consistent with basic science work showing that esophageal remodeling and deposition of fibrosis are key pathogenic features of EoE.[51,52] The hypothesis is that in children, eosinophilic inflammation in the esophagus manifests with white plaques or exudates, decreased vascularity or mucosa edema, and linear furrows, but without esophageal rings or strictures, and causes symptoms such as pain, heartburn, and failure to thrive. However, with ongoing inflammation, subepithelial collagen is deposited, esophageal rings, narrowing, and strictures develop, and symptoms become dysphagia predominant.

A retrospective cohort study of patients in Switzerland explored this issue by assessing diagnostic delay (how long patients experienced symptoms before the EoE diagnosis and before any treatment) as a proxy for ongoing inflammation.[53] There was a strong association between increasing diagnostic delay and the prevalence of strictures at diagnosis. For example, only 17% of those with less than 2 years of symptoms before diagnosis had strictures compared with 71% with more than 20 years of symptoms. These investigators calculated that for every increased decade of untreated EoE, there was a doubling of odds of having an esophageal stricture. Another study assessed the same issue by examining endoscopically defined phenotypes of EoE and noted nearly identical results, with the odds of having a fibrostenotic EoE phenotype doubling with each increasing decade of age.[48] These natural history data provide important information for patients, show long-term consequences of EoE, and support the need for treatment of this condition.

PREVALENCE

The prevalence of a condition is defined by how many total cases exist during a given time frame in a specified location and is a useful measure of the burden of that disease. EoE has been described in many places throughout the world, including North America, Europe, South America, Australia, Asia, and the Middle East, but the prevalence seems to be highest in the United States, Western Europe, and Australia compared with Japan or China.[17–22,54–62] There are no reported EoE cohorts in sub-Saharan Africa or India.

The prevalence of EoE depends on the population that is studied, the definition of EoE that was used (and whether the study was conducted before the recognition of proton pump inhibitor [PPI]-responsive esophageal eosinophilia [REE]),[13,14] and the study methodology (prospective vs retrospective), and this contributes to variation in the range of prevalence estimates (**Tables 1** and **2**). Although most prevalence estimates are derived from single centers with defined catchment areas,[15,16,18,20,58,59,63,64] there are some studies that have used either population-based techniques or national databases to attempt to generate more accurate or generalizable estimates.[17,21,22,65–67] Because EoE is chronic and nonfatal, studies universally report an increasing prevalence of EoE, regardless of the geographic location.[54,68]

Prevalence of EoE in the General Population

How common is EoE? In reviewing data assessing the prevalence of EoE in general populations (see **Table 1**), a reasonable answer is 0.5 to 1 cases/1000 persons. Most estimates in the United States range from 40 to 90 cases/100,000 persons.[15,18,19,22,63,65] The largest study in the United States examined administrative health claims data and found the prevalence to be 57/100,000, or approximately 152,000 cases, with a range from 39 to 153/100,000 (106,000–411,000 cases), based on the case definition that was used.[22,69] These findings are consistent with the most recent estimates from Australia (89/100,000),[58] Switzerland (43/100,000),[20] Spain (45/100,000),[59] and Canada (34/100,000).[67] In addition, these prevalence estimates are of the same order of magnitude of pediatric Crohn disease and ulcerative colitis, and are beginning to approach the prevalence of inflammatory bowel disease overall,[70] a remarkable observation, given that EoE was essentially unknown 2 decades ago.

However, several studies have provided estimates that are outside this range. In Northern Sweden, data from a population-based study assessing the prevalence of Barrett esophagus were reanalyzed, and a prevalence of 400/100,000 was found for EoE.[17] These patients were largely asymptomatic and, although they had esophageal

Table 1
Population-based estimates of the prevalence of EoE

Author	Location	Population	Time Frame	Prevalence (per 100,000)
Noel	Hamilton County, OH	Pediatric	2000–2003	43.0
Buckmeier			2000–2006	90.7
Cherian	Perth, Australia	Pediatric	1995, 1999, 2004	89.0
Straumann	Olten County, Switzerland	Adult	1989–2004	23.0
Hruz			1989–2009	42.8
Ronkainen	Northern Sweden	Adult	1998–2001	400
Prasad	Olmstead County, MN	Adult and pediatric	1976–2005	55.0
Gill	Huntington region, WV	Pediatric	1995–2004	73.0
Dalby	Southern Denmark	Pediatric	2005–2007	2.3
Spergel	United States	Adult and pediatric	2010	52.2
Ally	United States (military)	Adult and pediatric	2009	9.7
van Rhijn	Netherlands	Adult and pediatric	1996–2010	4.1
Syed	Calgary, Canada	Adult and pediatric	2004–2008	33.7
Arias	Castilla-La Mancha region, Spain	Adult and pediatric	2005–2011	44.6
Dellon	United States	Adult and pediatric	2009–2011	56.7

Data from Refs.[15–22,58,59,63–67]

eosinophilia, they may not have met current diagnostic criteria for EoE.[13,14] A study in the US military found a prevalence of 10/100,000, but this might have been an underestimate because of the specialized population assessed or because of low sensitivity of the administrative code for EoE.[66,69] Studies from the Netherlands and the southern region of Denmark have also reported lower prevalences of EoE.[21,64] It is unknown if these results are because of practice patterns in those countries or a true difference in the prevalence of disease.

Prevalence of EoE in Patients Undergoing Endoscopy

Although these previous studies assessed the overall prevalence of EoE, depending on the specific patient population seen in health care settings, the prevalence may be orders of magnitude higher (see **Table 2**). For example, a prospective study, which collected esophageal biopsies on consecutive patients undergoing upper endoscopy for any indication, found that 6.5% of patients were diagnosed with EoE.[26] Other studies with a similar design found comparable rates, from 2.4% to 6.6%.[71,72] Given that approximately 6.9 million upper endoscopies are performed annually in the United States,[73] endoscopists should expect to commonly encounter EoE in the procedure suite.

EoE is even more common in patients undergoing upper endoscopy for symptoms of dysphagia. In 3 prospective studies conducted in this focused patient population, the prevalence of EoE ranged from 12% to 22%.[25,74,75] However, not every patient in these studies with a finding of esophageal eosinophilia would meet current diagnostic guidelines with exclusion of PPI-REE, because patients were enrolled before the recognition of this phenomenon. A recent study conducted in an esophageal referral center reported an EoE prevalence of 23% for patients undergoing endoscopy for dysphagia, after excluding those patients with PPI-REE.[76] In that study,

Table 2
Prevalence of EoE in selected patient populations undergoing endoscopy

Author	Population	Time Frame	Prevalence (per 100)
Patients undergoing endoscopy for any reason			
Veerappan	Adults	2007	6.5
Joo	Adults	2009	6.6
Sealock	Adults (VA population)	n/a	2.4
Patients undergoing endoscopy for dysphagia			
Prasad	Adults	2005–2006	15
Mackenzie	Adults	2005–2007	12
Ricker	Adults (nonobstructive dysphagia only)	2007–2009	22
Dellon	Adults	2009–2011	23
Patients undergoing endoscopy for food bolus impaction			
Desai	Adults	2000–2003	55
Kerlin	Adults	n/a	50
Sperry	Adults and pediatric	2002–2009	46
Hurtado	Pediatric	2005–2009	63
Patients undergoing endoscopy for refractory reflux			
Liacouras	Pediatric	1993–1995	3
Rodrigro	Adult	2002–2005	0.2
Veerappan	Adult	2007	8
Sa	Adult	2006–2008	1
Poh	Adult	n/a	1
Foroutan	Adult	2006	8
Garcia-Campean	Adult	2007–2009	4
Dellon	Adult	2009–2011	2
Patients undergoing endoscopy for noncardiac chest pain			
Achem	Adult	2006–2007	6
Patients undergoing endoscopy for abdominal pain			
Thakkar	Pediatric	2007–2010	4
Patients with refractory aerodigestive symptoms			
Hill	Pediatric	2003–2013	4

Abbreviation: n/a, not applicable.
Data from Refs.[25,26,41,42,61,71,72,74–87]

esophageal eosinophilia itself was seen in 40% of those undergoing upper endoscopy for dysphagia, before a PPI trial was conducted. Given that approximately 20% of all upper endoscopies performed are for an indication of dysphagia,[73] EoE must be highly suspected in this population.

In the most extreme form of dysphagia (esophageal food bolus impaction requiring a visit to an emergency department and urgent endoscopy), EoE is now the most frequent condition identified. In this setting, between 46% and 63% of patients with food impaction have EoE.[77–80] However, these data are limited because less than half of patients with food or foreign body impactions have esophageal biopsies to evaluate for esophageal eosinophilia,[78,80] so EoE in this setting may still be underdiagnosed. If patients have a bolus impaction and no biopsies are obtained, it is reasonable to perform a follow-up procedure to identify the underlying cause.

The prevalence of EoE in patients undergoing endoscopy for other upper GI symptoms has also been described. For patients with heartburn-predominant symptom who do not respond clinically to PPI therapy (PPI-refractory reflux), EoE has been identified as the cause 1% to 8% of the time.[26,42,61,76,81–84] In adults with noncardiac chest pain, 1 study found that EoE was the cause in 6%.[85] In children undergoing upper endoscopy for abdominal pain, the frequency of EoE was 4%,[86] and in children undergoing multispecialty evaluation for refractory aerodigestive symptoms, it was also 4%.[87]

Although these epidemiologic data are useful for understanding how common EoE is, building a differential diagnosis for patients undergoing endoscopy, and measuring the burden of disease attributable to EoE, they also imply a practical point. Because EoE is common in patients undergoing endoscopic procedures, practitioners should strongly consider the diagnosis and obtain esophageal biopsies to evaluate for it. Currently, guidelines recommend obtaining biopsies for all patients presenting with dysphagia, regardless of the endoscopic appearance.[12–14] There is also a recent analysis that suggests if the clinical probability of EoE is at least 8% to 10%, obtaining biopsies in patients with PPI-refractory reflux is also cost-effective.[88]

INCIDENCE

The incidence of a condition is how many new cases occur during a given time frame in a specified location, and is a measure of the number of people newly affected by a disease. The incidence of a condition can be low (a few new cases), but the prevalence can be relatively high if the condition is chronic and does not affect longevity. In addition, the incidence of a condition can be approximately equivalent to the prevalence for a condition that is either short-lived or highly morbid.

To study the incidence of a condition, it is necessary not only to detect all new (incident) cases but to ensure that existing (prevalent) cases are not falsely counted as new cases. In EoE, this goal has been accomplished primarily at referral centers in regions in which the patient population and catchment area are well defined,[15,19,20,59,64] but there are some emerging regional and national data as well.[21,67] Most of the reports estimate the incidence of EoE from 6 to 13 cases/100,000 persons (**Table 3**). The

Table 3 Population-based estimates of the incidence of EoE				
Author	Location	Population	Time Frame	Incidence (per 100,000)
Noel	Hamilton County, OH	Pediatric	2003	12.8
Hruz	Olten County, Switzerland	Adult	2007–2009	7.4
Prasad	Olmstead County, MN	Adult and pediatric	2001–2005	9.5
Dalby	Southern Denmark	Pediatric	2005–2007	1.6
van Rhijn	Netherlands	Adult and pediatric	2010	1.3
Syed	Calgary, Canada	Adult and pediatric	2004–2008	11
Arias	Castilla-La Mancha region, Spain	Adult and pediatric	2005–2011	6.4

The estimated incidence of the most recent time point in each study is presented.
Data from Refs.[15,19–21,59,64,67]

2 studies that have reported lower incidence, from the Netherlands and southern Denmark, were the same ones that reported lower prevalence.[21,64]

Increasing Incidence and Risk Factors

Studies are consistent in showing that the incidence of EoE has been increasing rapidly. In a report from Hamilton County, Ohio, the incidence of EoE was noted to increase from 9 to 12.8/100,000 over a 3-year period.[15] In a report from Olmstead County, Minnesota, no EoE cases were seen before 1990, but the incidence increased from 0.35 to 9.5/100,000 over a 15-year period.[19] Similar increases have been reported in Switzerland (1.2–7.4/100,000 over a 20-year period)[20] and in the Netherlands (0.01–1.3/100,000 over 14 years).[21] This increasing incidence has also been reflected in temporal trends in the relative prevalence of dysphagia causes, with EoE becoming a more frequent cause of dysphagia over time.[89]

Why is EoE Increasing?

Although these marked changes in EoE incidence account for its increasing prevalence, they also beg the question of why the incidence is itself increasing. Although the answer is not known, there are several hypotheses.[90] One explanation is simply that EoE is increasing because of increasing recognition; the condition was always there but given the research and clinical interest in the condition, practitioners are more aware of EoE, have a higher degree of suspicion when performing endoscopy, take more esophageal biopsies, and are therefore more likely to make the diagnosis. The exponential increase in the number of publications related to EoE is a testament to the increased interest in EoE (from 0 to 1 publication per year before 2000, to >200 publications in 2013). Some data that support this theory show that the increase in incidence rates relatively closely matches the increase in endoscopy volume or biopsy rates.[67,91] However, there are other studies in which biopsy rates do increase 2 to 3 times over the study period, but the incidence of EoE outpaces that increase by several-fold, indicating that increased recognition is not the only explanation.[11,19,89,92] In addition, in studies in which archived pathology samples have been retrieved and reanalyzed, cases of probable EoE identified in the early 1980s and 1990s occur at lower rates than are currently being observed.[93,94]

There are other epidemiologic clues that provide insight. Recent data suggest that the prevalence of EoE steadily increases as age increases, peaks in the 35-year to 45-year age range, and then decreases (**Fig. 1**).[22] This is a counterintuitive observation for a chronic and nonfatal disease (in which prevalence would be expected to continue to increase as age increases) and suggests a possible cohort effect. It is interesting to speculate whether something might have changed in the environment 40 to 50 years ago that began to affect children born after that time, but did not affect older individuals. In contrast, genetic changes would not be expected to affect a new disease over a relatively short time frame. This time frame is also consistent with decades-long symptom duration before EoE diagnosis in some older patients with EoE.[23,48,90,95]

Allergen and Hygiene Hypotheses

There are several etiologic risk factors that have been either identified or hypothesized to contribute to the increase of EoE (**Box 1**). One possibility relates to EoE as an allergic disease (see also the article on allergic mechanisms elsewhere in this issue). All allergic diseases, including asthma, atopic dermatis, allergic rhinitis, and food allergies, have been increasing in recent decades.[96] One global explanation for this increase is the hygiene hypothesis, which holds that because the environment in developed counties has become more sterile, human immune systems are exposed

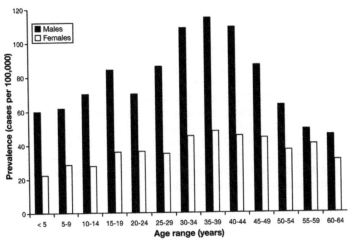

Fig. 1. Prevalence of EoE (cases per 100,000) in the United States as stratified by sex and by 5-year increments of age, in a study of administrative health claims data. (*From* Dellon ES, Jensen ET, Martin CF, et al. Prevalence of Eosinophilic Esophagitis in the United States. Clin Gastroenterol Hepatol 2013. [Epub ahead of print]; with permission.)

to a smaller variety of antigens, and tolerance is less likely to develop.[96] Thus, EoE as an allergen-mediated/immune-mediated disease would be increasing in parallel with other allergic diseases.

Environmental Hypotheses

Related to the hygiene hypothesis are theories that changing environmental factors are contributing to the increase in EoE. One factor is aeroallergens. There have been clear links in humans between pollen and other aeroallergen exposure either triggering EoE or correlating with EoE disease activity.[97–99] In addition, many studies have shown a link between the season of the year and EoE diagnosis, with EoE more commonly being diagnosed in summer or autumn, times of potentially higher aeroallergen activity.[11,19,100,101] Other environmental exposures such as air pollution or industrial exposures have yet to be formally assessed.

Box 1
Potential etiologic risk factors for EoE

- Aeroallergens
- Food allergens
- *Helicobacter pylori* (protective)
- PPIs
- Cold or arid climates
- Population density (urban vs rural locations)
- Early life factors (antibiotic use; cesarean section)
- Connective tissue disorders

Data from Refs.[4,45,65,97–100,102–105,108,109,112,123,126]

Geographic risk factors have also been reported. Several studies have used a large nationwide pathology database containing hundreds of thousands of patients undergoing endoscopy with esophageal biopsy, and representing more than 14,000 cases of esophageal eosinophilia and EoE.[102,103] Prevalence of esophageal eosinophilia was noted to vary by climate zone, with cases more commonly noted in arid and cold weather climates.[102] This was an interesting finding because the climate zone classification used is closely linked to types of vegetation, again raising the question of allergen exposure, and also because other autoimmune and allergic diseases have geographic variation with a north-south gradient. A related study showed that esophageal eosinophilia appeared to be more common in rural areas with low population density.[103] Although this theory may be counterintuitive (some allergic diseases such as asthma and atopic dermatitis are believed to be more common in urban areas), there are other studies on EoE that support this as well.[65,104] This hypothesis raises the question of whether vegetation or environmental exposures more likely to be found in rural areas are risk factors for EoE, but additional research is required to explore these possibilities.

Food allergens can also be considered environmental exposures. It is well established that foods can trigger EoE and that allergen-free elemental formula or elimination of certain food allergens from the diet can result in clinical, endoscopic, and histologic remission (see also the article on dietary therapy for EoE elsewhere in this issue).[4,5,45,105,106] However, it is less clear why foods that have been tolerated for much of human history are now allergic triggers in EoE. Whether this situation is because of recent changes in agricultural practices, decreased variety of foods, genetic modification of crops, pesticides, antibiotic or hormone use in livestock, or other factors, such as packaging and transport of foods, remains to be determined.

Helicobacter pylori Hypothesis

When thinking about reasons that EoE may be increasing, it is possible that something being removed from the environment could also play a role. *Helicobacter pylori* is 1 such factor. Since its formal characterization in the early 1980s and subsequent association with peptic ulcer disease and gastric cancer, the prevalence of *H pylori* has markedly decreased in the United States with ongoing treatment of this pathogen.[107] In a study examining more than 165,000 paired esophageal and gastric biopsy samples, there was a strong inverse relationship between *H pylori* and esophageal eosinophilia; those who were more likely to have esophageal eosinophilia or EoE were less likely to have *H pylori*.[108] This relationship has also been noted in 2 smaller studies in EoE[17,109] and is consistent with the observation that *H pylori* is inversely associated with other atopic disorders, such as asthma and eczema.[110] The mechanism by which *H pylori* may be protective of EoE is not known, but it has been hypothesized that the infection polarizes the immune system toward a Th1 response, and the lack of infection might allow a Th2 response, less tolerance, and increased atopy.[108]

PPI Hypothesis

Another potential ecologic association to explain the increase in EoE is the parallel increase in use of PPI medications over the past 3 decades. This increase in use has also been noted in infants as a treatment of reflux and colic, which represents a major change in practice during a time when the immune system is developing.[111] Although there is no direct evidence that PPI use has caused EoE in an individual patient, there are some intriguing mechanistic reasons that this could be a concern, especially given the multitude of effects that PPIs have outside their antisecretory action.[112,113] Specifically, PPIs can increase upper GI tract permeability, potentially creating a new route of antigen exposure, and their use has also been associated with the development of new food-specific IgE antibodies.[112,114–116] However, these data are balanced by 2 important points. First, many patients who are diagnosed with EoE have never taken a PPI previously. Second, convincing data show that PPIs have antiinflammatory/anti-eosinophil effects both in vitro[117] and in vivo; at least 30% to 40% of individuals with esophageal eosinophilia have symptomatic and histologic resolution after a PPI trial.[76,118,119] Because of this situation, a PPI trial is now a required part of the EoE diagnostic algorithm.[12–14] Therefore, before PPIs can be considered to be a cause of EoE, direct evidence is required.

Early Life Exposure Hypotheses

A new area of investigation has started to examine early life exposures that might predispose to development of EoE. Antibiotic exposure in early life increases the odds of developing other allergic diseases such as asthma or atopic dermatitis and inflammatory bowel disease, especially Crohn disease.[120–122] There are recent pilot data suggesting the same may be true in EoE, in which exposures during the first year of life were assessed and the subsequent odds of pediatric EoE determined.[123] In this study, infants who received antibiotics were markedly more likely to have EoE than controls who did not, and there was also a trend for increased EoE in infants delivered by cesarean section, those who were born prematurely, and those who had nonexclusive breastfeeding. All of these factors could theoretically affect the early life microbiome, perturbations of which have been hypothesized to be a determinant of atopic disease.[124] Novel research techniques in EoE have begun to characterize the esophageal microbiome, but this has yet to be fully explored as a risk factor for EoE.[125]

Other Hypotheses

Another set of risk factors for EoE that have been recently identified are connective tissue and autoimmune disorders. A report in a large cohort of patients with EoE found a subset with coexisting diseases such as Ehlers-Danlos, Marfan, and Loeys-Dietz syndromes, in which EoE was significantly increased compared with expected rates in the general population.[126] Moreover, this association suggested potential genetic links that could be used to learn more about the pathogenesis of EoE. In a preliminary study using administrative data, a similar relationship between EoE and connective tissue disorders was noted, and there was also a relationship with autoimmune diseases.[127]

SUMMARY

The epidemiology of EoE has become increasingly well understood over the past decade. The disease is well characterized clinically, and those features have informed diagnostic guidelines. EoE can affect patients of any age, but there is a male predominance, it is more common in whites, and there is a strong association with atopic diseases. EoE is chronic, relapses are frequent with cessation of treatment, and new data suggest that unopposed inflammation and persistent symptoms with diagnostic delay increase the risk of fibrostenotic complications. The prevalence of EoE is increasing substantially, and it is now the most common cause of food impaction in patients presenting to the emergency department, and is frequently encountered in the endoscopy suite. Approximately 0.5 to 1 in 1000 people are estimated to have EoE, a prevalence that is beginning to approach that of inflammatory bowel disease. Incidence estimates suggest that there are 1/10,000 new cases per year, and the increase in incidence is outpacing the increase in recognition and endoscopy volume. The reasons for this evolving epidemiology are not yet fully delineated, but possibilities include changes in food allergens, increasing aeroallergens and other environmental factors, the decrease of *H pylori*, and early life exposures that may affect the microbiome. The study of the epidemiology of EoE has now shifted from case description to risk factor ascertainment, and new etiologic hypotheses have been raised that present exciting avenues for future epidemiologic and pathogenic research in this condition, with the goal of preventing the occurrence of EoE.

REFERENCES

1. Landres RT, Kuster GG, Strum WB. Eosinophilic esophagitis in a patient with vigorous achalasia. Gastroenterology 1978;74:1298–301.
2. Attwood SE, Smyrk TC, Demeester TR, et al. Esophageal eosinophilia with dysphagia. A distinct clinicopathologic syndrome. Dig Dis Sci 1993;38: 109–16.
3. Straumann A, Spichtin HP, Bernoulli R, et al. Idiopathic eosinophilic esophagitis: a frequently overlooked disease with typical clinical aspects and discrete endoscopic findings. Schweiz Med Wochenschr 1994;124:1419–29 [in German].
4. Kelly KJ, Lazenby AJ, Rowe PC, et al. Eosinophilic esophagitis attributed to gastroesophageal reflux: improvement with an amino acid-based formula. Gastroenterology 1995;109:1503–12.
5. Liacouras CA, Spergel JM, Ruchelli E, et al. Eosinophilic esophagitis: a 10-year experience in 381 children. Clin Gastroenterol Hepatol 2005;3:1198–206.
6. Assa'ad AH, Putnam PE, Collins MH, et al. Pediatric patients with eosinophilic esophagitis: an 8-year follow-up. J Allergy Clin Immunol 2007;119:731–8.
7. Straumann A, Spichtin HP, Grize L, et al. Natural history of primary eosinophilic esophagitis: a follow-up of 30 adult patients for up to 11.5 years. Gastroenterology 2003;125:1660–9.
8. Gonsalves N, Policarpio-Nicolas M, Zhang Q, et al. Histopathologic variability and endoscopic correlates in adults with eosinophilic esophagitis. Gastrointest Endosc 2006;64:313–9.
9. Aceves SS, Newbury RO, Dohil R, et al. Distinguishing eosinophilic esophagitis in pediatric patients: clinical, endoscopic, and histologic features of an emerging disorder. J Clin Gastroenterol 2007;41:252–6.
10. Spergel JM, Brown-Whitehorn TF, Beausoleil JL, et al. 14 years of eosinophilic esophagitis: clinical features and prognosis. J Pediatr Gastroenterol Nutr 2009;48:30–6.
11. Dellon ES, Gibbs WB, Fritchie KJ, et al. Clinical, endoscopic, and histologic findings distinguish eosinophilic esophagitis from gastroesophageal reflux disease. Clin Gastroenterol Hepatol 2009;7:1305–13.
12. Furuta GT, Liacouras CA, Collins MH, et al. Eosinophilic esophagitis in children and adults: a systematic review and consensus recommendations for diagnosis and treatment. Gastroenterology 2007;133:1342–63.
13. Liacouras CA, Furuta GT, Hirano I, et al. Eosinophilic esophagitis: updated consensus recommendations for children and adults. J Allergy Clin Immunol 2011;128:3–20.e6.
14. Dellon ES, Gonsalves N, Hirano I, et al. ACG Clinical Guideline: evidence based approach to the diagnosis and management of esophageal eosinophilia and eosinophilic esophagitis. Am J Gastroenterol 2013;108:679–92.
15. Noel RJ, Putnam PE, Rothenberg ME. Eosinophilic esophagitis. N Engl J Med 2004;351:940–1.

16. Straumann A, Simon HU. Eosinophilic esophagitis: escalating epidemiology? J Allergy Clin Immunol 2005;115:418–9.
17. Ronkainen J, Talley NJ, Aro P, et al. Prevalence of oesophageal eosinophils and eosinophilic oesophagitis in adults: the population-based Kalixanda study. Gut 2007;56:615–20.
18. Buckmeier BK, Rothenberg ME, Collins MH. The incidence and prevalence of eosinophilic esophagitis. J Allergy Clin Immunol 2008;121(Suppl 2):S71 [abstract: 271].
19. Prasad GA, Alexander JA, Schleck CD, et al. Epidemiology of eosinophilic esophagitis over three decades in Olmsted County, Minnesota. Clin Gastroenterol Hepatol 2009;7:1055–61.
20. Hruz P, Straumann A, Bussmann C, et al. Escalating incidence of eosinophilic esophagitis: a 20-year prospective, population-based study in Olten County, Switzerland. J Allergy Clin Immunol 2011;128:1349–50.e5.
21. van Rhijn BD, Verheij J, Smout AJ, et al. Rapidly increasing incidence of eosinophilic esophagitis in a large cohort. Neurogastroenterol Motil 2013;25:47–52.e5.
22. Dellon ES, Jensen ET, Martin CF, et al. Prevalence of eosinophilic esophagitis in the United States. Clin Gastroenterol Hepatol 2013. [Epub ahead of print].
23. Kapel RC, Miller JK, Torres C, et al. Eosinophilic esophagitis: a prevalent disease in the United States that affects all age groups. Gastroenterology 2008; 134:1316–21.
24. Dellon ES, Aderoju A, Woosley JT, et al. Variability in diagnostic criteria for eosinophilic esophagitis: a systematic review. Am J Gastroenterol 2007;102:2300–13.
25. Mackenzie SH, Go M, Chadwick B, et al. Clinical trial: eosinophilic esophagitis in patients presenting with dysphagia: a prospective analysis. Aliment Pharmacol Ther 2008;28:1140–6.
26. Veerappan GR, Perry JL, Duncan TJ, et al. Prevalence of eosinophilic esophagitis in an adult population undergoing upper endoscopy: a prospective study. Clin Gastroenterol Hepatol 2009;7:420–6.
27. Franciosi JP, Tam V, Liacouras CA, et al. A case-control study of sociodemographic and geographic characteristics of 335 children with eosinophilic esophagitis. Clin Gastroenterol Hepatol 2009;7:415–9.
28. Sperry SL, Woosley JT, Shaheen NJ, et al. Influence of race and gender on the presentation of eosinophilic esophagitis. Am J Gastroenterol 2012;107:215–21.
29. Bohm M, Malik Z, Sebastiano C, et al. Mucosal eosinophilia: prevalence and racial/ethnic differences in symptoms and endoscopic findings in adults over 10 years in an urban hospital. J Clin Gastroenterol 2012;46:567–74.
30. Sharma HP, Mansoor DK, Sprunger AC, et al. Racial disparities in the presentation of pediatric eosinophilic esophagitis. J Allergy Clin Immunol 2011;127: AB110.
31. Moawad FJ, Veerappan GR, Dias JA, et al. Race may play a role in the clinical presentation of eosinophilic esophagitis. Am J Gastroenterol 2012;107:1263.
32. Konikoff MR, Noel RJ, Blanchard C, et al. A randomized, double-blind, placebo-controlled trial of fluticasone propionate for pediatric eosinophilic esophagitis. Gastroenterology 2006;131:1381–91.
33. Dohil R, Newbury R, Fox L, et al. Oral viscous budesonide is effective in children with eosinophilic esophagitis in a randomized, placebo-controlled trial. Gastroenterology 2010;139:418–29.
34. Straumann A, Conus S, Degen L, et al. Budesonide is effective in adolescent and adult patients with active eosinophilic esophagitis. Gastroenterology 2010;139:1526–37, 37.e1.

35. Alexander JA, Jung KW, Arora AS, et al. Swallowed fluticasone improves histologic but not symptomatic responses of adults with eosinophilic esophagitis. Clin Gastroenterol Hepatol 2012;10:742–9.e1.

36. Assa'ad AH, Gupta SK, Collins MH, et al. An antibody against IL-5 reduces numbers of esophageal intraepithelial eosinophils in children with eosinophilic esophagitis. Gastroenterology 2011;141:1593–604.

37. Gupta SK, Collins MH, Lewis JD, et al. Efficacy and safety of oral budesonide suspension (OBS) in pediatric subjects with eosinophilic esophagitis (EoE): results from the double-blind, placebo-controlled PEER study. Gastroenterology 2011;140(Suppl 1):S179.

38. Spergel JM, Rothenberg ME, Collins MH, et al. Reslizumab in children and adolescents with eosinophilic esophagitis: results of a double-blind, randomized, placebo-controlled trial. J Allergy Clin Immunol 2012;129:456–63, 63.e1–3.

39. Noel RJ, Putnam PE, Collins MH, et al. Clinical and immunopathologic effects of swallowed fluticasone for eosinophilic esophagitis. Clin Gastroenterol Hepatol 2004;2:568–75.

40. DeBrosse CW, Franciosi JP, King EC, et al. Long-term outcomes in pediatric-onset esophageal eosinophilia. J Allergy Clin Immunol 2011;128:132–8.

41. Menard-Katcher P, Marks KL, Liacouras CA, et al. The natural history of eosinophilic oesophagitis in the transition from childhood to adulthood. Aliment Pharmacol Ther 2013;37:114–21.

42. Liacouras CA, Wenner WJ, Brown K, et al. Primary eosinophilic esophagitis in children: successful treatment with oral corticosteroids. J Pediatr Gastroenterol Nutr 1998;26:380–5.

43. Helou EF, Simonson J, Arora AS. 3-yr-follow-up of topical corticosteroid treatment for eosinophilic esophagitis in adults. Am J Gastroenterol 2008;103:2194–9.

44. Straumann A, Conus S, Degen L, et al. Long-term budesonide maintenance treatment is partially effective for patients with eosinophilic esophagitis. Clin Gastroenterol Hepatol 2011;9:400–9.e1.

45. Markowitz JE, Spergel JM, Ruchelli E, et al. Elemental diet is an effective treatment for eosinophilic esophagitis in children and adolescents. Am J Gastroenterol 2003;98:777–82.

46. Prieto R, Richter JE. Eosinophilic esophagitis in adults: an update on medical management. Curr Gastroenterol Rep 2013;15:324.

47. Hirano I. Therapeutic end points in eosinophilic esophagitis: is elimination of esophageal eosinophils enough? Clin Gastroenterol Hepatol 2012;10:750–2.

48. Dellon ES, Kim HP, Sperry SL, et al. A phenotypic analysis shows that eosinophilic esophagitis is a progressive fibrostenotic disease. Gastrointest Endosc 2013. [Epub ahead of print].

49. Straumann A. The natural history and complications of eosinophilic esophagitis. Thorac Surg Clin 2011;21:575–87.

50. Kim HP, Vance RB, Shaheen NJ, et al. The prevalence and diagnostic utility of endoscopic features of eosinophilic esophagitis: a meta-analysis. Clin Gastroenterol Hepatol 2012;10:988–96.e5.

51. Aceves SS, Newbury RO, Dohil R, et al. Esophageal remodeling in pediatric eosinophilic esophagitis. J Allergy Clin Immunol 2007;119:206–12.

52. Chehade M, Sampson HA, Morotti RA, et al. Esophageal subepithelial fibrosis in children with eosinophilic esophagitis. J Pediatr Gastroenterol Nutr 2007;45:319–28.

53. Schoepfer AM, Safroneeva E, Bussmann C, et al. Delay in diagnosis of eosino-philic esophagitis increases risk for stricture formation in a time-dependent manner. Gastroenterology 2013;145:1230–6.e2.
54. Sealock RJ, Rendon G, El-Serag HB. Systematic review: the epidemiology of eosinophilic oesophagitis in adults. Aliment Pharmacol Ther 2010;32: 712–9.
55. Fujishiro H, Amano Y, Kushiyama Y, et al. Eosinophilic esophagitis investigated by upper gastrointestinal endoscopy in Japanese patients. J Gastroenterol 2011;46:1142–4.
56. Kinoshita Y, Furuta K, Ishimaura N, et al. Clinical characteristics of Japanese patients with eosinophilic esophagitis and eosinophilic gastroenteritis. J Gastroenterol 2013;48(3):333–9.
57. Shi YN, Sun SJ, Xiong LS, et al. Prevalence, clinical manifestations and endo-scopic features of eosinophilic esophagitis: a pathological review in China. J Dig Dis 2012;13:304–9.
58. Cherian S, Smith NM, Forbes DA. Rapidly increasing prevalence of eosinophilic oesophagitis in Western Australia. Arch Dis Child 2006;91:1000–4.
59. Arias A, Lucendo AJ. Prevalence of eosinophilic oesophagitis in adult patients in a central region of Spain. Eur J Gastroenterol Hepatol 2013;25:208–12.
60. Hasosah MY, Sukkar GA, Alsahafi AF, et al. Eosinophilic esophagitis in Saudi children: symptoms, histology and endoscopy results. Saudi J Gastroenterol 2011;17:119–23.
61. Foroutan M, Norouzi A, Molaei M, et al. Eosinophilic esophagitis in patients with refractory gastroesophageal reflux disease. Dig Dis Sci 2010;55:28–31.
62. Fujiwara Y, Sugawa T, Tanaka F, et al. A multicenter study on the prevalence of eosinophilic esophagitis and PPI-responsive esophageal eosinophilic infiltra-tion. Intern Med 2012;51:3235–9.
63. Gill R, Durst P, Rewalt M, et al. Eosinophilic esophagitis disease in children from West Virginia: a review of the last decade (1995-2004). Am J Gastroenterol 2007;102:2281–5.
64. Dalby K, Nielsen RG, Kruse-Andersen S, et al. Eosinophilic oesophagitis in in-fants and children in the region of Southern Denmark: a prospective study of prevalence and clinical presentation. J Pediatr Gastroenterol Nutr 2010;51: 280–2.
65. Spergel JM, Book WM, Mays E, et al. Variation in prevalence, diagnostic criteria, and initial management options for eosinophilic gastrointestinal diseases in the United States. J Pediatr Gastroenterol Nutr 2011;52:300–6.
66. Ally M, Maydonovitch C, McAllister D, et al. The prevalence of eosinophilic esophagitis in the United States military healthcare population. Am J Gastroen-terol 2012;107(Suppl 1):S1 [abstract: 2].
67. Syed AA, Andrews CN, Shaffer E, et al. The rising incidence of eosinophilic oe-sophagitis is associated with increasing biopsy rates: a population-based study. Aliment Pharmacol Ther 2012;36:950–8.
68. Soon IS, Butzner JD, Kaplan GG, et al. Incidence and prevalence of eosinophilic esophagitis in children. J Pediatr Gastroenterol Nutr 2013;57:72–80.
69. Rybnicek DA, Hathorn KE, Pfaff ER, et al. Administrative coding is specific, but not sensitive, for identifying eosinophilic esophagitis. Dis Esophagus 2013. [Epub ahead of print].
70. Kappelman MD, Rifas-Shiman SL, Kleinman K, et al. The prevalence and geographic distribution of Crohn's disease and ulcerative colitis in the United States. Clin Gastroenterol Hepatol 2007;5:1424–9.

71. Sealock RJ, Kramer JR, Verstovsek G, et al. The prevalence of oesophageal eosinophilia and eosinophilic oesophagitis: a prospective study in unselected patients presenting to endoscopy. Aliment Pharmacol Ther 2013;37:825–32.
72. Joo MK, Park JJ, Kim SH, et al. Prevalence and endoscopic features of eosinophilic esophagitis in patients with esophageal or upper gastrointestinal symptoms. J Dig Dis 2012;13:296–303.
73. Peery AF, Dellon ES, Lund J, et al. Burden of gastrointestinal disease in the United States: 2012 update. Gastroenterology 2012;143:1179–87.e1–3.
74. Prasad GA, Talley NJ, Romero Y, et al. Prevalence and predictive factors of eosinophilic esophagitis in patients presenting with dysphagia: a prospective study. Am J Gastroenterol 2007;102:2627–32.
75. Ricker J, McNear S, Cassidy T, et al. Routine screening for eosinophilic esophagitis in patients presenting with dysphagia. Therap Adv Gastroenterol 2011;4:27–35.
76. Dellon ES, Speck O, Woodward K, et al. Clinical and endoscopic characteristics do not reliably differentiate PPI-responsive esophageal eosinophilia and eosinophilic esophagitis in patients undergoing upper endoscopy: a prospective cohort study. Am J Gastroenterol 2013;108:1854–60.
77. Desai TK, Stecevic V, Chang CH, et al. Association of eosinophilic inflammation with esophageal food impaction in adults. Gastrointest Endosc 2005;61:795–801.
78. Hurtado CW, Furuta GT, Kramer RE. Etiology of esophageal food impactions in children. J Pediatr Gastroenterol Nutr 2011;52:43–6.
79. Kerlin P, Jones D, Remedios M, et al. Prevalence of eosinophilic esophagitis in adults with food bolus obstruction of the esophagus. J Clin Gastroenterol 2007;41:356–61.
80. Sperry SL, Crockett SD, Miller CB, et al. Esophageal foreign-body impactions: epidemiology, time trends, and the impact of the increasing prevalence of eosinophilic esophagitis. Gastrointest Endosc 2011;74:985–91.
81. Rodrigo S, Abboud G, Oh D, et al. High intraepithelial eosinophil counts in esophageal squamous epithelium are not specific for eosinophilic esophagitis in adults. Am J Gastroenterol 2008;103:435–42.
82. Sa CC, Kishi HS, Silva-Werneck AL, et al. Eosinophilic esophagitis in patients with typical gastroesophageal reflux disease symptoms refractory to proton pump inhibitor. Clinics (Sao Paulo) 2011;66:557–61.
83. Poh CH, Gasiorowska A, Navarro-Rodriguez T, et al. Upper GI tract findings in patients with heartburn in whom proton pump inhibitor treatment failed versus those not receiving antireflux treatment. Gastrointest Endosc 2010;71:28–34.
84. Garcia-Compean D, Gonzalez Gonzalez JA, Marrufo Garcia CA, et al. Prevalence of eosinophilic esophagitis in patients with refractory gastroesophageal reflux disease symptoms: a prospective study. Dig Liver Dis 2011;43:204–8.
85. Achem SR, Almansa C, Krishna M, et al. Oesophageal eosinophilic infiltration in patients with noncardiac chest pain. Aliment Pharmacol Ther 2011;33:1194–201.
86. Thakkar K, Chen L, Tatevian N, et al. Diagnostic yield of oesophagogastroduodenoscopy in children with abdominal pain. Aliment Pharmacol Ther 2009;30:662–9.
87. Hill CA, Ramakrishna J, Fracchia MS, et al. Prevalence of eosinophilic esophagitis in children with refractory aerodigestive symptoms. JAMA Otolaryngol Head Neck Surg 2013;139:903–6.

88. Miller SM, Goldstein JL, Gerson LB. Cost-effectiveness model of endoscopic biopsy for eosinophilic esophagitis in patients with refractory GERD. Am J Gastroenterol 2011;106:1439–45.
89. Kidambi T, Toto E, Ho N, et al. Temporal trends in the relative prevalence of dysphagia etiologies from 1999-2009. World J Gastroenterol 2012;18:4335–41.
90. Bonis PA. Putting the puzzle together: epidemiological and clinical clues in the etiology of eosinophilic esophagitis. Immunol Allergy Clin North Am 2009;29: 41–52.
91. Vanderheyden AD, Petras RE, DeYoung BR, et al. Emerging eosinophilic (allergic) esophagitis: increased incidence or increased recognition? Arch Pathol Lab Med 2007;131:777–9.
92. Dellon ES, Gibbs WB, Woosley JT, et al. Increasing incidence of eosinophilic esophagitis: a persistent trend after accounting for procedure indication and biopsy rate. Gastroenterology 2008;134(Suppl 1):S1972 [abstract: 289].
93. DeBrosse CW, Collins MH, Buckmeier Butz BK, et al. Identification, epidemiology, and chronicity of pediatric esophageal eosinophilia, 1982-1999. J Allergy Clin Immunol 2010;126:112–9.
94. Whitney-Miller CL, Katzka D, Furth EE. Eosinophilic esophagitis: a retrospective review of esophageal biopsy specimens from 1992 to 2004 at an adult academic medical center. Am J Clin Pathol 2009;131:788–92.
95. Garrean CP, Gonsalves N, Hirano I. Epidemiologic implications of symptom onset in adults with eosinophilic esophagitis. Gastroenterology 2009; 136(Suppl 1). AB S1875.
96. Okada H, Kuhn C, Feillet H, et al. The 'hygiene hypothesis' for autoimmune and allergic diseases: an update. Clin Exp Immunol 2010;160:1–9.
97. Wolf WA, Jerath MR, Dellon ES. De-novo onset of eosinophilic esophagitis after large volume allergen exposures. J Gastrointestin Liver Dis 2013;22:205–8.
98. Fogg MI, Ruchelli E, Spergel JM. Pollen and eosinophilic esophagitis. J Allergy Clin Immunol 2003;112:796–7.
99. Moawad FJ, Veerappan GR, Lake JM, et al. Correlation between eosinophilic oesophagitis and aeroallergens. Aliment Pharmacol Ther 2010;31:509–15.
100. Almansa C, Krishna M, Buchner AM, et al. Seasonal distribution in newly diagnosed cases of eosinophilic esophagitis in adults. Am J Gastroenterol 2009;104: 828–33.
101. Wang FY, Gupta SK, Fitzgerald JF. Is there a seasonal variation in the incidence or intensity of allergic eosinophilic esophagitis in newly diagnosed children? J Clin Gastroenterol 2007;41:451–3.
102. Hurrell JM, Genta RM, Dellon ES. Prevalence of esophageal eosinophilia varies by climate zone in the United States. Am J Gastroenterol 2012;107:698–706.
103. Jensen ET, Hoffman K, Shaheen NJ, et al. Esophageal eosinophilia and eosinophilic esophagitis are increased in rural areas with low population density: results from a national pathology database. Am J Gastroenterol 2013;108(Suppl 1):S8 [abstract: 22].
104. Elitsur Y, Aswani R, Lund V, et al. Seasonal distribution and eosinophilic esophagitis: the experience in children living in rural communities. J Clin Gastroenterol 2013;47:287–8.
105. Peterson KA, Byrne KR, Vinson LA, et al. Elemental diet induces histologic response in adult eosinophilic esophagitis. Am J Gastroenterol 2013;108:759–66.
106. Gonsalves N, Yang GY, Doerfler B, et al. Elimination diet effectively treats eosinophilic esophagitis in adults; food reintroduction identifies causative factors. Gastroenterology 2012;142:1451–9.e1.

107. Blaser MJ. *Helicobacter pylori* and esophageal disease: wake-up call? Gastroenterology 2010;139:1819–22.

108. Dellon ES, Peery AF, Shaheen NJ, et al. Inverse association of esophageal eosinophilia with *Helicobacter pylori* based on analysis of a US pathology database. Gastroenterology 2011;141:1586–92.

109. Furuta K, Adachi K, Aimi M, et al. Case-control study of association of eosinophilic gastrointestinal disorders with *Helicobacter pylori* infection in Japan. J Clin Biochem Nutr 2013;53:60–2.

110. Chen Y, Blaser MJ. Inverse associations of *Helicobacter pylori* with asthma and allergy. Arch Intern Med 2007;167:821–7.

111. Hassall E. Over-prescription of acid-suppressing medications in infants: how it came about, why it's wrong, and what to do about it. J Pediatr 2012;160:193–8.

112. Merwat SN, Spechler SJ. Might the use of acid-suppressive medications predispose to the development of eosinophilic esophagitis? Am J Gastroenterol 2009;104:1897–902.

113. Kedika RR, Souza RF, Spechler SJ. Potential anti-inflammatory effects of proton pump inhibitors: a review and discussion of the clinical implications. Dig Dis Sci 2009;54:2312–7.

114. Mullin JM, Valenzano MC, Whitby M, et al. Esomeprazole induces upper gastrointestinal tract transmucosal permeability increase. Aliment Pharmacol Ther 2008;28:1317–25.

115. Untersmayr E, Bakos N, Scholl I, et al. Anti-ulcer drugs promote IgE formation toward dietary antigens in adult patients. FASEB J 2005;19:656–8.

116. Untersmayr E, Scholl I, Swoboda I, et al. Antacid medication inhibits digestion of dietary proteins and causes food allergy: a fish allergy model in BALB/c mice. J Allergy Clin Immunol 2003;112:616–23.

117. Cheng E, Zhang X, Huo X, et al. Omeprazole blocks eotaxin-3 expression by oesophageal squamous cells from patients with eosinophilic oesophagitis and GORD. Gut 2013;62:824–32.

118. Molina-Infante J, Ferrando-Lamana L, Ripoll C, et al. Esophageal eosinophilic infiltration responds to proton pump inhibition in most adults. Clin Gastroenterol Hepatol 2011;9:110–7.

119. Molina-Infante J, Katzka DA, Gisbert JP. Review article: proton pump inhibitor therapy for suspected eosinophilic oesophagitis. Aliment Pharmacol Ther 2013;37:1157–64.

120. Hviid A, Svanstrom H, Frisch M. Antibiotic use and inflammatory bowel diseases in childhood. Gut 2011;60:49–54.

121. Marra F, Lynd L, Coombes M, et al. Does antibiotic exposure during infancy lead to development of asthma?: a systematic review and metaanalysis. Chest 2006;129:610–8.

122. Wang JY, Liu LF, Chen CY, et al. Acetaminophen and/or antibiotic use in early life and the development of childhood allergic diseases. Int J Epidemiol 2013;42:1087–99.

123. Jensen ET, Kappelman MD, Kim HP, et al. Early life exposures as risk factors for pediatric eosinophilic esophagitis: a pilot and feasibility study. J Pediatr Gastroenterol Nutr 2013;57:67–71.

124. Brown EM, Arrieta MC, Finlay BB. A fresh look at the hygiene hypothesis: how intestinal microbial exposure drives immune effector responses in atopic disease. Semin Immunol 2013;25:378–87.

125. Fillon SA, Harris JK, Wagner BD, et al. Novel device to sample the esophageal microbiome–the esophageal string test. PLoS One 2012;7:e42938.

126. Abonia JP, Wen T, Stucke EM, et al. High prevalence of eosinophilic esophagitis in patients with inherited connective tissue disorders. J Allergy Clin Immunol 2013;132:378–86.

127. Jensen ET, Martin CF, Shaheen NJ, et al. High prevalence of co-existing autoimmune conditions among patients with eosinophilic esophagitis. Gastroenterology 2013;144(Suppl 1):S491 (Su1852).

Eosinophilic Esophagitis
Clinical Presentation in Children

Chris A. Liacouras, MD[a],*, Jonathan Spergel, MD[b], Laura M. Gober, MD[c]

KEYWORDS

- Eosinophil • Esophagitis • EoE • Children • Pediatric

KEY POINTS

- Symptoms of eosinophilic esophagitis (EoE) vary by age. They range from failure to thrive in toddlers, to abdominal pain in school age children, to dysphagia in adolescents.
- Symptom overlap exists between EoE and other disorders, including gastroesophageal reflux disease, asthma, and primary eating disorders.
- Diagnosis is made by clinical history combined with results of upper endoscopy with biopsy.

INTRODUCTION

Our understanding of eosinophilic esophagitis (EoE) has evolved over the past 30 years from isolated case reports of patients with prominent esophageal eosinophilia (often misclassified as gastroesophageal reflux [GERD]) to a well-defined clinical disorder. In the past, EoE was described differently, including allergic esophagitis, primary EoE, or idiopathic EoE. We now know that EoE is a distinct disease. It is defined as a clinicopathologic diagnosis characterized by a localized eosinophilic inflammation of the esophagus (with no other gastrointestinal involvement), symptoms of esophageal dysfunction, the presence of 15 or more eosinophils in the most severely involved high-powered field (HPF) isolated to the esophagus, and failure to respond to adequate proton-pump inhibitor (PPI) therapy. Other recognized causes of esophageal eosinophilia should be excluded before making the diagnosis (**Box 1**).

DEMOGRAPHICS

EoE is characterized by eosinophilia of the esophagus, an organ typically devoid of eosinophils, without infiltration in other parts of the gastrointestinal tract.[1,2] First

[a] Division of Gastroenterology, Hepatology and Nutrition, The Children's Hospital of Philadelphia, Perelman School of Medicine, University of Pennsylvania, 3401 Civic Center Boulevard, Philadelphia, PA 19104, USA; [b] Division of Allergy, Immunology, and Infectious Diseases, The Children's Hospital of Philadelphia, Perelman School of Medicine, University of Pennsylvania, 3401 Civic Center Boulevard, Philadelphia, PA 19104, USA; [c] Division of Allergy, Immunology, and Infectious Diseases, Center for Pediatric Eosinophilic Disorders, The Children's Hospital of Philadelphia, 3401 Civic Center Boulevard, Philadelphia, PA 19104, USA
* Corresponding author.
E-mail address: liacouras@email.chop.edu

Gastroenterol Clin N Am 43 (2014) 219–229
http://dx.doi.org/10.1016/j.gtc.2014.02.012
0889-8553/14/$ – see front matter © 2014 Elsevier Inc. All rights reserved.

Box 1
Causes of esophageal eosinophilia

- EoE
- GERD
- PPI-responsive esophageal eosinophilia
- Celiac disease
- Eosinophilic gastroenteritis
- Crohn disease
- Hypereosinophilic syndrome
- Achalasia
- Vasculitis
- Pemphigus
- Connective tissue disease
- Infection
- Graft-versus-host disease

---

described in 1993, EoE has been increasing in incidence and prevalence in Western nations with an estimated annual incidence equal to Crohn disease.[3–8] The increase in EoE mirrors the increased prevalence of allergic diseases (asthma, allergic rhinitis, atopic dermatitis, and food allergy) over the last few decades. Data from the CDC National Health Information Survey (NHIS) confirm the increase in all atopic diseases.[9,10] The reported prevalence of asthma increased from 3% in 1990% to 7.7% in 2007.[11] An estimated 25% to 30% of the population in industrialized countries has atopic dermatitis, food allergy, or allergic rhinitis.[12] EoE has now been reported in every continent.[12–15] Five to 10% of pediatric patients and 6% of adult patients with poorly controlled GERD are thought to have EoE.[16–18] In our cohort at The Children's Hospital of Philadelphia, the authors have seen a 70-fold increase, from 1994 to 2011.[19] In Olten Country, Switzerland, this increase has also been observed in the adult population with increased prevalence from 2 per 100,000 in 1989 to 23 per 100,000 in 2004.[5] Patients who have EoE typically are male (by a 3:1 ratio)[8,19] and 75% have a personal history of atopy.[19–22] Like other atopic diseases, such as asthma and eczema, EoE is a chronic disease. Most patients will continue to have the disease into adulthood. In a 12-year study of adults, no patients had remission.[23] In a 14-year study of pediatric patients, only 2% had remission of disease.[19]

CLINICAL PRESENTATION: GENERAL CONSIDERATIONS

EoE should be suspected in patients describing symptoms consistent with GERD but not responding to adequate reflux medications. Presentation in children varies depending on the age of the child. Characteristic symptoms in infants and young children are feeding difficulties, failure to thrive, and classic GERD symptoms. In contrast, school-aged children are more likely to present with vomiting, abdominal pain, and regurgitation. Dysphagia and food impaction are more prevalent in adolescents and adults.[1,19,20,22,24–26] One study looked at age of presenting symptoms over a 14-year span and found feeding difficulties or failure to thrive in young children (median age 2.8 years), vomiting and GERD symptoms in older children (median age

5.1 years), abdominal pain in young adolescents (median age 9.0 years), and dysphagia and food impaction (median age 11.1 years) in older adolescents.[19] Food impaction can be a presenting symptom especially if dysphagia is intermittent and mild in nature. In adults, the percent of patients who present with dysphagia and who are diagnosed with EoE has risen by 15% from 1999 to 2009.[27] In addition, adult reports have also suggested that the probability of developing fibrostenosis increases over time (especially when not properly treated).[28] It is easy to postulate that chronic untreated inflammation in children may lead to the esophageal dysfunction and dysphagia seen in older adolescents and adults. In addition, a select cohort of patients with abdominal pain on initial presentation who refused therapy all returned 6 years later with symptoms changed to dysphagia.[19] Mechanical obstruction can be the cause for dysphagia.[29] It is unclear whether variable presentations represent different disease phenotypes or the natural history of the untreated disease.

VOMITING AND PAIN

Vomiting is a common symptom in younger children. It can be mistaken for GERD but, unlike GERD, vomiting associated with EoE usually is not diagnosed before 6 months of life. It can be sporadic in occurrence and not associated with meals. If occurring after ingestion of particular foods, vomiting can be mistaken for food protein-induced enterocolitis or IgE-mediated food allergy especially in children with other food allergies. Although vomiting can present early on in infancy, especially in a highly atopic child, it is more likely after the introduction of solid food into the diet. Some children may induce vomiting if they have dysphagia and feel something is stuck in their throat.

Children may complain of abdominal pain, in particular localizing to the epigastrium despite only having esophageal disease. Adolescents and adults are more likely to localize pain to the chest or complain of heartburn. The pain, which is spasmodic, can be severe enough to lead patients to seek emergency evaluation and lead to cardiac evaluation.

DYSPHAGIA AND FOOD IMPACTION

Dysphagia associated with EoE is intermittent and some patients may experience it for more than 2 years before presentation.[29,30] How patients report dysphagia varies, as can be expected, especially in different age groups. Patients may describe difficultly initiating swallowing, food going down the esophagus too slowly, or food being stuck in the throat. Food impaction can lead to patient anxiety. Patients gradually learn techniques for compensating for dysphagia, including taking small bites, eating slowly with excessive chewing, and drinking fluids after each bite. Some may even jump up and down to help food pass. Patients may also avoid certain food textures or types (eg, meat) due to difficulty swallowing these in the past. In younger children and infants, it is unclear if symptoms such as gagging, choking, feeding difficulties, and food aversions are secondary to current dysphagia and the associated pain or due to previous negative feeding experiences and the related anxiety toward eating. In adolescents, patients with EoE have been misdiagnosed with eating disorders because of symptoms of food-related anxiety, vomiting, and food aversion. Barium radiographic studies are extremely useful in patients who complain of dysphagia. These studies can demonstrate fixed strictures, small caliber esophagus, transient or fixed rings, or a normal esophagus (suggesting that dysphagia is due to secondary esophageal dysmotility). These findings are especially important for the gastroenterologist before an endoscopy is performed.

EoE patients with dysphagia may have a mechanical obstruction. Strictures can be seen, even in infants.[1] Strictures are, however, less common in children who usually do not have radiographic evidence of obvious mechanical obstruction.[29] One study found that 8 out of 18 children found to have Schatzki rings via radiographic images had EoE. Those having EoE did not have rings on endoscopy but, most likely, had a focal spasm at time of imaging. In contrast, strictures, rings, narrowing of the esophagus, and Schatzki rings have all been described in adults with EoE and dysphagia.[31] A biopsy should be performed on patients with mechanical obstruction, including foreign bodies (eg, food, coins), to rule out EoE.

One active area of research in EoE, as well as other atopic conditions, is tissue remodeling. In atopic dermatitis, skin can become lichenified and thick over time.[32] In poorly controlled asthmatics, a permanent decline in lung function may occur.[33] Patients with EoE can have narrowing of the esophagus or stricture formation secondary to untreated EoE.[25,26,33] However, narrowing occurs in only a very small percentage of adult patients because strictures are only seen in 5% to 15% of adult series and these are usually only in patients with longstanding untreated disease.[23,34] This progression of complications is attributed to fibrous remodeling associated with the natural history of untreated EoE.[35] Delayed diagnosis of EoE is associated with an increased risk of stricture formation in a time-dependent manner.[36] Children with untreated EoE have basement membrane thickening and increased vascular activation, similar to changes seen in airway remodeling with increased SMAD2/3 and transforming growth factor (TGF)-β.[37,38]

CORRELATION OF SYMPTOMS WITH ENDOSCOPY AND HISTOLOGY

The appearance of mucosal rings, furrowing, strictures, and white plaques are often seen on visual inspection.[20,23–26,39] However, up to one-third of patients with active EoE may have a normal appearing esophagus.[25] There is poor correlation between biopsies and symptoms. Patients can have normal biopsies and still have symptoms and the converse. For example, in the largest clinical trial for EoE with 240 subjects, there was no correlation between symptoms and eosinophils found on esophageal biopsies. Subjects on placebo had symptom resolution without improvement in esophageal eosinophilia.[22] Currently, serial endoscopies of the esophagus are unavoidable for EoE because there are no other available testing options. One study followed 330 subjects with at least 1 year of clinical follow-up (average 3.2 years). These subjects had 2526 total biopsies with an average of 4.5 esophagogastroduodenoscopies (EGDs) per subject. At time of presentation, 144 subjects also required lower endoscopies.[19] Disease burden, including financial, would be eased if there was a reliable, easily obtainable (eg, blood, stool) biomarker for EoE that would lessen the frequency of EGDs.

OTHER CLINICAL PRESENTATIONS

In children with asthma, chest pain and cough may be mistaken for an asthma exacerbation; however when these patients do not respond to aggressive asthma treatment, after asking a careful history, EoE should be considered. The diagnosis of EoE has also been made in children with airway anomalies such as subglottic stenosis and laryngeal cleft.[40]

Eosinophilic gastroenteritis is eosinophilic inflammation at extraesophageal gastrointestinal sites. This entity usually does not respond to dietary therapies and it is treated with corticosteroids. EoE has also been described in conjunction with other gastrointestinal disorders such as Crohn disease and celiac disease. The prevalence of EoE in children with confirmed celiac disease is 1% to 4%.[41,42] In general, EoE is not typically in remission with removal of gluten-containing foods alone.

Connective tissue disorders (CTDs) have been recently associated with a greater risk for EoE. A recent retrospective study noted an eightfold increase in EoE (1.3% prevalence) in patients with CTDs at their institution.[43] This included patients with Marfan syndrome, Ehlers-Danlos syndrome, joint hypermobility syndrome, and Loeys-Dietz syndrome. Patients had dysmorphic scaphocephalic facial features, hypermobility of hands and large joints, and high rate of atopic diseases. Esophageal biopsies from EoE patients with CTDs were indistinguishable from those without CTDs but this cohort was more likely to have significant eosinophilic gastrointestinal inflammatory disease affecting other sites such as stomach, duodenum, and colon. On a molecular level, the EoE transcriptome for EoE-CTD was not unique. However, two genes (CD200R1 and SAMSN1) had higher expression and two genes (PTGFRN and COL8A2) had lower expression in this group. This association may further support that TGF-β signaling plays a role in EoE pathogenesis and help target future pharmacotherapies.

EoE has been described in neurologic disorders such as seizure disorders, cerebral palsy, migraines, and Chiari malformation. Certain antiepileptic drugs have been linked to the development of EoE in the setting of a hypersensitivity reaction involving other organ systems.[44] There is no evidence for a causal relationship between EoE and neurodevelopmental disorders such as pervasive developmental delays or sensory integration disorders.

PSYCHOSOCIAL DYSFUNCTION

A recent retrospective study at a tertiary care EoE program evaluated patients and families for psychosocial dysfunction.[45] Most children (69%) evaluated suffered from difficulties in at least one area assessed (sleep, social, school, anxiety, and depression). Children who had pain or eating difficulties were more likely to have difficulties across multiple assessed areas. Anxiety (41%) and depression (28%) increased with age. Children with gastrostomy tubes had more social (64%), school (26%), and psychological adjustment (44%) disorders. Adjustment problems were more likely in older children, whereas sleep problems (33%) were seen almost exclusively in younger children. In addition, 48% of families and children had concerns about feeding refusal or poor appetite, predominantly in younger children. Another study found that caregivers (98% were mothers) of children with eosinophilic gastrointestinal disorders reported stress and psychological distress from caring for their child.[46] These studies support the need for psychosocial evaluation and support for children with EoE as well as their families.

GROWTH AND NUTRITIONAL CONCERNS

Long-term elimination diets pose significant challenges to patients and families, so nonadherence must be ruled out. In particular, milk and wheat generally are the most difficult allergens to remove because they make up a large part of children's diets. Their removal also results in the greatest nutritional impact and has a significant affect on quality of life of children and their families. In children, a nutritionist needs to be closely involved with family when multiple foods are removed to assess risk of malnutrition and calcium, iron, vitamin D, vitamin E, and zinc deficiencies.[47] Children with milk allergy or children with two or more food allergies were shorter, based on height-for-age percentiles than those with only one food allergy (not cow's milk). In addition, children with cow's milk allergy or multiple food allergies consumed less dietary calcium than did children without cow's milk allergy and/or one food allergy.[48]

A frequent barrier in children with EoE is acceptance of amino acid formulas whenever a strict amino acid based diet is warranted. The use of amino acids as the main protein source renders the formulas significantly less palatable than their intact protein counterparts are. Flavors of these formulas have improved in recent years, although this remains, as expected, largely a matter of the child's opinion. If elemental formulas are essential, enteral tube feeds may be inevitable and should be managed in conjunction with an experienced dietician. Micronutrient supplementation may be required, depending up the volume of formula consumed. Fiber supplementation may be required because elemental formulas do not contain dietary fiber; these are especially useful for children with constipation, or those dependent on elemental formula with little solid food in diet for a prolonged period.

Not all patients require elemental formulas for treatment of their EoE. Dietary restriction may be based on individual testing or empiric removal of foods. A history is obtained from the family and then testing to foods in the child's diet is recommended. One approach involves using skin prick testing (identifying IgE-mediated reactions) and patch testing (identifying non–IgE-mediated reactions) in guiding food removal; upwards of 75% improve symptomatically and histologically with this approach.[49] Another approach is empiric removal of foods. Empiric removal of the six most common food allergens (milk, soy, egg, peanut, tree nuts, wheat, and seafood) has also been used with reported success of 74% in one study.[50] However, removal of the most common food allergens did not reduce eosinophils to a normal range (13.6 eosinophils per HPF).[50] When effective, elimination diets (based on a combination of skin prick testing and patch testing) reduced counts to 1.1 eosinophils per HPF.[49,51] Elemental diets reduced eosinophil counts to 0 eosinophils per HPF.[25] Even with elemental diets there is a small percentage (<10%) of patients who do not have resolution of esophageal eosinophilia. In these patients, it is important to review adherence to diet and compliance with reflux medications, and to rule out other causes of eosinophilia in the gastrointestinal tract, including aeroallergens.

ATOPIC COMORBIDITIES

Children with EoE have a higher rate of atopy compared with normal children. Approximately 30% to 50% of children with EoE have asthma compared with 10% in the normal population. Similarly, 50% to 75% have allergic rhinitis compared with 30% in normal children. In addition, 10% to 20% of children with EoE have IgE-mediated food allergy (urticaria and anaphylaxis) compared with 1% to 5% in normal children. These data suggest EoE has a superatopic phenotype. However, it does not appear to be IgE-mediated because skin testing or specific IgE do not identify foods, and murine models of EoE do not require IgE to produce symptoms or esophageal eosinophilia.[19] These rates of atopy (asthma, allergic rhinitis, and atopic dermatitis) are approximately three times higher than what is expected in the general population. Other studies of pediatric and adult patients with EoE have confirmed the higher prevalence of environmental and/or food allergies, approximately 50% higher than the general population.[20,21,52] Similar to asthma and atopic dermatitis,[53–56] 14% of patients with EoE have a single nucleotide polymorphism (SNP) inferring a possible genetic component.[16] Furthermore, there is a strong familial association with EoE.[57–59]

ROLE OF ALLERGENS IN PEDIATRIC EoE

In almost all cases of pediatric EoE, an underlying food allergy has been found to be the culprit. Convincing work from Kelly and colleagues[14] revealed the use of an elemental diet and a few basic foods in 10 patients with refractory EoE, six of whom had Nissen fundoplications. All children improved and eight of the original children had complete resolution on biopsy. Other studies have corroborated this data showing success rates of 98% with elemental diets.[25,60]

A few studies have suggested that aeroallergens may play a causative role in the development of EoE in humans. A seasonal variation in cases of newly diagnosed EoE has been described, with fewer cases diagnosed in the winter when the air contains less pollen.[61] During pollen season there are increased numbers of eosinophils in subjects with allergic rhinitis compared with normal controls, although the number of eosinophils observed was lower than values typically seen in patients who have EoE.[62] In a case report, full disease control was achieved only during seasons without pollen and symptoms and esophageal eosinophilia worsened during seasons with pollen.[19] There are various case reports of immunotherapy for birch pollen and dust mite aeroallergens leading to symptomatic improvement of EoE.[63,64] Food allergies were still the primary cause of disease in these patients. However, in a few patients, during pollen season in the spring or fall, biopsy-confirmed exacerbation of disease without change in diet have been documented. In these patients, disease control was improved during seasons without pollen and on proper dietary therapy.[19] Assuming that environmental allergens cause EoE, the mechanism of action could be either that direct deposition of pollens onto the esophageal mucosa cause esophageal eosinophilia or that aeroallergens stimulate eotaxin secretion leading to eosinophil migration into the esophagus. Eotaxin overexpression was noted in subjects with EoE.[16] Intranasal steroid therapy has decreased nasal secretion of eotaxin in subjects who have allergic rhinitis,[65] thus aggressive treatment of allergic rhinitis with intranasal steroids is highly recommended in patients with EoE.[66]

More recently, sublingual immunotherapy to aeroallergens has been shown to induce EoE.[67] Oral immunotherapy (OIT) has shown to be effective for treatment of IgE-mediated food allergies but one of the reported side effects is the development of EoE in patients having undergone OIT to milk and egg. This confirms that IgE-mediated food allergy and EoE have different disease mechanisms.[68–70] In these cases, EoE resolved once the food was removed again from the diet.

SUMMARY

The prevalence of EoE is increasing in children. Characteristic symptoms in infants and young children are feeding difficulties, failure to thrive, and classic GERD symptoms in contrast to school-aged children who are more likely to present with vomiting, abdominal pain, and regurgitation. Dysphagia and food impaction are more prevalent in adolescents and adults. Atopic comorbidities, growth or nutritional deficiencies, psychosocial impact, and recently recognized associations with CTDs are concerns in pediatric patients with EoE. Although food elimination diets can effectively treat most children with this disease, there is a lack of allergy testing with high specificity to identify foods that trigger the disease. Food reintroduction can be difficult because endoscopies are required to identify trigger foods. Earlier research studies failed to correlate noninvasive biomarkers with biopsy findings. Currently, in asymptomatic children with abnormal biopsies, the standard of care is to treat because of the risk of tissue remodeling and fibrosis resulting in stricture formation with potential need for dilatation.

REFERENCES

1. Furuta GT, Liacouras CA, Collins MH, et al. Eosinophilic esophagitis in children and adults: a systematic review and consensus recommendations for diagnosis and treatment. Gastroenterology 2007;133(4):1342–63.

2. Liacouras CA, Furuta GT, Hirano I, et al. Eosinophilic esophagitis: updated consensus recommendations for children and adults. J Allergy Clin Immunol 2011;128(1):3–20.

3. Prasad GA, Alexander JA, Schleck CD, et al. Epidemiology of eosinophilic esophagitis over three decades in Olmsted County, Minnesota. Clin Gastroenterol Hepatol 2009;7(10):1055–61.

4. Noel RJ, Putnam PE, Rothenberg ME. Eosinophilic esophagitis. N Engl J Med 2004;351(9):940–1.

5. Straumann A, Simon HU. Eosinophilic esophagitis: escalating epidemiology? J Allergy Clin Immunol 2005;115(2):418–9.

6. Hruz P, Straumann A, Bussmann C, et al. Escalating incidence of eosinophilic esophagitis: a 20-year prospective, population-based study in Olten County, Switzerland. J Allergy Clin Immunol 2011;128(6):1349–50.

7. Cherian S, Smith NM, Forbes DA. Rapidly increasing prevalence of eosinophilic oesophagitis in Western Australia. Arch Dis Child 2006;91(12):1000–4.

8. van Rhijn BD, Verheij J, Smout AJ, et al. Rapidly increasing incidence of eosinophilic esophagitis in a large cohort. Neurogastroenterol Motil 2013;25(1): 47–52.

9. Branum AM, Lukacs SL. Food allergy among U.S. children: trends in prevalence and hospitalizations. NCHS Data Brief 2008;10:1–8.

10. Mannino DM, Homa DM, Pertowski CA, et al. Surveillance for asthma—United States, 1960–1995. MMWR CDC Surveill Summ 1998;47(1):1–27.

11. Brim SN, Rudd RA, Funk RH, et al. Asthma prevalence among US children in underrepresented minority populations: American Indian/Alaska Native, Chinese, Filipino, and Asian Indian. Pediatrics 2008;122(1):217–22.

12. Kiyohara C, Tanaka K, Miyake Y. Genetic susceptibility to atopic dermatitis. Allergol Int 2008;57(1):39–56.

13. Riou PJ, Nicholson AG, Pastorino U. Esophageal rupture in a patient with idiopathic eosinophilic esophagitis. Ann Thorac Surg 1996;62(6):1854–6.

14. Kelly KJ, Lazenby AJ, Rowe PC, et al. Eosinophilic esophagitis attributed to gastroesophageal reflux: improvement with an amino acid-based formula. Gastroenterology 1995;109(5):1503–12.

15. Straumann A, Spichtin HP, Bernoulli R, et al. Idiopathic eosinophilic esophagitis: a frequently overlooked disease with typical clinical aspects and discrete endoscopic findings. Schweiz Med Wochenschr 1994;124(33):1419–29.

16. Blanchard C, Wang N, Stringer KF, et al. Eotaxin-3 and a uniquely conserved gene-expression profile in eosinophilic esophagitis. J Clin Invest 2006;116(2): 536–47.

17. Markowitz JE, Liacouras CA. Ten years of eosinophilic oesophagitis: small steps or giant leaps? Dig Liver Dis 2006;38(4):251–3.

18. Fox VL, Nurko S, Furuta GT. Eosinophilic esophagitis: it's not just kid's stuff. Gastrointest Endosc 2002;56(2):260–70.

19. Spergel JM, Brown-Whitehorn TF, Beausoleil JL, et al. 14 years of eosinophilic esophagitis: clinical features and prognosis. J Pediatr Gastroenterol Nutr 2009;48(1):30–6.

20. Assa'ad AH, Putnam PE, Collins MH, et al. Pediatric patients with eosinophilic esophagitis: an 8-year follow-up. J Allergy Clin Immunol 2007;119(3): 731–8.

21. Simon D, Marti H, Heer P, et al. Eosinophilic esophagitis is frequently associated with IgE-mediated allergic airway diseases. J Allergy Clin Immunol 2005;115(5): 1090–2.

22. Spergel JM, Brown-Whitehorn TF, Cianferoni A, et al. Identification of causative foods in children with eosinophilic esophagitis treated with an elimination diet. J Allergy Clin Immunol 2012;130(2):461–7.
23. Straumann A, Spichtin HP, Grize L, et al. Natural history of primary eosinophilic esophagitis: a follow-up of 30 adult patients for up to 11.5 years. Gastroenterology 2003;125(6):1660–9.
24. Orenstein SR, Shalaby TM, Di Lorenzo C, et al. The spectrum of pediatric eosinophilic esophagitis beyond infancy: a clinical series of 30 children. Am J Gastroenterol 2000;95(6):1422–30.
25. Liacouras CA, Spergel JM, Ruchelli E, et al. Eosinophilic esophagitis: a 10-year experience in 381 children. Clin Gastroenterol Hepatol 2005;3(12):1198–206.
26. Baxi S, Gupta SK, Swigonski N, et al. Clinical presentation of patients with eosinophilic inflammation of the esophagus. Gastrointest Endosc 2006;64(4):473–8.
27. Kidambi T, Toto E, Ho N, et al. Temporal trends in the relative prevalence of dysphagia etiologies from 1999–2009. World J Gastroenterol 2012;18(32): 4335–41.
28. Dellon ES, Kim HP, Sperry SL, et al. A phenotypic analysis shows that eosinophilic esophagitis is a progressive fibrostenotic disease. Gastrointest Endosc 2013;79(4):57–85.
29. Khan S, Orenstein SR, Di Lorenzo C, et al. Eosinophilic esophagitis: strictures, impactions, and dysphagia. Dig Dis Sci 2003;48(1):22–9.
30. Nurko S, Teitelbaum JE, Husain K, et al. Association of Schatzki ring with eosinophilic esophagitis in children. J Pediatr Gastroenterol Nutr 2004;38(4):436–41.
31. Vasilopoulos S, Murphy P, Auerbach A, et al. The small-caliber esophagus: an unappreciated cause of dysphagia for solids in patients with eosinophilic esophagitis. Gastrointest Endosc 2002;55(1):99–106.
32. Bieber T. Atopic dermatitis. N Engl J Med 2008;358(14):1483–94.
33. Hoshino M, Nakamura Y, Sim J, et al. Bronchial subepithelial fibrosis and expression of matrix metalloproteinase-9 in asthmatic airway inflammation. J Allergy Clin Immunol 1998;102(5):783–8.
34. Attwood SE, Smyrk TC, Demeester TR, et al. Esophageal eosinophilia with dysphagia. A distinct clinicopathologic syndrome. Dig Dis Sci 1993;38(1): 109–16.
35. Aceves SS, Ackerman SJ. Relationships between eosinophilic inflammation, tissue remodeling, and fibrosis in eosinophilic esophagitis. Immunol Allergy Clin North Am 2009;29:197–211.
36. Schoepfer AM, Safroneeva E, Bussmann C, et al. Delay in diagnosis of eosinophilic esophagitis increases risk for stricture formation in a time-dependent manner. Gastroenterology 2013;145(6):1230–6.
37. Aceves SS, Furuta GT, Spechler SJ. Integrated approach to treatment of children and adults with eosinophilic esophagitis. Gastrointest Endosc Clin N Am 2008;18(1):195–217.
38. Aceves SS, Newbury RO, Dohil R, et al. Esophageal remodeling in pediatric eosinophilic esophagitis. J Allergy Clin Immunol 2007;119(1):206–12.
39. Siafakas CG, Ryan CK, Brown MR, et al. Multiple esophageal rings: an association with eosinophilic esophagitis: case report and review of the literature. Am J Gastroenterol 2000;95(6):1572–5.
40. Goldstein NA, Putnam PE, Dohar JE. Laryngeal cleft and eosinophilic gastroenteritis: report of 2 cases. Arch Otolaryngol Head Neck Surg 2000;126(2):227–30.
41. Leslie C, Mews C, Charles A, et al. Celiac disease and eosinophilic esophagitis: a true association. J Pediatr Gastroenterol Nutr 2010;50(4):397–9.

42. Ooi CY, Day AS, Jackson R, et al. Eosinophilic esophagitis in children with celiac disease. J Gastroenterol Hepatol 2008;23(7):1144–8.

43. Abonia JP, Wen T, Stucke EM, et al. High prevalence of eosinophilic esophagitis in patients with inherited connective tissue disorders. J Allergy Clin Immunol 2013;132:378–86.

44. Balatsinou C, Milano A, Caldarella MP, et al. Eosinophilic esophagitis is a component of the anticonvulsant hypersensitivity syndrome: description of two cases. Dig Liver Dis 2008;40(2):145–8.

45. Harris RF, Menard-Katcher C, Atkins D, et al. Psychosocial dysfunction in children and adolescents with eosinophilic esophagitis. J Pediatr Gastroenterol Nutr 2013;57(4):500–5.

46. Taft TH, Ballou S, Keefer L. Preliminary evaluation of maternal caregiver stress in pediatric eosinophilic gastrointestinal disorders. J Pediatr Psychol 2012;37: 523–32.

47. Spergel JM, Shuker M. Nutritional management of eosinophilic esophagitis. Gastrointest Endosc Clin N Am 2008;18(1):179–94.

48. Christie L, Hine RJ, Parker JG, et al. Food allergies in children affect nutrient intake and growth. J Am Diet Assoc 2002;102:1648–51.

49. Spergel JM, Beausoleil JL, Mascarenhas M, et al. The use of skin prick tests and patch tests to identify causative foods in eosinophilic esophagitis. J Allergy Clin Immunol 2002;109(2):363–8.

50. Kagalwalla AF, Sentongo TA, Ritz S, et al. Effect of six-food elimination diet on clinical and histologic outcomes in eosinophilic esophagitis. Clin Gastroenterol Hepatol 2006;4(9):1097–102.

51. Spergel JM, Brown-Whitehorn T. The use of patch testing in the diagnosis of food allergy. Curr Allergy Asthma Rep 2005;5(1):86–90.

52. Roy-Ghanta S, Larosa DF, Katzka DA. Atopic characteristics of adult patients with eosinophilic esophagitis. Clin Gastroenterol Hepatol 2008;6(5): 531–5.

53. Weidinger S, O'Sullivan M, Illig T, et al. Filaggrin mutations, atopic eczema, hay fever, and asthma in children. J Allergy Clin Immunol 2008;121(5):1203–9.

54. Weiss ST, Raby BA, Rogers A. Asthma genetics and genomics 2009. Curr Opin Genet Dev 2009;19(3):279–82.

55. Flory JH, Sleiman PM, Christie JD, et al. 17q12-21 variants interact with smoke exposure as a risk factor for pediatric asthma but are equally associated with early-onset versus late-onset asthma in North Americans of European ancestry. J Allergy Clin Immunol 2009;124(3):605–7.

56. Steinke JW, Rich SS, Borish L. 5. Genetics of allergic disease. J Allergy Clin Immunol 2008;121(Suppl 2):S384–7.

57. Meyer GW. Eosinophilic esophagitis in a father and a daughter. Gastrointest Endosc 2005;61(7):932.

58. Patel SM, Falchuk KR. Three brothers with dysphagia caused by eosinophilic esophagitis. Gastrointest Endosc 2005;61(1):165–7.

59. Zink DA, Amin M, Gebara S, et al. Familial dysphagia and eosinophilia. Gastrointest Endosc 2007;65(2):330–4.

60. Markowitz JE, Spergel JM, Ruchelli E, et al. Elemental diet is an effective treatment for eosinophilic esophagitis in children and adolescents. Am J Gastroenterol 2003;98(4):777–82.

61. Wang FY, Gupta SK, Fitzgerald JF. Is there a seasonal variation in the incidence or intensity of allergic eosinophilic esophagitis in newly diagnosed children? J Clin Gastroenterol 2007;41(5):451–3.

62. Onbasi K, Sin AZ, Doganavsargil B, et al. Eosinophil infiltration of the oesopha-geal mucosa in patients with pollen allergy during the season. Clin Exp Allergy 2005;35(11):1423–31.
63. De Swert L, Veereman G, Bublin M, et al. Eosinophilic gastrointestinal disease suggestive of pathogenesis-related class 10 (PR-10) protein allergy resolved af-ter immunotherapy. J Allergy Clin Immunol 2013;131(2):600–2.
64. Ramirez RM, Jacobs RL. Eosinophilic esophagitis treated with immunotherapy to dust mites. J Allergy Clin Immunol 2013;132(2):503–4.
65. Greiff L, Petersen H, Mattsson E, et al. Mucosal output of eotaxin in allergic rhinitis and its attenuation by topical glucocorticosteroid treatment. Clin Exp Al-lergy 2001;31(8):1321–7.
66. Fogg MI, Ruchelli E, Spergel JM. Pollen and eosinophilic esophagitis. J Allergy Clin Immunol 2003;112(4):796–7.
67. Miehlke S, Alpan O, Schröder S, et al. Induction of eosinophilic esophagitis by sublingual pollen immunotherapy. Case Rep Gastroenterol 2013;7(3):363–8.
68. Narisety SD, Skripak JM, Steele P, et al. Open-label maintenance after milk oral immunotherapy for IgE-mediated cow's milk allergy. J Allergy Clin Immunol 2009;124(3):610–2.
69. Sanchez-Garcia S, Rodriguez del Rio P, Escudero C, et al. Possible eosinophilic esophagitis induced by milk oral immunotherapy. J Allergy Clin Immunol 2012; 124(4):1155–7.
70. Ridolo E, De Angelis GL, Dall'aglio P. Eosinophilic esophagitis after specific oral tolerance induction for egg protein. Ann Allergy Asthma Immunol 2011;106(1): 73–4.

Clinical Presentation of Eosinophilic Esophagitis in Adults

Gary W. Falk, MD, MS

KEYWORDS

- Eosinophilic esophagitis • Esophageal eosinophilia • Endoscopy
- Narrow-caliber esophagus • PPI-responsive esophageal eosinophilia
- Gastroesophageal reflux disease • Dysphagia

KEY POINTS

- Eosinophilic esophagitis (EoE) has protean symptoms in adults.
- Diagnostic delay in EoE is common and is associated with endoscopic features of fibrosis and remodeling.
- No endoscopic or clinical parameters differentiate EoE from PPI-responsive esophageal eosinophilia.
- The sensitivity of endoscopic findings of EoE is problematic, emphasizing the importance of obtaining biopsies in individuals in whom EoE is a diagnostic consideration.
- Patients with EoE have concerns about the impact of the disease on quality of life.

INTRODUCTION

Eosinophilic esophagitis (EoE) is an increasingly recognized immune antigen-mediated esophageal disease found in both children and adults. It is defined as a clinicopathologic entity characterized by symptoms of esophageal dysfunction accompanied by an eosinophil-predominant esophageal inflammation that occurs in the absence of other causes of esophageal eosinophilia.[1] As such, symptoms are central to the diagnosis of EoE. Classic symptoms of EoE in adults include dysphagia to solids and food bolus impaction, but a variety of other symptoms are also encountered, some of which are uncommon and not widely recognized. Despite the increasing awareness of EoE among practicing physicians, a long delay from onset

Disclosure: The author is a consultant for Aptalis and Olympus.
Grant Support: Aptalis, Meritage.
Division of Gastroenterology, Hospital of the University of Pennsylvania, University of Pennsylvania Perelman School of Medicine, 9 Penn Tower, One Convention Avenue, Philadelphia, PA 19104, USA
E-mail address: gary.falk@uphs.upenn.edu

http://dx.doi.org/10.1016/j.gtc.2014.02.009
0889-8553/14/$ – see front matter © 2014 Elsevier Inc. All rights reserved.
gastro.theclinics.com

of symptoms to diagnosis remains an important clinical problem, in part because of altered eating behaviors on the part of patients that may result in a delay in seeking medical attention. Furthermore, this diagnostic delay seems to be associated with complications related to ongoing esophageal remodeling. A variety of endoscopic features are associated with EoE but the performance characteristics of these features are problematic. EoE needs to be distinguished from proton pump inhibitor (PPI)–responsive esophageal eosinophilia (PPI-REE), but there are currently no endoscopic or clinical features that allow that distinction. This article summarizes current knowledge of the clinical and endoscopic presentation of EoE in adults.

DYSPHAGIA

Dysphagia is the most common symptom in adults with EoE.[1,2] Dysphagia may be either chronic or intermittent and is seen in 25% to 100% of adult patients with EoE.[3] Two recent studies provide perhaps the best estimate of the magnitude of this problem using modern consensus definitions of EoE that exclude PPI-REE. A Swiss EoE database study of 200 patients with EoE found dysphagia to be present in 95% of patients before the diagnosis of EoE.[4] The median diagnostic delay from onset of symptoms to initial diagnosis of EoE was 6 years. Dellon and colleagues[5] took the issue of dysphagia a step further and examined the relationship between the presence of dysphagia and the endoscopic phenotype of EoE in the University of North Carolina EoE database. Dysphagia was present in 83% of the adult cohort. From the inflammatory to the mixed inflammatory/fibrostenotic to the fibrostenotic endoscopic phenotypes (described later), dysphagia increased from 36% to 77% to 92% of the patients respectively. Symptoms in each of these phenotypes were similarly present before the diagnosis of EoE for a mean of 5.3, 8.3, and 8.4 years respectively. Both of these studies highlight the importance of the diagnostic delay that is so common in EoE as well as the cardinal symptom of dysphagia. What accounts for this diagnostic delay? Although initially part of the problem was likely the lack of physician awareness and recognition, it also may be related to patient reporting of symptoms. Symptoms of dysphagia may be minimized by patients because of a variety of adaptive behaviors to lessen this symptom, including eating more slowly, using liquid chasers with a meal, and chewing food more carefully.[6] Thus, elucidating these behavioral modifications is crucial in the clinical assessment of these patients.

How common is EoE in patients undergoing endoscopy for unexplained dysphagia? This question is difficult to answer because 2 studies that addressed this question did not use current consensus criteria for the diagnosis of EoE, thereby allowing an answer only to the issue of esophageal eosinophilia and not EoE. Esophageal eosinophilia was found in 15% to 16% of patients undergoing endoscopy for unexplained dysphagia.[7,8] Esophageal eosinophilia was encountered in 5% to 10% of these patients with dysphagia despite an endoscopically normal-appearing esophagus.

What accounts for dysphagia in EoE? Several different mechanisms have been proposed, with the most important being esophageal remodeling. This process of progressive fibrosis may lead to fixed rings, strictures, decreased esophageal distensibility, and narrow-caliber esophagus.[9] Dysphagia may also be caused by dysmotility related to alterations in neuromuscular function of the esophagus, leading to dysfunction of longitudinal muscle contraction.[10] A wide spectrum of esophageal motility abnormalities have also been described in EoE; notably weak peristalsis and failed peristalsis.[11] However, the relationship between these abnormalities and dysphagia remains unclear. Overall, it seems that esophageal remodeling is likely the key driver of the symptom of dysphagia.

FOOD BOLUS IMPACTION

Food bolus impaction is another common clinical manifestation of EoE in adults. It can either precede the diagnosis of EoE or be an ongoing manifestation of the disease. The symptom is characterized by either a sense of food sticking for a period of time before eventual passage or sticking to the point of requiring endoscopic removal. Food bolus impaction warranting endoscopic removal is encountered in 33% to 54% of adult patients with EoE.[1,2] A study of 251 patients in the Swiss EoE database, diagnosed by consensus criteria, found that 87 patients (35%) had one or more food bolus impactions that required endoscopic removal.[12] Studies of unselected consecutive patients presenting with food bolus impaction in the community and in tertiary care settings find EoE by consensus criteria in 12% to 42% of patients.[13,14] However, this may underestimate the magnitude of the problem because many patients with a food bolus impaction do not have esophageal biopsies obtained at the time of bolus removal or are not on PPI therapy. When considering esophageal foreign body impactions more broadly, patients with EoE are more likely to be younger, white men with a food bolus impaction than patients without known EoE.[14] Food bolus impaction is more likely to be found in the fibrostenotic and mixed endoscopic phenotypes of EoE compared with the inflammatory phenotype.[5] It is also more associated with lower esophageal distensibility than in patients who only have solid food dysphagia.[15] It is clear from the studies to date that multiple episodes of food bolus impaction are characteristic of EoE in adults.

CHEST PAIN

Unexplained chest pain unrelated to swallowing may be encountered in a subset of patients with EoE. The large natural history studies of Dellon[3] and Schoepfer and colleagues[4] found chest pain in 13% and 36% of patients respectively. It is unclear whether this symptom is caused by underlying inflammation, gastroesophageal reflux disease (GERD), acid hypersensitivity, or some other cause.[2]

GASTROESOPHAGEAL REFLUX–TYPE SYMPTOMS

The classic GERD symptoms of heartburn and acid regurgitation have been described in 7% to 100% of patients with EoE.[16] EoE is found in approximately 1% to 9% of patients with GERD symptoms refractory to PPI therapy.[17–19] Given the different treatment implications of the two diseases, it is important to differentiate the clinical presentation of the two entities as well as that of PPI-REE, as described later. Clinical features that tend to distinguish EoE from GERD include male gender, younger age, atopy, dysphagia, and prior food impaction, although there is clear overlap between the two entities.[20,21]

PPI-RESPONSIVE ESOPHAGEAL EOSINOPHILIA

The entity of PPI-REE has recently been described.[22] PPI-REE is defined as symptoms of esophageal dysfunction, with many patients having endoscopic features of EoE, with esophageal eosinophilia that responds to PPI therapy.[1] PPI-REE is viewed as being separate from the esophageal eosinophilia seen in the setting of erosive esophagitis and typical GERD symptoms. The cause of this entity is poorly understood at present and it may represent an atypical presentation of GERD, a variant of allergic EoE that responds to PPI therapy, or a separate entity.[23] Experimental models suggest that PPIs reduce cytokine-stimulated eotaxin-3 expression, a mechanism that may explain a reduction in eosinophils independent of reduced acid secretion.[24]

At present there are no clinical, endoscopic, histologic, or pH testing criteria that allow the distinction of PPI-REE from EoE.[1,23] The Chapel Hill group recently examined consecutive patients referred for endoscopy, of whom 66 were found to have esophageal eosinophilia and dysphagia when naive to PPI therapy. PPI-REE was found in 24 of these patients (36%), whereas the other 40 were classified as having EoE.[25] On univariate analysis, the patients with PPI-REE were older, and were even more male predominant and less likely to have endoscopic features of EoE such as rings, narrowing, or furrowing than patients with EoE. However, none of these features reliably separated the two groups after multivariable analysis. Furthermore, there was no difference in the absolute number of eosinophils before PPI therapy between the two groups. Given the treatment implications inherent in the two entities, an increased understanding of the significance of this entity is eagerly awaited.

PERFORATION AND INTRAMURAL DISSECTION

Patients with previously undiagnosed EoE may present acutely with spontaneous esophageal rupture (Boerhaave syndrome). Esophageal perforation typically occurs in the setting of a food bolus impaction followed by induced vomiting. Symptoms suggesting perforation include chest and epigastric pain after vomiting. To date, a limited number of patients have presented in this manner, often in the setting of prior unrecognized esophageal symptoms.[26-28] Another complication seen as a presentation of EoE is esophageal dissection between the mucosal and submucosal layers. Patients with dissection may have hematemesis in addition to chest pain and dysphagia.[29-31] Although both of these complications may precede the diagnosis of EoE, they may also result from endoscopy and instrumentation, including food bolus removal and dilation.[32]

ALLERGIC DIATHESIS

Because EoE is a chronic immune/antigen-mediated disease, features of atopy including asthma, allergic rhinitis, atopic dermatitis, food allergies, and environmental allergies are commonly seen in adults with EoE. The overall magnitude of the problem is difficult to ascertain given the evolving definition of EoE and early studies that did not require exclusion of GERD or PPI-REE. However, several recent studies using consensus-based definitions for EoE describe atopy in 60% to 96% of adult patients.[33-36] In addition, oral allergy syndrome, characterized by oropharyngeal pruritus with or without angioedema of the lip, tongue, palate, and posterior oropharynx after ingestion of uncooked fruits and vegetables, may be encountered in these patients, although the magnitude of this problem remains unclear.[34]

Aeroallergens have also been implicated in EoE, because several studies have found a seasonal predilection for the diagnosis of EoE coinciding with peak pollen season, extending from the spring to early fall.[36-38] However, given that atopy is not a universal finding, it is unclear what the presence or absence of atopy means in terms of disease presentation, treatment, and natural history.

MISCELLANEOUS SYMPTOMS

The clinical presentation of adults is different from that encountered in children. Nevertheless, a variety of clinical findings more characteristic of pediatric EoE may also be seen in adults, including abdominal pain, nausea, vomiting, and failure to thrive.[5] The frequency of these symptoms is difficult to estimate, but practitioners should be aware that nonspecific symptoms such as these may be the only clinical manifestation of EoE in selected adults.

ENDOSCOPIC APPEARANCE

Patients with EoE have a wide variety of endoscopic findings. These findings include concentric rings (fixed or transient) (**Fig. 1**), longitudinal furrows (**Figs. 2** and **3**), white exudates (plaques) (**Fig. 4**), loss of vascularity (also referred to as edema or mucosal pallor) (**Figs. 5** and **6**), strictures, narrow-caliber esophagus (see **Fig. 1**), crepe-paper esophagus (mucosal fragility or laceration with passage of an adult diagnostic endoscope), and even a normal-appearing esophagus.

Concentric rings may be observed focally in esophageal segments or may involve the length of the esophagus. The cause of these esophageal rings is not completely understood and it is thought that rings may represent an intermittent contraction of the deep muscle layer, may represent eosinophilic infiltration, or may be a consequence of esophageal remodeling.[39] Longitudinal furrows typically involve the full length of the esophagus and observations with endoscopic ultrasonography suggest that furrows may be related to thickening of the mucosal and submucosal layers.[40] White exudates vary in size from 1 mm to 3 mm and are typically scattered along the length of the esophagus, giving the esophagus a speckled appearance that may be confused with Candida esophagitis. This finding corresponds with collections of eosinophils or even microabscesses in the mucosa.[41] Mucosal inflammation may be associated with a loss of the normal vascular pattern. This appearance may be caused by expansion of the basal layer of the mucosa accompanied by edema.[39] Focal strictures, in the absence of narrow-caliber esophagus or concentric rings, may be encountered anywhere in the esophagus. Narrow-caliber esophagus is defined as a narrow, fixed internal diameter of the esophagus.[42] This feature may not be appreciated on endoscope insertion, but is characterized by extensive linear abrasions or mucosal rents best seen on withdrawal of the endoscope.[43] The term crepe-paper esophagus was first suggested by Straumann and colleagues[44] in a 2003 case series of 5 men. The mucosa of the esophagus is characterized as fragile, delicate, and inelastic, and tears with little pressure. Normal endoscopy may be encountered in patients with EoE as well. In a study of 376 patients with unexplained dysphagia at the Mayo Clinic, 10 of 102 patients (9.8%) with a normal-appearing esophagus had EoE on biopsies.[8]

How common are the endoscopic features of EoE? A recent meta-analysis of various endoscopic features of EoE found the pooled prevalence of the endoscopic

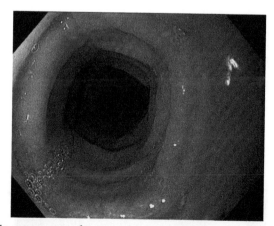

Fig. 1. Endoscopic appearance of concentric rings associated with narrow-caliber esophagus. A diagnostic adult endoscope could not pass distally.

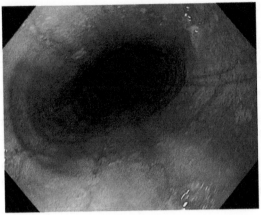

Fig. 2. Endoscopic appearance of longitudinal furrows.

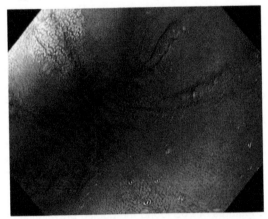

Fig. 3. Endoscopic appearance of longitudinal furrows with narrow band imaging.

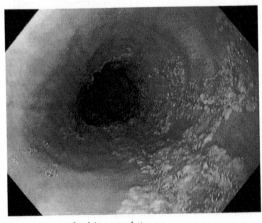

Fig. 4. Endoscopic appearance of white exudate.

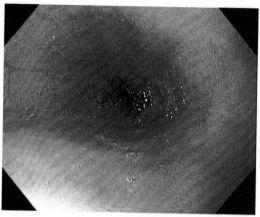

Fig. 5. Endoscopic appearance of decreased vascularity.

features of EoE as follows: linear furrows, 48%; decreased vascularity, 41%; rings, 44%; white exudates, 27%; stricture, 21%; narrow-caliber esophagus, 9%; and normal endoscopy, in 17%.[45] However, the sensitivity of these findings is problematic, varying from 15% to 48%, although specificity varies from 90% to 95%. However, the use of electronic chromoendoscopy techniques such as narrow band imaging does not seem to improve the recognition of endoscopic features of EoE.[46] All of this serves to highlight the importance of obtaining biopsy specimens in individuals with suspected EoE.

In an effort to provide a better and more consistent endoscopic description of EoE, Hirano and colleagues[47] developed an endoscopic classification system that incorporates 4 major endoscopic features of EoE: rings, furrows, exudates, and edema (loss of vascularity), along with the additional feature of strictures and crepe-paper esophagus (**Box 1**). This system has moderate to good interobserver variability characteristics, and may provide a common language for EoE akin to the Los Angeles classification for GERD and the Prague classification for Barrett esophagus.

The information presented earlier, as well as a better understanding of both the natural history of EoE and its underlying pathophysiology, has led to the conceptual

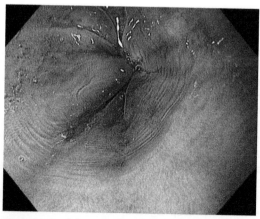

Fig. 6. Endoscopic appearance of decreased vascularity by narrow band imaging.

Box 1
New EoE endoscopic classification system

1. Major features
   a. Fixed rings
      i. Grade 0: none
      ii. Grade 1: mild (subtle circumferential ridges)
      iii. Grade 2: moderate (distinct rings that do not impair passage of standard adult diagnostic endoscope)
      iv. Grade 3: (distinct rings that do not allow passage of standard adult diagnostic endoscope)
   b. Exudates
      i. Grade 0: none
      ii. Grade 1: mild (involving <10% of the esophageal surface area)
      iii. Grade 2: severe (involving >10% of the esophageal surface area)
   c. Furrows
      i. Grade 0: absent
      ii. Grade 1: present
   d. Edema (loss of vascularity)
      i. Grade 0: distinct vascularity present
      ii. Grade 1: loss of clarity or absence of vascular markings
   e. Stricture
      i. Grade 0: absent
      ii. Grade 1: present
2. Minor features
   a. Crepe-paper esophagus (mucosal fragility or laceration after passage of a diagnostic endoscope)
      i. Grade 0: absent
      ii. Grade 1: present

---

model of endoscopic phenotypes of the disease. The inflammatory phenotype is characterized by linear furrows, white exudates, or a normal-appearing esophagus; the fibrostenotic phenotype by rings, narrowing, or strictures; and the mixed phenotype characterized by a combination of these findings.[5] These findings have potential implications in the understanding of the natural history of the disease because the patients with the inflammatory phenotype are typically younger, have less food impactions, less need for dilation, and a shorter duration of symptoms before diagnosis. In contrast, the frequency of the fibrostenotic phenotype increases with increasing age. Work in Switzerland by Schoepfer and colleagues[4] similarly found that the endoscopic phenotype of EoE changed with increasing delay in diagnosis: the frequency of the inflammatory phenotype decreased, whereas the fibrostenotic phenotypes increased with increasing length of diagnostic delay. Also noted was an increase in the prevalence of esophageal strictures with increased duration of diagnostic delay.

QUALITY OF LIFE

EoE has an impact on quality of life, but little is known about this in adults. In an effort to address this knowledge gap, the Northwestern group interviewed 24 adults in order to better understand the patient experience and provide preliminary data to develop a formal disease-specific quality-of-life questionnaire.[48] Six distinct themes reflected the patient experience with EoE: (1) relief on receiving the diagnosis that explained their symptoms; (2) concerns about EoE as a new disease, including its unknown natural history; (3) concerns about dysphagia episodes, including unpredictability and how to handle it; (4) impact of the disease on eating habits; (5) concerns about available therapy; and (6) concerns about social relationships. None of these areas had been addressed adequately in existing quality-of-life instruments. This work has led to the development and validation of a new Adult Eosinophilic Esophagitis Quality of Life Questionnaire, which focuses on 5 factors, including eating/diet impact, social impact, emotional impact, disease anxiety, and choking anxiety.[49] This instrument provides a valid and reliable disease-specific instrument that should be especially useful in therapeutic trials and should help enhance the understanding of this disease in the future.

SUMMARY

The clinical manifestations of EoE are protean. It is hoped that increased awareness of this disease by both patients and physicians will lead to a decrease in the long diagnostic delay that is so typical of this disease at present. It is hoped that early recognition and diagnosis combined with more effective and targeted therapies can alter the natural history of EoE, which recent studies suggest leads to an inexorable progression to complications associated with esophageal remodeling. More information is needed about PPI-REE, including implications on diagnosis and management of these patients. The development of disease-specific quality-of-life measures along with disease-specific symptom questionnaires should enhance ongoing efforts to develop new treatment approaches to EoE.

REFERENCES

1. Dellon ES, Gonsalves N, Hirano I, et al. ACG clinical guideline: evidenced based approach to the diagnosis and management of esophageal eosinophilia and eosinophilic esophagitis (EoE). Am J Gastroenterol 2013;108:679–92.
2. Liacouras CA, Furuta GT, Hirano I, et al. Eosinophilic esophagitis: updated consensus recommendations for children and adults. J Allergy Clin Immunol 2011;128:3–20.
3. Dellon ES. Diagnosis and management of eosinophilic esophagitis. Clin Gastroenterol Hepatol 2012;10:1066–78.
4. Schoepfer AM, Safroneeva E, Bussmann C, et al. Delay in diagnosis of eosinophilic esophagitis increases risk for stricture formation in a time-dependent manner. Gastroenterology 2013;145:1230–6.
5. Dellon ES, Kim HP, Sperry SL, et al. A phenotypic analysis shows that eosinophilic esophagitis is a progressive fibrostenotic disease. Gastrointest Endosc 2014;79:577–85.
6. Lucendo AJ, Sánchez-Cazalilla M. Adult versus pediatric eosinophilic esophagitis: important differences and similarities for the clinician to understand. Expert Rev Clin Immunol 2012;8:733–45.

7. Mackenzie SH, Go M, Chadwick B, et al. Eosinophilic oesophagitis in patients presenting with dysphagia–a prospective analysis. Aliment Pharmacol Ther 2008;28:1140–6.

8. Prasad GA, Talley NJ, Romero Y, et al. Prevalence and predictive factors of eosinophilic esophagitis in patients presenting with dysphagia: a prospective study. Am J Gastroenterol 2007;102:2627–32.

9. Kwiatek MA, Hirano I, Kahrilas PJ, et al. Mechanical properties of the esophagus in eosinophilic esophagitis. Gastroenterology 2011;140:82–90.

10. Korsapati H, Babaei A, Bhargava V, et al. Dysfunction of the longitudinal muscles of the oesophagus in eosinophilic oesophagitis. Gut 2009;58:1056–62.

11. Roman S, Hirano I, Kwiatek MA, et al. Manometric features of eosinophilic esophagitis in esophageal pressure topography. Neurogastroenterol Motil 2011;23:208–14.

12. Straumann A, Bussmann C, Zuber M, et al. Eosinophilic esophagitis: analysis of food impaction and perforation in 251 adolescent and adult patients. Clin Gastroenterol Hepatol 2008;6:598–600.

13. Desai TK, Stecevic V, Chang CH, et al. Association of eosinophilic inflammation with esophageal food impaction in adults. Gastrointest Endosc 2005;61:795–801.

14. Sperry SL, Crockett SD, Miller CB, et al. Esophageal foreign-body impactions: epidemiology, time trends, and the impact of the increasing prevalence of eosinophilic esophagitis. Gastrointest Endosc 2011;74:985–91.

15. Nicodème F, Hirano I, Chen J, et al. Esophageal distensibility as a measure of disease severity in patients with eosinophilic esophagitis. Clin Gastroenterol Hepatol 2013;11:1101–7.

16. Furuta GT, Liacouras CA, Collins MH, et al. Eosinophilic esophagitis in children and adults: a systematic review and consensus recommendations for diagnosis and treatment. Gastroenterology 2007;133:1342–63.

17. Poh CH, Gasiorowska A, Navarro-Rodriguez T, et al. Upper GI tract findings in patients with heartburn in whom proton pump inhibitor treatment failed versus those not receiving antireflux treatment. Gastrointest Endosc 2010;71:28–34.

18. García-Compeán D, González González JA, Marrufo García CA, et al. Prevalence of eosinophilic esophagitis in patients with refractory gastroesophageal reflux disease symptoms: a prospective study. Dig Liver Dis 2011;43:204–8.

19. Foroutan M, Norouzi A, Molaei M, et al. Eosinophilic esophagitis in patients with refractory gastroesophageal reflux disease. Dig Dis Sci 2010;55:28–31.

20. Dellon ES, Gibbs WB, Fritchie KJ, et al. Clinical, endoscopic, and histologic findings distinguish eosinophilic esophagitis from gastroesophageal reflux disease. Clin Gastroenterol Hepatol 2009;7:1305–13.

21. Mulder DJ, Hurlbut DJ, Noble AJ, et al. Clinical features distinguish eosinophilic and reflux-induced esophagitis. J Pediatr Gastroenterol Nutr 2013;56:263–70.

22. Molina-Infante J, Ferrando-Lamana L, Ripoll C, et al. Esophageal eosinophilic infiltration responds to proton pump inhibition in most adults. Clin Gastroenterol Hepatol 2011;9:110–7.

23. Molina-Infante J, Katzka DA, Gisbert JP. Review article: proton pump inhibitor therapy for suspected eosinophilic oesophagitis. Aliment Pharmacol Ther 2013;37:1157–64.

24. Cheng E, Zhang X, Huo X, et al. Omeprazole blocks eotaxin-3 expression by oesophageal squamous cells from patients with eosinophilic oesophagitis and GORD. Gut 2013;62:824–32.

25. Dellon ES, Speck O, Woodward K, et al. Clinical and endoscopic characteristics do not reliably differentiate PPI-responsive esophageal eosinophilia and eosinophilic

esophagitis in patients undergoing upper endoscopy: a prospective cohort study. Am J Gastroenterol 2013;108:1854–60.

26. Lucendo AJ, Friginal-Ruiz AB, Rodríguez B. Boerhaave's syndrome as the primary manifestation of adult eosinophilic esophagitis. Two case reports and a review of the literature. Dis Esophagus 2011;24:E11–5.

27. Cohen MS, Kaufman A, DiMarino AJ Jr, et al. Eosinophilic esophagitis presenting as spontaneous esophageal rupture (Boerhaave's syndrome). Clin Gastroenterol Hepatol 2007;5:A24.

28. Riou PJ, Nicholson AG, Pastorino U. Esophageal rupture in a patient with idiopathic eosinophilic esophagitis. Ann Thorac Surg 1996;62:1854–6.

29. Liguori G, Cortale M, Cimino F, et al. Circumferential mucosal dissection and esophageal perforation in a patient with eosinophilic esophagitis. World J Gastroenterol 2008;14:803–4.

30. Sgrò A, Betalli P, Battaglia G, et al. An unusual complication of eosinophilic esophagitis in an adolescent: intramural esophageal dissection. Endoscopy 2012;44(Suppl 2):E419–20.

31. Predina JD, Anolik RB, Judy B, et al. Intramural esophageal dissection in a young man with eosinophilic esophagitis. Ann Thorac Cardiovasc Surg 2012;18:31–5.

32. Moawad FJ, Cheatham JG, DeZee KJ. Meta-analysis: the safety and efficacy of dilation in eosinophilic oesophagitis. Aliment Pharmacol Ther 2013;38:713–20.

33. Penfield JD, Lang DM, Goldblum JR, et al. The role of allergy evaluation in adults with eosinophilic esophagitis. J Clin Gastroenterol 2010;44:22–7.

34. Roy-Ghanta S, Larosa DF, Katzka DA. Atopic characteristics of adult patients with eosinophilic esophagitis. Clin Gastroenterol Hepatol 2008;6:531–5.

35. Straumann A, Spichtin HP, Grize L, et al. Natural history of primary eosinophilic esophagitis: a follow-up of 30 adult patients for up to 11.5 years. Gastroenterology 2003;125:1660–9.

36. Almansa C, Krishna M, Buchner AM, et al. Seasonal distribution in newly diagnosed cases of eosinophilic esophagitis in adults. Am J Gastroenterol 2009;104:828–33.

37. Prasad GA, Alexander JA, Schleck CD, et al. Epidemiology of eosinophilic esophagitis over three decades in Olmsted County, Minnesota. Clin Gastroenterol Hepatol 2009;7:1055–61.

38. Moawad FJ, Veerappan GR, Lake JM, et al. Correlation between eosinophilic oesophagitis and aeroallergens. Aliment Pharmacol Ther 2010;31:509–15.

39. Fox VL. Eosinophilic esophagitis: endoscopic findings. Gastrointest Endosc Clin N Am 2008;18:45–57.

40. Fox VL, Nurko S, Furuta GT. Eosinophilic esophagitis: it's not just kid's stuff. Gastrointest Endosc 2002;56:260–70.

41. Straumann A, Spichtin HP, Bucher KA, et al. Eosinophilic esophagitis: red on microscopy, white on endoscopy. Digestion 2004;70:109–16.

42. Potter JW, Saeian K, Staff D, et al. Eosinophilic esophagitis in adults: an emerging problem with unique esophageal features. Gastrointest Endosc 2004;59:355–61.

43. Vasilopoulos S, Murphy P, Auerbach A, et al. The small-caliber esophagus: an unappreciated cause of dysphagia for solids in patients with eosinophilic esophagitis. Gastrointest Endosc 2002;55:99–106.

44. Straumann A, Rossi L, Simon HU, et al. Fragility of the esophageal mucosa: a pathognomonic endoscopic sign of primary eosinophilic esophagitis? Gastrointest Endosc 2003;57:407–12.

45. Kim HP, Vance RB, Shaheen NJ, et al. The prevalence and diagnostic utility of endoscopic features of eosinophilic esophagitis: a meta-analysis. Clin Gastroenterol Hepatol 2012;10:988–96.

46. Peery AF, Cao H, Dominik R, et al. Variable reliability of endoscopic findings with white-light and narrow-band imaging for patients with suspected eosinophilic esophagitis. Clin Gastroenterol Hepatol 2011;9:475–80.
47. Hirano I, Moy N, Heckman MG, et al. Endoscopic assessment of the oesophageal features of eosinophilic oesophagitis: validation of a novel classification and grading system. Gut 2013;62:489–95.
48. Taft TH, Kern E, Keefer L, et al. Qualitative assessment of patient-reported outcomes in adults with eosinophilic esophagitis. J Clin Gastroenterol 2011;45:769–74.
49. Taft TH, Kern E, Kwiatek MA, et al. The adult eosinophilic oesophagitis quality of life questionnaire: a new measure of health-related quality of life. Aliment Pharmacol Ther 2011;34:790–8.

Eosinophilic Esophagitis
Interactions with Gastroesophageal Reflux Disease

Edaire Cheng, MD[a],*, Rhonda F. Souza, MD[b],
Stuart Jon Spechler, MD[b]

KEYWORDS

- Gastroesophageal reflux disease • Eosinophilic esophagitis • Proton pump inhibitors
- PPI-responsive esophageal eosinophilia

KEY POINTS

- Eosinophilic esophagitis (EoE) and gastroesophageal reflux disease (GERD) are not mutually exclusive disorders, and their interactions can be complex.
- The notion that EoE and GERD can be distinguished by the response to proton pump inhibitor (PPI) therapy has been challenged by the recognition of patients with PPI-responsive esophageal eosinophilia who show a clinical and histologic response to PPIs, even although they have no evidence of GERD.
- In addition to inhibiting gastric acid production, PPIs have acid-independent, anti-inflammatory effects.
- Both the acid-inhibitory and the anti-inflammatory effects of PPIs might benefit patients with EoE as well as patients with GERD.
- For patients with esophageal symptoms and eosinophilia, we believe that a clinical or histologic response to PPIs does not rule in GERD and does not rule out EoE.

INTRODUCTION

Heartburn and dysphagia are frequent symptoms of both eosinophilic esophagitis (EoE) and gastroesophageal reflux disease (GERD), and esophageal biopsies in both disorders can show epithelial infiltration by eosinophils. Therefore, it can

Funding: NIH, K08DK099383; R01CA134571; R01DK63621; Office of Medical Research, Departments of Veterans Affairs.
[a] Departments of Pediatrics and Internal Medicine, Esophageal Diseases Center, Children's Medical Center, VA North Texas Health Care System, University of Texas Southwestern Medical Center, 5323 Harry Hines Boulevard, Dallas, TX 75390, USA; [b] Department of Internal Medicine, Esophageal Diseases Center, Children's Medical Center, VA North Texas Health Care System, Harold C. Simmons Comprehensive Cancer Center, University of Texas Southwestern Medical Center, 5323 Harry Hines Boulevard, Dallas, TX 75390, USA
* Corresponding author. Department of Pediatrics, University of Texas Southwestern Medical Center, 5323 Harry Hines Boulevard, Dallas, TX 75390.
E-mail address: edaire.cheng@utsouthwestern.edu

sometimes be difficult to distinguish EoE from GERD. EoE was not described as a distinct clinicopathologic disorder until 1993,[1] and confusion with GERD delayed appreciation that EoE was a burgeoning new esophageal ailment. Throughout the 1990s, pathologists and clinicians often attributed esophageal eosinophilia to GERD and were either unaware of EoE or did not consider it seriously in the differential diagnosis.[2] It was not until well into the new millennium, when several reports had accumulated describing patients with esophageal symptoms and eosinophilia refractory to antireflux therapy, but responsive to elemental diets and steroids, that clinicians generally became aware that EoE was a bona fide new disorder distinct from GERD.[3–6]

In 2007, a consensus report from the First International Gastrointestinal Eosinophil Research Subcommittee defined EoE as a primary clinicopathologic disorder of the esophagus characterized by esophageal or upper gastrointestinal symptoms, an esophageal biopsy showing 15 or more per high power field, and the absence of pathologic GERD as shown by a normal esophageal pH monitoring study or lack of response to high-dose proton pump inhibitors (PPIs).[7] This definition, which implied that EoE and GERD were mutually exclusive conditions, was formulated in an attempt to eliminate confusion between the two. However, other authorities soon challenged this definition, contending that the interactions between EoE and GERD could be complex and that the notion of establishing a clear distinction between them was too simplistic.[8]

Several investigators chose simply to ignore the 2007 consensus definition and to include patients with abnormal acid reflux in their series of patients with EoE.[9–11] Others attempted to use clinical, endoscopic, histologic, and immunohistochemical features to distinguish GERD from EoE, with variable success.[12–19] However, some of the histologic and immunohistochemical differences described in those studies might have resulted merely from differences between GERD and EoE study patients in their number of esophageal eosinophils rather than from differences in the disorders underlying the esophageal eosinophilia.[20] In 2011, another consensus group (with the benefit of information on EoE pathogenesis not available in 2007) proposed a conceptual definition for EoE as "a chronic, immune/antigen-mediated esophageal disease characterized clinically by symptoms related to esophageal dysfunction and histologically by eosinophil-predominant inflammation."[21] This conceptual definition does not even mention GERD and does not imply that GERD and EoE are mutually exclusive disorders.

PROPOSED MECHANISMS UNDERLYING AN ASSOCIATION BETWEEN ESOPHAGEAL EOSINOPHILIA AND GERD

Four major mechanisms might explain an association between esophageal eosinophilia and GERD: (1) GERD causes esophageal eosinophilia in the absence of EoE, (2) GERD and EoE coexist but are unrelated, (3) EoE contributes to or causes GERD, (4) GERD contributes to or causes EoE.[8]

GERD Causes Esophageal Eosinophilia in the Absence of EoE

Since 1982, it has been appreciated that esophageal eosinophilia can be a manifestation of GERD.[22] This eosinophilia is usually mild, with fewer than 7 eosinophils per high power field, and may occur because refluxed gastric juice stimulates the esophagus to produce substances that attract eosinophils. In cultures of human esophageal microvascular endothelial cells, acid exposure has been shown to induce the expression of vascular cell adhesion molecule 1, an adhesion molecule recognized by ligands on the eosinophil cell surface.[23,24] Studies using a preparation of human esophageal mucosa have found that acid stimulates the release of platelet activating factor (PAF), a phospholipid that can attract and activate eosinophils.[25] Esophageal squamous epithelial cells in culture secrete interleukin 8 (IL-8) when they are exposed to acidified bile salts,[26,27] and HET-1A esophageal epithelial cells exposed to acid show upregulation of eotaxin-1, eotaxin-2, eotaxin-3, and macrophage inflammatory protein 1α (MIP-1α).[28] Eotaxins and MIP-1α bind eosinophil chemokine receptors (CCR3 and CCR1, respectively), which play a key role in eosinophil chemotaxis.[29] In patients with reflux esophagitis, furthermore, esophageal mucosal biopsy specimens show increased levels of eosinophil chemoattractants such as IL-8 and RANTES (regulated upon activation normal T cell expressed and secreted).[30] It is not known which, if any, of these factors underlie the esophageal eosinophilia of GERD.

GERD and EoE Coexist but Are Unrelated

Because approximately 20% of adults in Western countries have GERD,[31,32] it would expected that, by chance alone, 20% of Western adults with EoE should have GERD. This might not be the case if GERD were to protect the esophagus from EoE, but there is no evidence for such a protective effect. Some studies have suggested that pathologic acid reflux is inordinately common in EoE.[11,33] For example, 24-hour esophageal pH monitoring showed abnormal acid reflux in 10 (42%) of 24 adults with EoE in 1 study,[33] and in 14 (56%) of 25 in another.[11] Some studies have suggested that, unlike in adults, abnormal acid reflux is uncommon in pediatric patients with EoE.[34–36] However, the accuracy of esophageal pH monitoring as a test for GERD in children is not well established.[37] Further confounding interpretation of reports on the frequency of GERD in EoE is inconsistency among investigators regarding the criteria used to define EoE. According to the 2007 consensus statement, the frequency of abnormal acid reflux in EoE should be 0%, because, by the 2007 definition, an abnormal esophageal pH monitoring study would preclude the diagnosis.[7] The 2011 consensus definition has no such preclusion.[21]

EoE Contributes to or Causes GERD

Eosinophils produce several substances that might contribute to GERD by promoting gastroesophageal reflux and by impairing the ability of the esophagus to clear itself of noxious refluxed material. For example, eosinophils produce vasoactive intestinal peptide and PAF, which can reduce lower esophageal sphincter pressure and thereby predispose to reflux.[38,39] Eosinophils also secrete IL-6, a cytokine that weakens esophageal muscle contraction. This weak muscle contraction might impair peristalsis and delay esophageal acid clearance.[40,41] Furthermore, esophageal eosinophils can induce tissue remodeling with subepithelial fibrosis, and such fibrosis also conceivably might contribute to GERD by interfering with lower esophageal sphincter function and peristalsis.[42]

In addition to secreting substances that can promote reflux and delay esophageal acid clearance, eosinophils also produce cytotoxic substances that might render the esophageal epithelium more permeable and susceptible to injury by refluxed gastric material.[43–46] For example, major basic protein has been shown to disrupt barrier function in monolayers of human colonic carcinoma cells.[46] Eosinophil infiltration of the bronchial mucosa of asthmatic patients is associated with damage to cellular tight junctions and dilation of the intercellular spaces.[47] Similar changes are found in the esophageal mucosa of patients with GERD, presumably as the result of acid-peptic damage to tight junctions. This tight junction damage increases mucosal permeability, which enables acid and other noxious molecules to reach nociceptors located deep in the epithelium, and these nociceptors might convey the sensation of heartburn.[48] Perhaps increased mucosal permeability caused by cytotoxic eosinophil products underlies the hypersensitivity to esophageal acid perfusion that has been described in patients with EoE.[49]

GERD Contributes to or Causes EoE

Although increased mucosal permeability caused by eosinophilia might contribute to GERD, it is also possible that increased esophageal mucosal permeability caused by GERD predisposes to the development of EoE. The normal esophageal mucosa is highly impermeable to large molecules like food allergens,[50] which typically have a molecular weight between 3 and 90 kDa.[51] For example, Tobey and colleagues[50] found that the normal rabbit esophagus was virtually impermeable to epidermal growth factor, a peptide with a molecular weight of 6 kDa, and to dextrans with a molecular weight of 4 kDa. However, after exposure to acid and pepsin, the rabbit esophageal mucosa became permeable to epidermal growth factor and to dextrans as large as 20 kDa. By increasing esophageal permeability, therefore, GERD could render the squamous epithelium permeable to allergens that might cause EoE.

As discussed earlier, GERD might contribute to esophageal eosinophilia by inducing the expression of eosinophil chemoattractants. Refluxed gastric material also can cause the release of mast cell products and other substances that attract noneosinophil immune cells to the esophagus,[26,52] and it is conceivable that this immune response might contribute to the development of EoE. In addition, refluxed material can activate receptors that exacerbate EoE symptoms and inflammation. For example, reflux-induced activation of transient receptor potential cation channel, subfamily vanilloid member 1 (TRPV1) on esophageal neurons might contribute to the acid hypersensitivity that has been described in EoE patients,[49] and activated TRPV1 has been linked to the release of eosinophil chemoattractants (IL-8, PAF, eotaxin-1, eotaxin-2, eotaxin-3, and MIP-1α) and other inflammatory mediators such as substance P and calcitonin gene-related peptide.[28,53] Also, the proteinase-activated receptor 2 on esophageal epithelial cells can be activated by refluxed proteolytic enzymes to cause production of IL-8.[54–57]

PPI-RESPONSIVE ESOPHAGEAL EOSINOPHILIA

Recent reports have described patients with a condition called PPI-responsive esophageal eosinophilia (PPI-REE).[11,21,58–65] These patients have typical EoE symptoms and endoscopic abnormalities, no evidence of GERD by endoscopy or by esophageal pH/impedance monitoring, and nevertheless show a clinical and histologic response to PPI therapy. Studies in pediatric and adult patients with esophageal eosinophilia suggest that approximately 50% respond to PPIs,[11,58,60–65] and that no clinical or endoscopic feature independently distinguishes PPI responders from nonresponders.[64,65] In some pediatric patients initially found to have PPI-REE, Dohil and colleagues[59] observed the subsequent reaccumulation of eosinophils and other inflammatory cells in the esophagus over a period of 3 to 12 months despite ongoing PPI treatment. Thus, PPI-REE may be a transient condition. PPIs also might help to control esophageal symptoms, even if they do not cause resolution of esophageal eosinophilia. For example, Levine and colleagues[61] found that PPI treatment of children with EoE failed to resolve their esophageal inflammation, but nevertheless resulted in long-term symptomatic improvement.

It is possible that patients with PPI-REE simply have GERD that is not detected by conventional diagnostic tests but that benefits from the acid-suppressive effects of PPIs. Alternatively, these patients may have EoE or a related allergen-mediated process that responds to therapeutic effects of PPIs that are independent of gastric acid suppression (see later discussion). The relative contributions of these acid-suppressive and acid-independent PPI actions are not clear.

POTENTIAL ACID-DEPENDENT EFFECTS OF PPIS IN ESOPHAGEAL EOSINOPHILIA

PPIs target gastric H^+/K^+-adenosine triphosphatase (H^+/K^+-ATPase), the proton pump of the parietal cells responsible for gastric acid secretion. In the acidic environment of functioning parietal cells, PPIs are acid activated and covalently bind to cysteine residues on the H^+/K^+-ATPase, rendering the pumps inactive.[66] Without PPIs, the distal esophagus is exposed to refluxed acid for up to approximately 5% of the day in normal adults, and for 8% to 13% of the day in normal newborns and infants.[67,68] As discussed earlier, there are several mechanisms whereby acid reflux might contribute to esophageal eosinophilia and to esophageal infiltration by noneosinophil immune cells. Thus, patients who have EoE and no evidence of GERD still might benefit from acid suppression to control their normal acid reflux.[8] In addition, patients with EoE can have hypersensitivity to acid-induced esophageal pain.[49] Therefore, PPIs might provide symptomatic relief even for patients with normal esophageal acid exposure.

POTENTIAL ACID-INDEPENDENT, ANTI-INFLAMMATORY EFFECTS OF PPIS IN ESOPHAGEAL EOSINOPHILIA

PPIs might benefit patients with esophageal eosinophilia through effects that are entirely independent of gastric acid suppression. Th2 (T helper) cytokines such as IL-4 and IL-13, which can be overproduced in allergic disorders, stimulate esophageal epithelial cells to secrete the potent eosinophil chemoattractant eotaxin-3.[69–72] This mechanism is believed to contribute importantly to the esophageal eosinophilia of EoE. Two recent studies using esophageal epithelial cells in culture have shown that PPIs inhibit the Th2 cytokine-stimulated secretion of eotaxin-3.[72,73] This inhibition occurs with omeprazole in concentrations as low as 1 μM, which are readily achieved in blood with conventional oral dosing, and with lansoprazole, suggesting a PPI drug class effect.[74,75] Mechanistically, the inhibitory effect of PPIs seems to involve chromatin remodeling of the eotaxin-3 promoter, which blocks binding by its regulatory transcription factor STAT6 (signal transducer and activator of transcription 6), thereby reducing eotaxin-3 transcription (**Fig. 1**).

The PPIs are prodrugs that require acid activation to exert their antisecretory and anti-inflammatory effects.[72,73] This acid activation occurs readily in the acidic microenvironment of the functioning parietal cell, but it is not clear whether PPI acid activation can occur in the esophagus. Conceivably, gastroesophageal acid reflux might acidify the esophageal microenvironment sufficiently to achieve PPI acid activation. In addition, the Na^+/H^+ exchanger on esophageal epithelial cell membranes can extrude intracellular protons that accumulate in the setting of injury, thereby acidifying the microenvironment.[76] Eosinophils and neutrophils can also release protons from their exocytic granules and lysosomes into the microenvironment,[77–79] and microenvironment acidification has been well documented in the setting of inflammation.[80–82] Thus, there are several plausible mechanisms whereby PPIs might be activated in the diseased esophagus of EoE.

OTHER ANTI-INFLAMMATORY EFFECTS OF PPI

Several other potentially beneficial, acid-independent, anti-inflammatory effects of PPIs have been described (**Box 1**).[83] For example, PPIs have antioxidant properties,

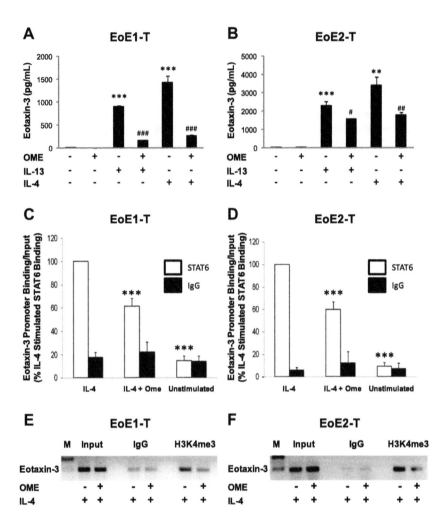

Fig. 1. (*A, B*) Omeprazole (OME) blocks cytokine-stimulated eotaxin-3 protein secretion (determined by enzyme-linked immunosorbent assay) in esophageal epithelial cells. EoE1-T and EoE2-T are nonneoplastic, telomerase-immortalized esophageal squamous epithelial cell lines established from patients with EoE. (*A*) EoE1-T and (*B*) EoE2-T were stimulated for 48 h with either IL-13 (50 ng/mL) or IL-4 (10 ng/mL) in the presence or absence of OME (50 μM). ** $P \leq .01$ and *** $P \leq .001$ compared with control; # $P \leq .05$, ## $P \leq .01$, and ### $P \leq .001$ compared with corresponding Th2 cytokine stimulation alone. (*C, D*) Omeprazole decreases transcription factor STAT6 binding to the eotaxin-3 promoter (determined by chromatin immunoprecipitation assay) in IL-4-stimulated (*C*) EoE1-T and (*D*) EoE2-T cells. *** $P \leq .001$ compared with IL-4 stimulation. Isotype matched IgG served as a control. (*E, F*) Omeprazole effects involve chromatin remodeling and reduced levels of histone 3 trimethylated lysine 4 (H3K4me3) bound to the eotaxin-3 promoter (determined by chromatin immunoprecipitation assay) in IL-4-stimulated (*E*) EoE1-T and (*F*) EoE2-T cells. Isotype matched IgG served as a control. M, marker. (*Adapted from [A, B]* Cheng E, Zhang X, Huo X, et al. Omeprazole blocks eotaxin-3 expression by esophageal squamous cells from patients with eosinophilic esophagitis and GORD. Gut 2013;62:829, with permission; and [*C–F*] *From* Zhang X, Cheng E, Huo X, et al. Omeprazole blocks STAT6 binding to the eotaxin-3 promoter in eosinophilic esophagitis cells. PLoS One 2012;7:e50037.)

Box 1
Potential mechanisms underlying beneficial PPI effects in esophageal eosinophilia

Acid-dependent effects

- Decrease acid-stimulated production of eosinophil chemoattractants by esophageal epithelial cells
- Decrease acid exposure that causes inflammatory cytokine production and esophageal damage
- Decrease acid exposure that causes increased esophageal permeability to potential allergens
- Decrease acid exposure that causes acid-induced pain

Acid-independent, anti-inflammatory effects

Effects on epithelial cells

- Inhibition of Th2 cytokine-stimulated eotaxin-3 expression
- Decrease production of proinflammatory cytokines

Antioxidant effects

- Direct scavenging of reactive oxygen species
- Increase bioavailability of protective sulfhydryl compounds
- Increase protective heme oxygenase 1 expression

Effects on inflammatory cells (neutrophils, monocytes)

- Inhibition of oxidative burst
- Impair phagocytosis of microorganisms
- Decrease expression of adhesion molecules
- Impair migration

Effects on endothelial cells

- Decrease expression of adhesion molecules
- Decrease production of proinflammatory cytokines

---

including their ability to scavenge hydroxyl radicals, to increase the bioavailability of sulfhydryl compounds, and to induce heme oxygenase 1.[84–88] PPIs can inhibit the oxidative burst, migration, and phagocytosis in neutrophils and monocytes.[89–91] In epithelial cells and endothelial cells, PPIs can decrease expression of adhesion molecule and proinflammatory cytokines (eg, IL-8, IL-6, tumor necrosis factor α),[83,92,93] and inhibit Th2 cytokine-driven STAT6 signaling.[94] These acid-independent, anti-inflammatory effects could benefit esophageal inflammation caused by GERD as well as by EoE.

PPI USE MIGHT PREDISPOSE TO THE DEVELOPMENT OF EoE

Although PPIs are used to treat esophageal eosinophilia, there are also intriguing data to suggest that PPIs might predispose to the development of celiac disease, food allergies, and EoE.[95,96] The human diet contains numerous proteins with the potential to evoke immunologic responses. Digestion of these potential food allergens normally begins in the stomach through the action of pepsin proteinases in acidic gastric juice.[95,97] By increasing the gastric pH to levels higher than 4, at which pepsin activity ceases, PPIs might enable food allergens to escape peptic digestion. In addition, PPIs have been shown to increase gastric mucosal permeability,[98,99] which might facilitate the absorption of undigested food allergens and their exposure to the immune cells that mediate allergy development. Also, gastric acid suppression by PPIs causes changes in the microbiome of the upper gastrointestinal tract, which conceivably could alter mucosal immune responses.[100,101]

There is experimental and clinical evidence that PPI treatment can have immunologic consequences. Untersmayr and colleagues[102] have shown that mice fed parvalbumin while treated with omeprazole develop parvalbumin-specific IgE antibodies, and that mice fed hazelnut extract while treated with omeprazole developed anaphylactogenic IgG1 antibodies and type I skin reactivity to hazelnut.[103] In 1 study of 152 allergy-free adults who were treated with acid-suppressive medications for 3 months, 10% showed an increase in blood IgE antibody levels and 15% developed new, food-specific IgE antibodies.[104]

PPIs were introduced into clinical practice in the United States in 1989, and the time course of their introduction and increasing usage parallels the emergence and increasing incidence of EoE. Although this association fits well with the hypothesis that PPIs play an etiologic role in EoE, a plausible association does not establish cause and effect. Further studies on the role of PPIs in the development of EoE clearly are warranted. Although it might seem paradoxic that a medication used to treat EoE also might cause EoE, there is no paradox because the proposed mechanisms are different. A remote exposure to PPIs (eg, in infancy or childhood) might trigger the food allergy that causes EoE, which might respond later to the anti-inflammatory effects of PPIs described earlier.

SUMMARY

GERD and EoE are not mutually exclusive disorders, and their interactions can be complex. The notion that GERD and EoE can be distinguished by the response to PPI treatment is based on the assumption that gastric acid suppression is the only important therapeutic effect of PPIs, and therefore only GERD can respond to PPIs. This assumption seems to be incorrect for 2 major reasons. First, there are multiple mechanisms whereby PPI-induced acid reduction might benefit patients with EoE. Second, PPIs have acid-independent, anti-inflammatory effects, which also might be beneficial both for GERD and for EoE. Because the PPIs have multiple effects, which might benefit both diseases, for patients who have esophageal symptoms and esophageal eosinophilia, we believe that a clinical or histologic response to PPIs does not rule in GERD and does not rule out EoE. For these reasons, we recommend a trial of PPI therapy for patients with symptomatic esophageal eosinophilia, even if the diagnosis of EoE seems clear-cut.

REFERENCES

1. Attwood SE, Smyrk TC, Demeester TR, et al. Esophageal eosinophilia with dysphagia. A distinct clinicopathologic syndrome. Dig Dis Sci 1993;38:109–16.
2. DeBrosse CW, Collins MH, Buckmeier Butz BK, et al. Identification, epidemiology, and chronicity of pediatric esophageal eosinophilia, 1982-1999. J Allergy Clin Immunol 2010;126:112–9.
3. Kelly KJ, Lazenby AJ, Rowe PC, et al. Eosinophilic esophagitis attributed to gastroesophageal reflux: improvement with an amino acid-based formula. Gastroenterology 1995;109:1503–12.
4. Liacouras CA, Wenner WJ, Brown K, et al. Primary eosinophilic esophagitis in children: successful treatment with oral corticosteroids. J Pediatr Gastroenterol Nutr 1998;26:380–5.

5. Ruchelli E, Wenner W, Voytek T, et al. Severity of esophageal eosinophilia predicts response to conventional gastroesophageal reflux therapy. Pediatr Dev Pathol 1999;2:15–8.
6. Teitelbaum JE, Fox VL, Twarog FJ, et al. Eosinophilic esophagitis in children: immunopathological analysis and response to fluticasone propionate. Gastroenterology 2002;122:1216–25.
7. Furuta GT, Liacouras CA, Collins MH, et al. Eosinophilic esophagitis in children and adults: a systematic review and consensus recommendations for diagnosis and treatment. Gastroenterology 2007;133:1342–63.
8. Spechler SJ, Genta RM, Souza RF. Thoughts on the complex relationship between gastroesophageal reflux disease and eosinophilic esophagitis. Am J Gastroenterol 2007;102:1301–6.
9. Rodrigo S, Abboud G, Oh D, et al. High intraepithelial eosinophil counts in esophageal squamous epithelium are not specific for eosinophilic esophagitis in adults. Am J Gastroenterol 2008;103:435–42.
10. Shah A, Kagalwalla AF, Gonsalves N, et al. Histopathologic variability in children with eosinophilic esophagitis. Am J Gastroenterol 2009;104:716–21.
11. Peterson KA, Thomas KL, Hilden K, et al. Comparison of esomeprazole to aerosolized, swallowed fluticasone for eosinophilic esophagitis. Dig Dis Sci 2010;55: 1313–9.
12. Parfitt JR, Gregor JC, Suskin NG, et al. Eosinophilic esophagitis in adults: distinguishing features from gastroesophageal reflux disease: a study of 41 patients. Mod Pathol 2006;19:90–6.
13. Bhattacharya B, Carlsten J, Sabo E, et al. Increased expression of eotaxin-3 distinguishes between eosinophilic esophagitis and gastroesophageal reflux disease. Hum Pathol 2007;38:1744–53.
14. Mueller S, Neureiter D, Aigner T, et al. Comparison of histological parameters for the diagnosis of eosinophilic oesophagitis versus gastro-oesophageal reflux disease on oesophageal biopsy material. Histopathology 2008;53:676–84.
15. Dellon ES, Gibbs WB, Fritchie KJ, et al. Clinical, endoscopic, and histologic findings distinguish eosinophilic esophagitis from gastroesophageal reflux disease. Clin Gastroenterol Hepatol 2009;7:1305–13 [quiz: 261].
16. Protheroe C, Woodruff SA, de Petris G, et al. A novel histologic scoring system to evaluate mucosal biopsies from patients with eosinophilic esophagitis. Clin Gastroenterol Hepatol 2009;7:749–55.e11.
17. Dellon ES, Chen X, Miller CR, et al. Tryptase staining of mast cells may differentiate eosinophilic esophagitis from gastroesophageal reflux disease. Am J Gastroenterol 2011;106:264–71.
18. Dellon ES, Chen X, Miller CR, et al. Diagnostic utility of major basic protein, eotaxin-3, and leukotriene enzyme staining in eosinophilic esophagitis. Am J Gastroenterol 2012;107:1503–11.
19. Mulder DJ, Hurlbut DJ, Noble AJ, et al. Clinical features distinguish eosinophilic and reflux-induced esophagitis. J Pediatr Gastroenterol Nutr 2013;56:263–70.
20. Sridhara S, Ravi K, Smyrk TC, et al. Increased numbers of eosinophils, rather than only etiology, predict histologic changes in patients with esophageal eosinophilia. Clin Gastroenterol Hepatol 2012;10:735–41.
21. Liacouras CA, Furuta GT, Hirano I, et al. Eosinophilic esophagitis: updated consensus recommendations for children and adults. J Allergy Clin Immunol 2011;128:3–20.e6 [quiz: 21–2].
22. Winter HS, Madara JL, Stafford RJ, et al. Intraepithelial eosinophils: a new diagnostic criterion for reflux esophagitis. Gastroenterology 1982;83:818–23.

23. Rafiee P, Theriot ME, Nelson VM, et al. Human esophageal microvascular endothelial cells respond to acidic pH stress by PI3K/AKT and p38 MAPK-regulated induction of Hsp70 and Hsp27. Am J Physiol Cell Physiol 2006;291:C931–45.

24. Barthel SR, Annis DS, Mosher DF, et al. Differential engagement of modules 1 and 4 of vascular cell adhesion molecule-1 (CD106) by integrins alpha4beta1 (CD49d/29) and alphaMbeta2 (CD11b/18) of eosinophils. J Biol Chem 2006; 281:32175–87.

25. Cheng L, Cao W, Behar J, et al. Acid-induced release of platelet-activating factor by human esophageal mucosa induces inflammatory mediators in circular smooth muscle. J Pharmacol Exp Ther 2006;319:117–26.

26. Souza RF, Huo X, Mittal V, et al. Gastroesophageal reflux might cause esophagitis through a cytokine-mediated mechanism rather than caustic acid injury. Gastroenterology 2009;137:1776–84.

27. Lampinen M, Rak S, Venge P. The role of interleukin-5, interleukin-8 and RANTES in the chemotactic attraction of eosinophils to the allergic lung. Clin Exp Allergy 1999;29:314–22.

28. Ma J, Altomare A, Guarino M, et al. HCl-induced and ATP-dependent upregulation of TRPV1 receptor expression and cytokine production by human esophageal epithelial cells. Am J Physiol Gastrointest Liver Physiol 2012;303:G635–45.

29. Luster AD, Rothenberg ME. Role of the monocyte chemoattractant protein and eotaxin subfamily of chemokines in allergic inflammation. J Leukoc Biol 1997;62: 620–33.

30. Isomoto H, Wang A, Mizuta Y, et al. Elevated levels of chemokines in esophageal mucosa of patients with reflux esophagitis. Am J Gastroenterol 2003;98: 551–6.

31. Locke GR 3rd, Talley NJ, Fett SL, et al. Prevalence and clinical spectrum of gastroesophageal reflux: a population-based study in Olmsted County, Minnesota. Gastroenterology 1997;112:1448–56.

32. Shaheen N, Provenzale D. The epidemiology of gastroesophageal reflux disease. Am J Med Sci 2003;326:264–73.

33. Remedios M, Campbell C, Jones DM, et al. Eosinophilic esophagitis in adults: clinical, endoscopic, histologic findings, and response to treatment with fluticasone propionate. Gastrointest Endosc 2006;63:3–12.

34. Sant'Anna AM, Rolland S, Fournet JC, et al. Eosinophilic esophagitis in children: symptoms, histology and pH probe results. J Pediatr Gastroenterol Nutr 2004; 39:373–7.

35. Steiner SJ, Gupta SK, Croffie JM, et al. Correlation between number of eosinophils and reflux index on same day esophageal biopsy and 24 hour esophageal pH monitoring. Am J Gastroenterol 2004;99:801–5.

36. Steiner SJ, Kernek KM, Fitzgerald JF. Severity of basal cell hyperplasia differs in reflux versus eosinophilic esophagitis. J Pediatr Gastroenterol Nutr 2006;42:506–9.

37. Vandenplas Y, Rudolph CD, Di Lorenzo C, et al. Pediatric gastroesophageal reflux clinical practice guidelines: joint recommendations of the North American Society for Pediatric Gastroenterology, Hepatology, and Nutrition (NASPGHAN) and the European Society for Pediatric Gastroenterology, Hepatology, and Nutrition (ESPGHAN). J Pediatr Gastroenterol Nutr 2009;49:498–547.

38. Cheng L, Harnett KM, Cao W, et al. Hydrogen peroxide reduces lower esophageal sphincter tone in human esophagitis. Gastroenterology 2005;129:1675–85.

39. Farre R, Auli M, Lecea B, et al. Pharmacologic characterization of intrinsic mechanisms controlling tone and relaxation of porcine lower esophageal sphincter. J Pharmacol Exp Ther 2006;316:1238–48.

40. Cao W, Cheng L, Behar J, et al. IL-1beta signaling in cat lower esophageal sphincter circular muscle. Am J Physiol Gastrointest Liver Physiol 2006;291: G672–80.
41. Cao W, Cheng L, Behar J, et al. Proinflammatory cytokines alter/reduce esophageal circular muscle contraction in experimental cat esophagitis. Am J Physiol Gastrointest Liver Physiol 2004;287:G1131–9.
42. Cheng E, Souza RF, Spechler SJ. Tissue remodeling in eosinophilic esophagitis. Am J Physiol Gastrointest Liver Physiol 2012;303:G1175–87.
43. Tai PC, Hayes DJ, Clark JB, et al. Toxic effects of human eosinophil products on isolated rat heart cells in vitro. Biochem J 1982;204:75–80.
44. Motojima S, Frigas E, Loegering DA, et al. Toxicity of eosinophil cationic proteins for guinea pig tracheal epithelium in vitro. Am Rev Respir Dis 1989;139:801–5.
45. Young JD, Peterson CG, Venge P, et al. Mechanism of membrane damage mediated by human eosinophil cationic protein. Nature 1986;321:613–6.
46. Furuta GT, Nieuwenhuis EE, Karhausen J, et al. Eosinophils alter colonic epithelial barrier function: role for major basic protein. Am J Physiol Gastrointest Liver Physiol 2005;289:G890–7.
47. Ohashi Y, Motojima S, Fukuda T, et al. Relationship between bronchial reactivity to inhaled acetylcholine, eosinophil infiltration and a widening of the intercellular space in patients with asthma. Arerugi 1990;39:1541–5.
48. Orlando RC. Pathophysiology of gastroesophageal reflux disease. J Clin Gastroenterol 2008;42:584–8.
49. Krarup AL, Villadsen GE, Mejlgaard E, et al. Acid hypersensitivity in patients with eosinophilic oesophagitis. Scand J Gastroenterol 2010;45:273–81.
50. Tobey NA, Hosseini SS, Argote CM, et al. Dilated intercellular spaces and shunt permeability in nonerosive acid-damaged esophageal epithelium. Am J Gastroenterol 2004;99:13–22.
51. Untersmayr E, Jensen-Jarolim E. The effect of gastric digestion on food allergy. Curr Opin Allergy Clin Immunol 2006;6:214–9.
52. Paterson WG. Role of mast cell-derived mediators in acid-induced shortening of the esophagus. Am J Physiol 1998;274:G385–8.
53. Yoshida N, Kuroda M, Suzuki T, et al. Role of nociceptors/neuropeptides in the pathogenesis of visceral hypersensitivity of nonerosive reflux disease. Dig Dis Sci 2013;58:2237–43.
54. Kandulski A, Wex T, Monkemuller K, et al. Proteinase-activated receptor-2 in the pathogenesis of gastroesophageal reflux disease. Am J Gastroenterol 2010; 105:1934–43.
55. Souza RF. Bringing GERD management up to PAR-2. Am J Gastroenterol 2010; 105:1944–6.
56. Yoshida N, Katada K, Handa O, et al. Interleukin-8 production via protease-activated receptor 2 in human esophageal epithelial cells. Int J Mol Med 2007;19:335–40.
57. Shan J, Oshima T, Chen X, et al. Trypsin impaired epithelial barrier function and induced IL-8 secretion through basolateral PAR-2: a lesson from a stratified squamous epithelial model. Am J Physiol Gastrointest Liver Physiol 2012;303:G1105–12.
58. Molina-Infante J, Ferrando-Lamana L, Ripoll C, et al. Esophageal eosinophilic infiltration responds to proton pump inhibition in most adults. Clin Gastroenterol Hepatol 2011;9:110–7.
59. Dohil R, Newbury RO, Aceves S. Transient PPI responsive esophageal eosinophilia may be a clinical sub-phenotype of pediatric eosinophilic esophagitis. Dig Dis Sci 2012;57(5):1413–9.

60. Dranove JE, Horn DS, Davis MA, et al. Predictors of response to proton pump inhibitor therapy among children with significant esophageal eosinophilia. J Pediatr 2009;154:96–100.
61. Levine J, Lai J, Edelman M, et al. Conservative long-term treatment of children with eosinophilic esophagitis. Ann Allergy Asthma Immunol 2012;108:363–6.
62. Moawad FJ, Veerappan GR, Dias JA, et al. Randomized controlled trial comparing aerosolized swallowed fluticasone to esomeprazole for esophageal eosinophilia. Am J Gastroenterol 2013;108:366–72.
63. Sayej WN, Patel R, Baker RD, et al. Treatment with high-dose proton pump inhibitors helps distinguish eosinophilic esophagitis from noneosinophilic esophagitis. J Pediatr Gastroenterol Nutr 2009;49:393–9.
64. Schroeder S, Capocelli KE, Masterson JC, et al. Effect of proton pump inhibitor on esophageal eosinophilia. J Pediatr Gastroenterol Nutr 2013;56:166–72.
65. Dellon ES, Speck O, Woodward K, et al. Clinical and endoscopic characteristics do not reliably differentiate PPI-responsive esophageal eosinophilia and eosinophilic esophagitis in patients undergoing upper endoscopy: a prospective cohort study. Am J Gastroenterol 2013;108:1854–60.
66. Sachs G, Shin JM, Howden CW. Review article: the clinical pharmacology of proton pump inhibitors. Aliment Pharmacol Ther 2006;23(Suppl 2):2–8.
67. Richter JE, Bradley LA, DeMeester TR, et al. Normal 24-hr ambulatory esophageal pH values. Influence of study center, pH electrode, age, and gender. Dig Dis Sci 1992;37:849–56.
68. Vandenplas Y, Goyvaerts H, Helven R, et al. Gastroesophageal reflux, as measured by 24-hour pH monitoring, in 509 healthy infants screened for risk of sudden infant death syndrome. Pediatrics 1991;88:834–40.
69. Straumann A, Bauer M, Fischer B, et al. Idiopathic eosinophilic esophagitis is associated with a T(H)2-type allergic inflammatory response. J Allergy Clin Immunol 2001;108:954–61.
70. Straumann A, Kristl J, Conus S, et al. Cytokine expression in healthy and inflamed mucosa: probing the role of eosinophils in the digestive tract. Inflamm Bowel Dis 2005;11:720–6.
71. Blanchard C, Wang N, Stringer KF, et al. Eotaxin-3 and a uniquely conserved gene-expression profile in eosinophilic esophagitis. J Clin Invest 2006;116:536–47.
72. Cheng E, Zhang X, Huo X, et al. Omeprazole blocks eotaxin-3 expression by oesophageal squamous cells from patients with eosinophilic oesophagitis and GORD. Gut 2013;62:824–32.
73. Zhang X, Cheng E, Huo X, et al. Omeprazole blocks STAT6 binding to the eotaxin-3 promoter in eosinophilic esophagitis cells. PLoS One 2012;7:e50037.
74. Li XQ, Andersson TB, Ahlstrom M, et al. Comparison of inhibitory effects of the proton pump-inhibiting drugs omeprazole, esomeprazole, lansoprazole, pantoprazole, and rabeprazole on human cytochrome P450 activities. Drug Metab Dispos 2004;32:821–7.
75. Cederberg C, Thomson AB, Mahachai V, et al. Effect of intravenous and oral omeprazole on 24-hour intragastric acidity in duodenal ulcer patients. Gastroenterology 1992;103:913–8.
76. Tobey NA, Koves G, Orlando RC. Human esophageal epithelial cells possess an Na+/H+ exchanger for H+ extrusion. Am J Gastroenterol 1998;93:2075–81.
77. Kurashima K, Numata M, Yachie A, et al. The role of vacuolar H(+)-ATPase in the control of intragranular pH and exocytosis in eosinophils. Lab Invest 1996;75:689–98.

78. Lafourcade C, Sobo K, Kieffer-Jaquinod S, et al. Regulation of the V-ATPase along the endocytic pathway occurs through reversible subunit association and membrane localization. PLoS One 2008;3:e2758.
79. Bankers-Fulbright JL, Kephart GM, Bartemes KR, et al. Platelet-activating factor stimulates cytoplasmic alkalinization and granule acidification in human eosinophils. J Cell Sci 2004;117:5749–57.
80. Dubos RJ. The micro-environment of inflammation or Metchnikoff revisited. Lancet 1955;269:1–5.
81. Hunt JF, Fang K, Malik R, et al. Endogenous airway acidification. Implications for asthma pathophysiology. Am J Respir Crit Care Med 2000;161:694–9.
82. Ward TT, Steigbigel RT. Acidosis of synovial fluid correlates with synovial fluid leukocytosis. Am J Med 1978;64:933–6.
83. Kedika RR, Souza RF, Spechler SJ. Potential anti-inflammatory effects of proton pump inhibitors: a review and discussion of the clinical implications. Dig Dis Sci 2009;54:2312–7.
84. Takagi T, Naito Y, Yoshikawa T. The expression of heme oxygenase-1 induced by lansoprazole. J Clin Biochem Nutr 2009;45:9–13.
85. Lapenna D, de Gioia S, Ciofani G, et al. Antioxidant properties of omeprazole. FEBS Lett 1996;382:189–92.
86. Blandizzi C, Fornai M, Colucci R, et al. Lansoprazole prevents experimental gastric injury induced by non-steroidal anti-inflammatory drugs through a reduction of mucosal oxidative damage. World J Gastroenterol 2005;11:4052–60.
87. Simon WA, Sturm E, Hartmann HJ, et al. Hydroxyl radical scavenging reactivity of proton pump inhibitors. Biochem Pharmacol 2006;71:1337–41.
88. Biswas K, Bandyopadhyay U, Chattopadhyay I, et al. A novel antioxidant and antiapoptotic role of omeprazole to block gastric ulcer through scavenging of hydroxyl radical. J Biol Chem 2003;278:10993–1001.
89. Wandall JH. Effects of omeprazole on neutrophil chemotaxis, super oxide production, degranulation, and translocation of cytochrome b-245. Gut 1992;33:617–21.
90. Agastya G, West BC, Callahan JM. Omeprazole inhibits phagocytosis and acidification of phagolysosomes of normal human neutrophils in vitro. Immunopharmacol Immunotoxicol 2000;22:357–72.
91. Ohara T, Arakawa T. Lansoprazole decreases peripheral blood monocytes and intercellular adhesion molecule-1-positive mononuclear cells. Dig Dis Sci 1999;44:1710–5.
92. Sasaki T, Yamaya M, Yasuda H, et al. The proton pump inhibitor lansoprazole inhibits rhinovirus infection in cultured human tracheal epithelial cells. Eur J Pharmacol 2005;509:201–10.
93. Yoshida N, Yoshikawa T, Tanaka Y, et al. A new mechanism for anti-inflammatory actions of proton pump inhibitors–inhibitory effects on neutrophil-endothelial cell interactions. Aliment Pharmacol Ther 2000;14(Suppl 1):74–81.
94. Cortes JR, Rivas MD, Molina-Infante J, et al. Omeprazole inhibits IL-4 and IL-13 signaling signal transducer and activator of transcription 6 activation and reduces lung inflammation in murine asthma. J Allergy Clin Immunol 2009;124:607–10, 610.e1.
95. Merwat SN, Spechler SJ. Might the use of acid-suppressive medications predispose to the development of eosinophilic esophagitis? Am J Gastroenterol 2009;104:1897–902.
96. Lebwohl B, Spechler SJ, Wang TC, et al. Use of proton pump inhibitors and subsequent risk of celiac disease. Dig Liver Dis 2013;46(1):36–40.

97. Roberts NB. Review article: human pepsins–their multiplicity, function and role in reflux disease. Aliment Pharmacol Ther 2006;24(Suppl 2):2–9.

98. Mullin JM, Valenzano MC, Whitby M, et al. Esomeprazole induces upper gastrointestinal tract transmucosal permeability increase. Aliment Pharmacol Ther 2008;28:1317–25.

99. Hopkins AM, McDonnell C, Breslin NP, et al. Omeprazole increases permeability across isolated rat gastric mucosa pre-treated with an acid secretagogue. J Pharm Pharmacol 2002;54:341–7.

100. Theisen J, Nehra D, Citron D, et al. Suppression of gastric acid secretion in patients with gastroesophageal reflux disease results in gastric bacterial overgrowth and deconjugation of bile acids. J Gastrointest Surg 2000;4:50–4.

101. Williams C, McColl KE. Review article: proton pump inhibitors and bacterial overgrowth. Aliment Pharmacol Ther 2006;23:3–10.

102. Untersmayr E, Scholl I, Swoboda I, et al. Antacid medication inhibits digestion of dietary proteins and causes food allergy: a fish allergy model in BALB/c mice. J Allergy Clin Immunol 2003;112:616–23.

103. Scholl I, Untersmayr E, Bakos N, et al. Antiulcer drugs promote oral sensitization and hypersensitivity to hazelnut allergens in BALB/c mice and humans. Am J Clin Nutr 2005;81:154–60.

104. Untersmayr E, Bakos N, Scholl I, et al. Anti-ulcer drugs promote IgE formation toward dietary antigens in adult patients. FASEB J 2005;19:656–8.

Histopathologic Features of Eosinophilic Esophagitis and Eosinophilic Gastrointestinal Diseases

Margaret H. Collins, MD

KEYWORDS

- Eosinophilic esophagitis • Pathology • Pediatric • Gastroesophageal reflux disease
- Proton pump inhibitor • Eosinophilic gastrointestinal disease

KEY POINTS

- Esophageal biopsies from patients who have eosinophilic esophagitis differ significantly from normal esophageal biopsies, and by definition exhibit eosinophil-rich inflammation, often with additional pathologic changes in the epithelium and lamina propria.
- Biopsy pathology is a specific but not sensitive marker for allergic disease affecting the esophagus.
- Eosinophilic esophagitis biopsy pathology correlates with genetic abnormalities.
- A schema is provided to evaluate mucosal biopsies from the remainder of the gastrointestinal tract, and it may provide the basis for eosinophilic gastrointestinal disease diagnosis and entry criteria for research studies.

INTRODUCTION

Eosinophilic esophagitis (EoE) is a chronic immune antigen-mediated disease (**Box 1**).[1–3] Patients who have EoE respond to antigen elimination, especially elimination of food antigens, consistent with disease associated with a T helper cell type 2 (Th2) reaction to swallowed antigen. The definition of EoE does not differ with patient age or gender, esophageal biopsy pathology does not vary with patient age or gender, and response to antigen elimination occurs in both children and adults of both genders. However, symptoms of EoE differ according to patient age: vomiting and failure to thrive are common among young children, and dysphagia is more typically the predominant symptom among affected adolescents and adults.

Disclosures: The author is a consultant for Meritage Pharma, Receptos Inc, and Aptalis Pharma; a TIGER Executive Committee member; and APFED Medical Advisory Panel president.
Division of Pathology and Laboratory Medicine, Cincinnati Children's Hospital Medical Center, ML1035, 3333 Burnet Avenue, Cincinnati, OH 45229, USA
E-mail address: margaret.collins@cchmc.org

Box 1
Criteria for biopsy evaluation for eosinophilic gastrointestinal disease. At least one feature should be present for diagnosis in at least one biopsy from each site

Eosinophilic esophagitis

- Greater than or equal to 15 intraepithelial eosinophils per HPF in at least one esophageal site[1–3]; additional sections should be obtained from nondiagnostic but highly suggestive biopsies, and fewer eosinophils than the recommended threshold value may not eliminate the diagnosis in patients who otherwise would qualify for the diagnosis

- Altered eosinophil character manifest as surface layering and abscesses

- Epithelial changes such as basal layer hyperplasia, dilated intercellular spaces

- Thickened lamina propria fibers

Eosinophilic gastritis

- Greater than or equal to 30 eosinophils per HPF in 5 HPF[43]

- Altered eosinophil behavior manifest as lamina propria sheets, eosinophilic glandulitis, eosinophilic gland abscesses

- Epithelial changes such as reduced mucin, increased nuclear/cytoplasmic ratio, increased epithelial mitotic activity

- Altered eosinophil distribution such as one or more per HPF in surface epithelium, or more than one per HPF in gland epithelium[4]; excess eosinophils in muscularis mucosa or submucosa; concentration of eosinophils in the subepithelial superficial lamina propria instead of deep lamina propria

Eosinophilic enteritis (eosinophilic duodenitis, jejunitis, or ileitis)

- More than twice the normal number of eosinophils in the lamina propria per HPF:
  - More than 52 eosinophils per HPF in duodenum
  - More than 56 per HPF in ileum

- Altered eosinophil behavior manifest as lamina propria sheets, eosinophilic cryptitis, eosinophilic crypt abscesses

- Epithelial changes such as reduced mucin, increased nuclear/cytoplasmic ratio, increased epithelial mitotic activity

- Altered eosinophil distribution such as:
  - More than 2 per HPF and more than 4 per HPF in surface epithelium in duodenum and ileum respectively
  - More than 6 per HPF and more than 4 per HPF in crypt epithelium in duodenum and ileum respectively[4]
  - Excess eosinophils in muscularis mucosa or submucosa
  - Concentration of eosinophils in the subepithelial superficial lamina propria instead of deep lamina propria

- Acute inflammatory cells are not present

Eosinophilic colitis

- More than twice the normal number of eosinophils in the lamina propria per HPF:
  - More than 100 per HPF in right colon
  - More than 84 per HPF in transverse and descending colon
  - More than 64 per HPF in rectosigmoid colon

- Altered eosinophil behavior manifest as lamina propria sheets, eosinophilic cryptitis, eosinophilic crypt abscesses

- Epithelial changes such as reduced mucin, increased nuclear/cytoplasmic ratio, increased epithelial mitotic activity
- Altered eosinophil distribution such as:
  - More than 3 per HPF, more than 4 per HPF, more than 2 per HPF in surface epithelium in right, transverse/descending, rectosigmoid colon respectively
  - More than 11 per HPF, more than 4 per HPF, more than 9 per HPF in crypt epithelium in right, transverse/descending, rectosigmoid colon respectively[4]
  - Excess eosinophils in muscularis mucosa or submucosa
  - Concentration of eosinophils in the subepithelial superficial lamina propria instead of deep lamina propria
- Acute inflammatory cells are not present

EoE is the only form of eosinophilic gastrointestinal (GI) disease (EGID) for which there are consensus criteria for diagnosis. Eosinophils normally reside in the mucosa of all parts of the GI tract except the esophagus.[4] Therefore eosinophil-related disorders are easier to recognize in the esophagus compared with the remainder of the GI tract.

HISTORY OF EoE PATHOLOGY

In 1982, eosinophils in esophageal biopsies were correlated with abnormal pH monitoring results.[5] Most of the patients had respiratory problems, but some had signs and symptoms consistent with esophageal disease. Eosinophils in proximal as well as distal esophageal biopsies were found in these patients whose clinical diagnosis was reflux esophagitis. In that report, the number of eosinophils cited in the text and illustrated in photographs was significantly fewer than 15 per high-power field (HPF): intraepithelial eosinophils were found in esophageal biopsies from 18 of 46 patients, fewer than 1 eosinophil per HPF was found in biopsies from 12 of 18 patients, and more than 1 per HPF was found in biopsies from 6 of 18 patients. Additional pathologic features were noted, including marked basal layer hyperplasia in some cases. These findings are consistent with reflux esophagitis or gastroesophageal reflux disease (GERD). Subsequent studies confirmed that intraepithelial eosinophil counts much higher than those indicated in this report occur in esophageal biopsies from some patients who have GERD.[1–3]

Esophageal biopsies containing eosinophil-rich inflammation were subsequently recognized with increasing frequency. However, marked eosinophilic inflammation in those biopsies was also attributed to reflux esophagitis or GERD, contributing to the delay in recognizing antigen-related esophageal disease. Several laboratories retrieved archived slides, going back to the 1970s, and identified the pathologic changes of EoE in esophageal biopsies.[6–9] Studies that included analyses of the number of biopsies containing numerous intraepithelial eosinophils compared with the total number of esophageal biopsies obtained in the time period studied documented that the prevalence, but not incidence, of biopsies potentially showing EoE increased over time.[7–9] Because EoE is a disease requiring correlation of pathology results with clinical findings, and older medical records are often not as complete as current records, retrospective studies cannot determine with certainty when EoE emerged; reports in the early and mid-1990s of esophageal disease that did not respond to anti-GERD therapy and that was significantly improved clinically and histologically by removing antigens from the diet began the series of studies that further defined EoE.[10,11]

In a unique follow-up survey at an average of 15 years after esophageal biopsies were obtained, individuals who had eosinophils in their biopsies were significantly more likely to report dysphagia compared with age-matched controls, and the probability of reporting dysphagia at follow-up increased with increasing peak eosinophil count.[12] Further, individuals whose biopsies had shown greater than or equal to 15 eosinophils per HPF were more likely to report physician-diagnosed food allergy, history of food impaction, and need for current care from a gastroenterologist compared with individuals whose biopsies had fewer than 15 eosinophils per HPF. Individuals whose prior biopsies had only 5 eosinophils per HPF were more likely than controls to report a history of food impaction, suggesting (similar to an early report of esophageal eosinophilic inflammation[5]) that fewer intraepithelial eosinophils than the current threshold value for EoE diagnosis may be clinically significant, and in addition that this may portend prolonged esophageal dysfunction. The incidence of pathologic alterations in epithelium and lamina propria increased with increasing intraepithelial eosinophil density.[12]

ESOPHAGEAL MUCOSA BIOPSY HISTOLOGY

The histology (ie, the normal appearance) of esophageal mucosa comprises several layers and components:

- Epithelium: the esophageal lumen is lined by nonkeratinized stratified squamous epithelium consisting of a superficial layer near the lumen; a spinous layer below the superficial layer; and the basal zone in the deepest part of the epithelium, overlying the lamina propria. In normal epithelium, the basal zone is not more than 3 cell layers thick, and does not occupy more than 15% of the total epithelial thickness. Intercellular spaces in the basal zone or spinous layer are not visible (**Fig. 1**).
- Intraepithelial inflammatory cells: lymphocytes are normal components of esophageal epithelium, and most of the intraepithelial lymphocytes are T cells.[13] Acute

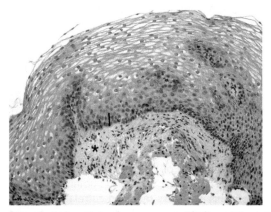

Fig. 1. Normal esophageal nonkeratinized squamous epithelium. Intraepithelial eosinophils are not seen. The basal zone (*bar*) occupies less than 15% of the total epithelial thickness. The lamina propria (*asterisk*) is composed of delicate collagen fibers. The underlying muscularis mucosa does not appear to be altered (hematoxylin-eosin, original magnification ×200).

inflammatory cells and eosinophils are not normally found in esophageal epithelium.

- Lamina propria: this layer of connective tissue is found below the squamous epithelium and superficial to the muscularis mucosa (see **Fig. 1**). Lamina propria is not seen in most endoscopically obtained biopsies and muscularis mucosa is even less commonly seen than lamina propria. Therefore less is known about the normal inflammatory component of these layers.[14]

EoE pathology involves all layers and components represented in biopsies:

- Epithelium: the epithelium in EoE biopsies may be acanthotic, meaning that the total epithelial thickness is increased. The thickening is caused by expansion of the basal zone, which can occupy virtually the entire epithelial thickness (**Fig. 2**A). In addition to acanthosis and basal zone hyperplasia, intercellular spaces are often dilated and intercellular bridges are seen (see **Fig. 2**B).
- Intraepithelial inflammatory cells: numerous intraepithelial eosinophils in esophageal biopsies are consistent with a Th2-mediated response to swallowed antigen (see **Fig. 2**; **Figs. 3–6**). The recommended threshold of eosinophilic inflammation for EoE diagnosis is a peak count of greater than or equal to 15 eosinophils per HPF. In addition to a numerical increase, eosinophils may show altered distribution in the form of surface exudate (see **Fig. 2**B), abscesses in exudate (see **Fig. 2**B) or in intact epithelium (see **Fig. 3**), surface layering (see **Fig. 4**), and prominence in the lamina propria (see **Fig. 6**). Extracellular eosinophil granules are common but may occur as a result of mechanical cellular disruption.[4,15] Lymphocytes, mainly T cells but also B cells, and mast cells are also increased in EoE biopsies but special stains are required to identify them.[13]
- Lamina propria: in contrast with normal lamina propria, lamina propria fibers in EoE are thick and dense (see **Figs. 2**A and **6**).[16,17] The lamina propria in EoE

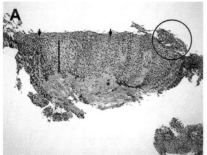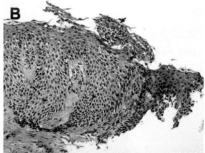

Fig. 2. (*A*) In contrast, in this biopsy from a patient who has EoE, numerous intraepithelial eosinophils are seen (*arrows*), primarily near the surface. The circle indicates a surface lesion that is densely inflamed with eosinophils. The basal zone occupies more than half of the total epithelial thickness (*bar*) and the total epithelial thickness is increased compared with the normal epithelium in **Fig. 1**: lower magnification (100×) was required to include the height of the EoE biopsy compared with the normal biopsy in **Fig. 1** (200×). The lamina propria (*asterisk*) is composed of dense, thick collagen fibers (hematoxylin-eosin, original magnification ×100). (*B*) A closer view of the right half of the image including the area demarcated by the circle in (*A*) shows eosinophils (*arrows*) admixed with detached and semi-detached epithelial cells, corresponding with the white specks (exudate) seen on the mucosa at endoscopy. In addition, intercellular spaces are dilated (*arrowheads*) and intercellular bridges are visible in the spaces (hematoxylin-eosin, original magnification ×200).

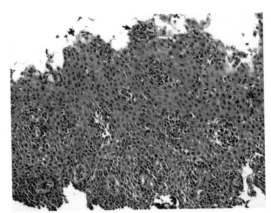

Fig. 3. Proper orientation is difficult to achieve for esophageal biopsies and tangential orientation is common, as seen here. Nevertheless, an aggregate of eosinophils forming an abscess (*arrow*) is easily identified (hematoxylin-eosin, original magnification ×200).

biopsies may also show eosinophilic[17] and chronic inflammation,[18] sometimes with numerous plasma cells (terminally differentiated B cells) (see **Fig. 6**). Esophageal lamina propria in adults may be more resistant to therapy compared with children: diet and topical steroid therapy reverse subepithelial collagen deposition in children[19] but prolonged topical steroid therapy results in reduced subepithelial collagen deposition that remains significantly increased compared with controls.[20]

In some patients, all EoE-related pathology results revert to normal histology with successful therapy.

DIAGNOSTIC PITFALLS

EoE may affect the esophagus in a patchy manner (see **Fig. 5**) and the possibility of biopsies yielding a false-negative diagnosis exists. Increasing the number of biopsies

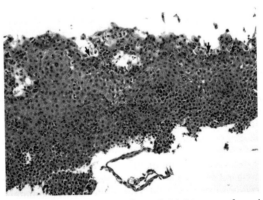

Fig. 4. Eosinophils (*arrows*) align near the surface of this biopsy, referred to as surface layering (hematoxylin-eosin, original magnification ×200).

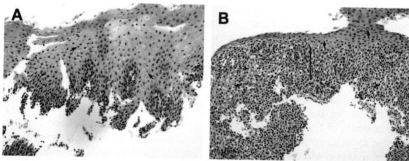

Fig. 5. (A) This biopsy from the distal esophagus shows few intraepithelial eosinophils (*arrows*) and mildly dilated intercellular spaces (*arrowhead*). Basal zone hyperplasia is difficult to evaluate because of orientation but is at most mild and focal (hematoxylin-eosin, original magnification ×200). (B). This biopsy from the midesophagus appears different from the biopsy from the distal esophagus in (A), but was obtained from the same patient whose biopsy is shown in (A), and at the same endoscopy. In this midesophageal biopsy, there are numerous intraepithelial eosinophils (*arrows*), basal zone expansion (*bar*), and dilated intercellular spaces (*arrowhead*). These images show the patchy nature of the infiltrate in some patients, and therefore the necessity to obtain biopsies from multiple sites in the esophagus to increase diagnostic yield. This type of variability may also be found among pieces obtained at the same site, emphasizing the need to obtain multiple biopsies at each site (hematoxylin-eosin, original magnification ×200).

increases the diagnostic yield, and a total of 5 or 6 esophageal biopsies is optimum to diagnose EoE using a threshold diagnostic value of 15 per HPF.[21,22] In practice, a threshold value is meaningful only in a clinical context; there may be patients who appear to have EoE whose biopsies do not have the recommended threshold eosinophil count. In such cases, pathologists should strongly consider examining additional sections because the eosinophil infiltrate may be patchy within and among biopsies obtained at the same site in the esophagus, as well as between biopsies obtained

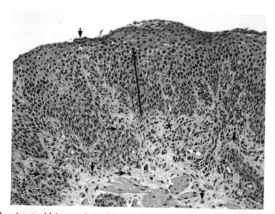

Fig. 6. In this well-oriented biopsy, basal zone expansion is prominent (*bar*), numerous intraepithelial eosinophils are present and there is a small focus of eosinophil surface layering (*arrow*), and intercellular spaces are dilated in many areas (*arrowheads*). The lamina propria shows thick fibers near the epithelium (*asterisk*) and contains numerous eosinophils (*arrows*) and plasma cells (*shaded arrows*) (hematoxylin-eosin, original magnification ×200).

from different sites. Expressing the eosinophil density as number per HPF is problematic because most studies, and pathologists, do not report the size of the HPF used to generate eosinophil counts; this problem can be resolved by expressing eosinophil density as number per unit area, such as square millimeter. Excellent interobserver variability for eosinophil density can be achieved among pathologists who agree on diagnostic criteria and adhere to uniform methods of evaluation.[23] Consensus recommendations for EoE diagnosis include recommendations about eosinophil inflammation but not about the other features of EoE disorders. A systematic method to evaluate aspects of EoE disorders in addition to eosinophil inflammation that could be adopted for diagnostic and research purposes would be advantageous for a variety of reasons, and is being developed.[24]

DIFFERENTIAL DIAGNOSIS

The pathologic alterations described earlier are highly characteristic of EoE, the chronic antigen-driven disease. However, similar alterations are found in esophageal biopsies from patients who have a variety of other diseases, and the characteristic pathology is therefore sensitive but not specific for the diagnosis of antigen-driven EoE. Perhaps the most important diseases that must be ruled out before diagnosing EoE are gastroesophageal reflux disease (GERD) and proton pump inhibitor (PPI)–responsive esophageal eosinophilia (PPIREE).[2,3] The prevalence of biopsies that resemble EoE among patients who have GERD will probably never be ascertained because most patients who have GERD symptoms do not undergo endoscopy. Nevertheless, biopsies from patients who have signs and symptoms of GERD, who do not respond to PPI therapy, and who have abnormal results of pH monitoring may appear identical to EoE biopsies. A reasonable estimate of the frequency of EoE-type pathology in GERD may be provided by a large study of adults with GERD that identified more than 15 eosinophils per HPF in 1.8% of esophageal biopsies (9 of 512) from patients at baseline.[25] PPIREE is currently an ill-defined entity, characterized by esophageal biopsies that resemble EoE in patients with or without abnormal pH monitoring results, who respond with reduced or resolved symptoms to PPI therapy, and whose esophageal biopsies show few or no eosinophils after PPI therapy.[26] The nature of PPIREE is not clear, but follow-up is required because the PPI response may be transient.[27] Additional diseases that may affect the esophagus and are associated with mucosal biopsy findings that resemble antigen-driven disease include achalasia, hypereosinophilic syndrome, inflammatory bowel disease, celiac disease, and drug reaction. Techniques such as endoscopic mucosal resection that yield significant amounts of deeper layers of the esophageal wall in addition to epithelium may identify eosinophilic inflammation in the deeper layers without significant epithelial eosinophilic inflammation in patients who have severe dysphagia[28]; these patients may be more properly classified as having eosinophilic gastroenteritis.

CLINICAL PHENOTYPES

As stated earlier, the typical clinical signs and symptoms of EoE vary according to patient age, with dysphagia being predominant among adolescents and adults; and vomiting, epigastric pain, and poor oral intake more common among young children. EoE was recently recognized as more frequent than expected among patients who have an inherited connective tissue disorder, characterized primarily by increased joint mobility.[29] In addition, patients who have phosphatase and tensin homolog (PTEN) abnormalities also have increased incidences of GI eosinophilia.[30]

MOLECULAR/GENETIC CORRELATIONS

Esophageal biopsies from patients who have EoE possess a unique transcriptome identified by genome-wide analysis.[31] Eotaxin-3 is the most upregulated gene and appears to be expressed by esophageal squamous epithelial cells following interleukin (IL)-13 stimulation.[32] Eotaxin-3 promotes eosinophil migration from the blood stream into tissue. Periostin is an extracellular matrix molecule that facilitates eosinophil adhesion to fibronectin.[33] Periostin expression is upregulated in eosinophilic esophagitis, and IL-13 stimulation increases periostin expression in primary esophageal fibroblasts. Desmoglein-1 is an intercellular adhesion molecule that is downregulated in EoE.[34] It appears to regulate esophageal epithelial cell adhesion and barrier function. Thymic stromal lymphopoietin (TSLP) is a proinflammatory cytokine and a gain-of-function single nucleotide polymorphism is associated with EoE.[35] TSLP appears to increase basophil responses in patients who have EoE.[36] A recently developed quantitative polymerase chain reaction–based array derived from the EoE transcriptome may be useful at diagnosis and for surveillance, and can be used with fresh tissue or formalin-fixed paraffin-embedded tissue.[37]

OTHER EGID

EGID occur anywhere in the GI tract and may affect multiple sites simultaneously (**Fig. 7**). Eosinophilic gastroenteritis, described before EGID, was identified based primarily on examination of bowel resections. The advent of improved anesthesia and more flexible endoscopes resulted in safer GI endoscopies and more readily obtained mucosa biopsies, and therefore currently many GI diseases are diagnosed based on examination of mucosal biopsies only. EGID diagnosis is challenging for several reasons. Resections are rarely performed for EGID and eosinophil infiltrates in deeper layers cannot be evaluated in mucosal biopsies; therefore negative mucosal biopsies do not rule out a diagnosis of eosinophilic gastroenteritis. Newer techniques for obtaining tissue endoscopically may overcome this limitation.[28] However, the entire small bowel is not examined endoscopically and therefore negative biopsies from duodenum, proximal jejunum, and distal ileum do not rule out EGID affecting the

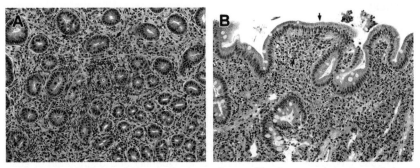

Fig. 7. (*A*) Eosinophilic gastritis typically shows sheets of lamina propria eosinophils (*arrow*), and increased numbers of intraepithelial eosinophils (*arrowheads*). Peak eosinophil count in this biopsy was more than 300 per HPF. Gastric gland epithelium typically shows reactive changes including reduced mucin and increased nuclear/cytoplasmic ratio (hematoxylin-eosin, original magnification ×200). (*B*) Eosinophilic duodenitis typically shows numerous eosinophils in lamina propria and surface epithelium (*arrows*), and the peak eosinophil count in this biopsy was greater than 100 per HPF. Additional alterations may include blunt villi as in this biopsy. The gastric and duodenal biopsies in this figure are from the same patient, who also had EoE.

unexamined, unsampled small bowel. Signs and symptoms of lower GI dysfunction are protean with multiple possible causes, and correlating clinical disease with specific portions of the lower GI tract is less easily accomplished than for patients who have dysphagia and a food impaction, which are definitive signs of esophageal dysfunction.

Features commonly found in EGID biopsies[38,39] include:

- Increased eosinophils. A numerical increase in eosinophils in mucosal biopsies is inherent in the diagnosis of EGID, but few studies report eosinophil density in normal mucosal biopsies.[4,40–44] An extreme numerical increase (>100 per HPF) by itself may merit a diagnosis of EGID.
- Altered eosinophil distribution. In normal GI biopsies, eosinophils appear as discrete cells sprinkled evenly in the deep lamina propria. In EGID biopsies, eosinophils appear as sheets in the lamina propria and eosinophils in abnormal locations may be found. These alterations should be considered meaningful signs of eosinophil-related disease.[38,39,45] Small numbers of intraepithelial eosinophils are normal[4] but markedly increased numbers of intraepithelial eosinophils, and certainly gland or crypt eosinophil abscesses, may indicate eosinophil-related disease even in the absence of excess lamina propria eosinophils.
- Eosinophil-related pathologic alterations, such as reactive epithelial changes (reduced mucin, increased mitotic activity, and so forth).
- Lack of acute inflammation. Acute inflammation in small bowel and colon biopsies that also show prominent eosinophil inflammation should prompt consideration of inflammatory bowel disease. Numerous eosinophils in colon biopsies may portend a poor prognosis in ulcerative colitis.[46]

SUMMARY

In the past decade, numerous advances in EoE include recognizing PPIREE and identifying a unique EoE transcriptome that has led to increased understanding of EoE pathogenesis and has provided the basis for potential therapeutic interventions. It is hoped that EoE will be the model for work on other forms of EGID.

REFERENCES

1. Furuta GT, Liacouras CA, Collins MH, et al. Eosinophilic esophagitis in children and adults: a systematic review and consensus recommendations for diagnosis and treatment. Gastroenterology 2007;133:1342–63.
2. Liacouras CA, Furuta GT, Hirano I, et al. Eosinophilic esophagitis: updated consensus recommendations for children and adults. J Allergy Clin Immunol 2011;128:3–20.
3. Dellon ES, Gonsalves N, Hirano I, et al. ACG clinical guideline: evidence based approach to the diagnosis and management of esophageal eosinophilia and eosinophilic esophagitis (EoE). Am J Gastroenterol 2013;108:679–92.
4. DeBrosse CW, Case JW, Putnam PE, et al. Quantity and distribution of eosinophils in the gastrointestinal tract of children. Pediatr Dev Pathol 2006;9:210–8.
5. Winter HS, Madara JL, Stafford RJ, et al. Intraepithelial eosinophils: a new diagnostic criterion for reflux esophagitis. Gastroenterology 1982;83:816–23.
6. Cherian S, Smith NM, Forbes DA. Rapidly increasing prevalence of eosinophilic oesophagitis in Western Australia. Arch Dis Child 2006;91:1000–4.
7. Vanderheyden AD, Petras RE, DeYoung BR, et al. Emerging eosinophilic (allergic) esophagitis: increased incidence or increased recognition? Arch Pathol Lab Med 2007;131:777–9.

8. Whitney-Miller CL, Katzka D, Furth EE. Eosinophilic esophagitis: a retrospective review of esophageal biopsy specimens from 1992 to 2004 at an adult academic medical center. Am J Clin Pathol 2009;131:788–92.

9. DeBrosse CW, Collins MH, Buckmeier Butz BK, et al. Identification, epidemiology, and chronicity of pediatric esophageal eosinophilia, 1982-1999. J Allergy Clin Immunol 2010;126:112–9.

10. Attwood SE, Smyrk TC, Demeester TR, et al. Esophageal eosinophilia with dysphagia: a distinct clinicopathologic syndrome. Dig Dis Sci 1993;38:109–16.

11. Kelly KJ, Lazenby AJ, Rowe PC, et al. Eosinophilic esophagitis attributed to gastroesophageal reflux: improvement with an amino-acid based formula. Gastroenterology 1995;109:1503–12.

12. DeBrosse CW, Franciosi JP, King EC, et al. Long-term outcomes in pediatric-onset esophageal eosinophilia. J Allergy Clin Immunol 2011;128:132–8.

13. Straumann A, Aceves SS, Blanchard C, et al. Pediatric and adult eosinophilic esophagitis: similarities and differences. Allergy 2012;67:477–90.

14. Appelman HD, Streutker C, Vieth M, et al. The esophageal mucosa and submucosa: immunohistology in GERD and Barrett's esophagus. Ann N Y Acad Sci 2013;1300:144–65.

15. Kato M, Kephart GM, Talley NJ, et al. Eosinophil infiltration and degranulation in normal human tissue. Anat Rec 1998;252:418–25.

16. Straumann A, Spichtin HP, Grize L, et al. Natural history of primary eosinophilic esophagitis: a follow-up of 30 adult patients for up to 11.5 years. Gastroenterology 2003;125:1660–9.

17. Aceves SS, Newbury RO, Dohil R, et al. Esophageal remodeling in pediatric eosinophilic esophagitis. J Allergy Clin Immunol 2007;119:206–12.

18. Vicario M, Blanchard C, Stringer KF, et al. Local B cells and IgE production in the oesophageal mucosa in eosinophilic oesophagitis. Gut 2010;59:12–20.

19. Lieberman JA, Morotti JA, Konstantinou GN, et al. Dietary therapy can reverse esophageal subepithelial fibrosis in patients with eosinophilic esophagitis: a historical cohort. Allergy 2012;67:1299–307.

20. Lucendo AJ, Arias A, De Rezende LC, et al. Subepithelial collagen deposition, profibrogenic cytokine gene expression, and changes after prolonged fluticasone propionate treatment in adult eosinophilic esophagitis: a prospective study. J Allergy Clin Immunol 2011;128:1037–46.

21. Gonsalves N, Policaropio-Nicolas M, Zhang Q, et al. Histopathologic variability and endoscopic correlates in adults with eosinophilic esophagitis. Gastrointest Endosc 2006;64:313–9.

22. Shah A, Kagalwalla AF, Gonsalves N, et al. Histopathologic variability in children with eosinophilic esophagitis. Am J Gastroenterol 2009;104:716–21.

23. Dellon ES, Fritchie KJ, Rubinas TC, et al. Inter- and intraobserver reliability and validation of a new method for determination of eosinophil counts in patients with esophageal eosinophilia. Dig Dis Sci 2010;55:1940–9.

24. Collins MH, Martin LJ, Alexander ES, et al. Histology scoring system is superior to eosinophil count to identify treated vs untreated eosinophilic esophagitis patients. J Allergy Clin Immunol 2012;129:AB96.

25. Fiocca R, Mastracci L, Engstrom C, et al. Long-term outcome of microscopic esophagitis in chronic GERD patients treated with esomeprazole or laparoscopic antireflux surgery in the LOTUS trial. Am J Gastroenterol 2010;105:1015–23.

26. Vazquez-Elizondo G, Ngamruengphong S, Khrisna M, et al. The outcome of patients with oesophageal eosinophilic infiltration after an eight-week trial of a proton pump inhibitor. Aliment Pharmacol Ther 2013;38:1312–9.

27. Dohil R, Newbury RO, Aceves SA. Transient PPI responsive esophageal eosino-philia may be a clinical sub-phenotype of pediatric eosinophilic esophagitis. Dig Dis Sci 2012;57:1413–9.
28. Benias PC, Matin A, Ascunce GI, et al. Esophageal obstruction as a result of iso-lated eosinophilic gastroenteritis. Gastroenterol Hepatol 2013;9:607–10.
29. Abonia JP, Wen T, Stucke EM, et al. High prevalence of eosinophilic esophagitis in patients with inherited connective tissue disorders. J Allergy Clin Immunol 2013;132:378–86.
30. Henderson CJ, Ngeow J, Collins MH, et al. Increased prevalence of eosinophilic gastrointestinal disorders (EGID) in pediatric PTEN hamartoma tumor syndromes (PHTS). J Pediatr Gastroenterol Nutr, in press.
31. Blanchard C, Wang N, Stringer KF, et al. Eotaxin-3 and a uniquely conserved gene-expression profile in eosinophilic esophagitis. J Clin Invest 2006;116: 536–47.
32. Blanchard C, Mingler MK, Vicario M, et al. IL-13 involvement in eosinophilic esophagitis: transcriptome analysis and reversibility with glucocorticoids. J Allergy Clin Immunol 2007;120:1292–300.
33. Blanchard C, Mingler MK, McBride M, et al. Periostin facilitates eosinophil tissue infiltration in allergic lung and esophageal responses. Mucosal Immunol 2008;1: 289–96.
34. Sherrill JD, Kc K, Wu D, et al. Desmoglein-1 regulates esophageal epithelial bar-rier function and immune responses in eosinophilic esophagitis. Mucosal Immu-nol, in press.
35. Sherrill JD, Gao PS, Stucke EM, et al. Variants of thymic stromal lymphopoietin and its receptor associate with eosinophilic esophagitis. J Allergy Clin Immunol 2010;126:160–5.
36. Noti M, Wojno ED, Kim BS, et al. Thymic stromal lymphopoietin-elicited basophil responses promote eosinophilic esophagitis. Nat Med 2013;19:1005–13.
37. Wen T, Stucke EM, Grotjan T, et al. Molecular diagnosis of eosinophilic esopha-gitis by gene expression profiling. Gastroenterology 2013;145:1289–99.
38. Collins MH. Histopathology associated with eosinophilic gastrointestinal dis-eases. Immunol Allergy Clin North Am 2009;29:109–17.
39. Hurrell JM, Genta RM, Melton SD. Histopathologic diagnosis of eosinophilic con-ditions in the gastrointestinal tract. Adv Anat Pathol 2011;18:335–48.
40. Lowichik A, Weinberg A. A quantitative evaluation of mucosal eosinophils in the pediatric gastrointestinal tract. Mod Pathol 1996;9:110–4.
41. Pascal RR, Gramlich TL, Parker KM, et al. Geographic variations in eosinophil concentration in normal colonic mucosa. Mod Pathol 1997;10:363–5.
42. Talley NJ, Walker MM, Aro P, et al. Non-ulcer dyspepsia and duodenal eosino-philia: an adult endoscopic population-based case-control study. Clin Gastroen-terol Hepatol 2007;5:1175–83.
43. Lwin T, Melton SD, Genta RM. Eosinophilic gastritis: histopathological character-ization and quantification of the normal gastric eosinophil content. Mod Pathol 2011;24:556–63.
44. Saad AG. Normal quantity and distribution of mast cells and eosinophils in the pediatric colon. Pediatr Dev Pathol 2011;14:294–300.
45. Clouse RE, Alpers DH, Hockenbery DM, et al. Pericrypt eosinophilic enterocolitis and chronic diarrhea. Gastroenterology 1992;103:168–76.
46. Ahrens R, Waddell A, Seidu L, et al. Intestinal macrophage/epithelial cell-derived CCL11/eotaxin-1 mediates eosinophil recruitment and function in pediatric ulcer-ative colitis. J Immunol 2008;181:7390–9.

Genetic and Epigenetic Underpinnings of Eosinophilic Esophagitis

Joseph D. Sherrill, PhD, Marc E. Rothenberg, MD, PhD*

KEYWORDS

- Genetic variant • Thymic stromal lymphopoietin • Eotaxin-3 • Epigenetics
- MicroRNA

KEY POINTS

- Eosinophilic esophagitis (EoE) is a complex, polygenic disorder.
- Disease risk variants and an altered esophageal transcriptional profile underlie the genetic origin of EoE.
- Emerging epigenetic modifications link environmental exposures to the genetic dysregulation in EoE.

INTRODUCTION

Early evidence for a genetic origin of eosinophilic esophagitis (EoE) came in the form of several epidemiologic studies showing a high prevalence of disease in specific genders and races, with nearly three-quarters of patients being men and almost all (≈90%) being of European descent, respectively.[1] Moreover, an increased disease risk is seen among familial cases, which typically demonstrate a non-Mendelian inheritance pattern.[2] Expression profiling from esophageal biopsies acquired during routine endoscopic procedures has provided molecular insight into genetic dysregulation occurring within the inflamed esophagus. These transcriptional changes affect both coding and noncoding (microRNA) transcripts and underscore consistent, disease-specific alterations in the levels of select molecules expressed by activated immune cells and structural cells of the esophagus.[3,4] These dysregulated transcripts and associated biologic pathways represent potential targets for novel therapeutics and diagnostic methods.[5]

In addition to the genetic elements, a role for environmental factors in EoE has been established through both clinical and basic research. Patients with EoE are often

Division of Allergy and Immunology, Department of Pediatrics, Cincinnati Children's Hospital Medical Center, University of Cincinnati College of Medicine, 3333 Burnet Avenue, Cincinnati, OH 45229, USA
* Corresponding author. Division of Allergy and Immunology, Cincinnati Children's Hospital Medical Center, 3333 Burnet Avenue, Cincinnati, OH 45229.
E-mail address: marc.rothenberg@cchmc.org

Gastroenterol Clin N Am 43 (2014) 269–280
http://dx.doi.org/10.1016/j.gtc.2014.02.003
0889-8553/14/$ – see front matter © 2014 Elsevier Inc. All rights reserved.

hypersensitized to multiple food antigens, making directed dietary modification one of the most effective therapies for EoE.[6] Several early life exposures, including Cesarean birth, antibiotics, and formula feeding, have been identified to influence the risk of pediatric EoE.[7] In addition, geographic location, industrialized environments, history of *Helicobacter pylori* infection, and seasonal variations in disease implicate environmental antigens.[8–11] These clinical findings have been supported through multiple basic research studies showing that epidermal and pulmonary exposure to various antigens can induce EoE-like symptoms in mice.[12–14] Emerging epigenetic data are now beginning to provide clues as to how these environmental factors may be intricately intertwined with the genetic dysregulation in EoE and thus act in a concerted fashion to affect disease pathophysiology.

GENETIC VARIANTS

Several candidate gene approaches have identified a handful of genetic risk variants in EoE. For instance, a common single-nucleotide variant (minor allele frequency [MAF] = 0.25 in the HapMap[15] population of European descent) located in the 3′ untranslated region of the chemokine (C-C motif) ligand 26 (*CCL26*) was overrepresented in patients with EoE in both a case-control and a family-based analysis.[4] Furthermore, 2 coding variants (R501X and 2282del4) in the epidermal barrier gene filaggrin (*FLG*), which is negatively regulated by interleukin (IL) 13 and is decreased in the esophageal mucosa of patients with EoE, associate with EoE risk.[16] Lastly, in a small cohort of patients with steroid-treated EoE, a genetic variant in the promoter of the transforming growth factor beta 1 (*TGF-β1*) gene, was associated with steroid unresponsiveness and correlated with increased TGF-β1–positive cells in the esophagus.[17] The genetic link between the TGF-β pathway and EoE identified in this study is remarkable given the evidence showing a high rate of EoE, other eosinophilic gastrointestinal disorders, and atopic disease in patients with connective tissue disorders,[18] such as Loeys-Dietz syndrome, which has been associated with variants in the TGF-β receptors 1 and 2 (**Table 1**).[19]

To identify disease risk variants in a more unbiased fashion, a genome-wide association study (GWAS) was performed in which 351 patients with EoE and 3,104 healthy controls were genotyped for more than 550,000 common variants. On chromosome 5q22, a single locus spanning the thymic stromal lymphopoietin (*TSLP*) and WD repeat domain 36 (*WDR36*) genes showed a significant association with EoE susceptibility.[20] TSLP is a potent Th2-promoting cytokine involved in the development of multiple allergic diseases.[21] Expression analyses showed increased *TSLP* in EoE and a genotypic effect of the top associated variant on *TSLP* expression, with patients carrying the risk allele having elevated *TSLP* expression.[20] In addition, *TSLP* risk genotypes correlated with increased levels of basophils, which have a key role in promoting EoE-like disease in mice, and with granulocyte-monocyte progenitor-like cells in the esophagus.[14,22]

A secondary candidate gene approach also identified variants within the *TSLP* locus that were significantly associated with EoE risk.[23] In this study assessing more than 700 variants in epithelial-derived genes linked to atopy, *TSLP* variants were the most significant genetic hits linked to EoE that, importantly, showed a stronger association with disease risk when compared with controls with atopic diseases (atopic dermatitis and asthma).[23] Moreover, a coding variant in the cytokine receptor–like factor 2 (*CRLF2*) gene, which encodes for the receptor for TSLP, showed a sex-specific association with EoE risk in men only.[23] These cumulative data support aberrant regulation affecting the TSLP pathway as a specific genetic origin in EoE. Given the

Table 1
Genetic and epigenetic modifications associated with EoE and related genetic disorders

		Target	Modification	Potential Biologic Effect
Genetic	Disease risk variants	CCL26	SNV in 3′ UTR	Enhanced mRNA stability; increased expression
		TGFB1	SNV in promoter	Increased expression; nonresponsiveness to topical steroid therapy
		FLG	Nonsense and missense SNVs	Loss of function; reduced barrier function
		TSLP	SNVs in promoter region and introns	Increased expression; correlates with esophageal levels of basophil and GMP-like cells
		CRLF2	Missense SNV	Male-specific association; enhanced TSLP signaling
		DSG1	Missense SNVs in patients with SAM syndrome[a]	Loss of function; reduced epithelial integrity; increased IL-5 and TSLP
		TGFBR1/TGFBR2	Missense SNVs in patients with LDS[b]	Increased TGF-β signaling; elevated CD4+ Th2 cells
		PTEN	Missense SNVs, insertions, and deletions in patients with PHTS[c]	Loss of function; hyperproliferation
	Transcriptome	CCL26	Increased expression (esophagus)	Promotes eosinophil trafficking into the esophagus
		POSTN	Increased expression (esophagus)	Increased eosinophil adhesion; promotes esophageal remodeling; increased TSLP expression
		DSG1	Decreased expression (esophagus)	Reduced barrier function; increased POSTN expression
Epigenetic	Histones	H3	Acetylated	Enhanced CCL26 promoter activity
		H3	Methylated (lysine 4)	Enhanced CCL26 promoter activity
	DNA	CCL26	Hypomethylation in promoter region	Enhanced CCL26 promoter activity
	MicroRNAs	miR-21	Increased expression (esophagus)	Skewed Th2 response; increased eosinophil survival
		miR-223	Increased expression (esophagus, blood)	Increased eosinophil progenitors
		miR-375	Decreased expression (esophagus)	Enhanced IL-13 transcriptional responses

Abbreviations: GMP, granulocyte-monocyte progenitor; LDS, Loeys-Dietz syndrome; PHTS, *PTEN* hamartoma tumor syndromes; SAM, severe atopic dermatitis, multiple allergies, and metabolic wasting; SNV, single-nucleotide variant; TSLP, thymic stromal lymphopoietin; UTR, untranslated region.

[a] EoE was a comorbidity in 1 of 3 patients with SAM syndrome.

[b] High prevalence of EoE and other eosinophilic gastrointestinal disorders (n = 6) in 58 patients with LDS.

[c] Significant enrichment of eosinophilic gastrointestinal disorders in patients with *PTEN* hamartoma tumor syndromes (odds ratio, 272; CI, 89–831; *P*<10⁻⁴).

Data from Refs. 3,4,14,16,17,19,20,22,23,27,37,40,45,46,50,51,54,56–59,62

established role of *TSLP* in the initiation of allergic diseases, the fact that *WDR36* was not differentially expressed in EoE underscores *TSLP* as the most likely gene involved in driving the esophageal inflammatory responses in EoE. Importantly, however, variants in *WDR36* have been linked with peripheral blood eosinophil levels and atopic asthma.[24] Thus, further studies are needed to identify the precise causal variants of EoE and to fully investigate a potential nonesophageal role for *WDR36* that may contribute to disease.

THE EoE TRANSCRIPTOME

A total of 574 highly dysregulated esophageal genes were identified, termed the *EoE transcriptome*, which distinguishes patients with EoE from healthy controls and, importantly, from patients with noneosinophilic forms of esophagitis.[4] Despite the patchiness of EoE and phenotypic diversity within the patients analyzed with EoE, the EoE transcriptome is surprisingly well conserved across patient age, gender, atopic status, and nonfamilial relationship.[4,25] A large-scale screen based on 94 signature EoE transcriptome genes has shown promise as a diagnostic tool capable of discriminating patients with EoE from those with noneosinophilic forms of esophagitis and patients with active EoE from those with EoE in remission (inactive EoE).[26] The cytokine IL-13 is capable of inducing an esophageal epithelial cell gene signature that represents 22% of the EoE transcriptome.[27] This article discusses 3 key genes within the EoE transcriptome, their regulation by IL-13, and their influence on disease pathophysiology.

Chemokine (C-C Motif) Ligand 26

Expression of *CCL26*, which encodes the eosinophil chemoattractant eotaxin-3, was upregulated 53-fold in EoE, making it the most highly induced gene of the EoE transcriptome. *CCL26* is believed to be the main driver for eosinophil recruitment into the esophagus, because the upregulation of *CCL26* was unique among other closely related chemokines from the eotaxin family (*CCL11* and *CCL24*)[4]; however, other studies have indicated that *CCL11* and *CCL24* are induced at low levels in EoE.[28,29] The levels of *CCL26* in patients with EoE correlated significantly with the esophageal levels of eosinophils and mast cells.[4] The induction of *CCL26* in patients with EoE was determined to be largely because of the influence of IL-13 on esophageal epithelial cells, as *CCL26* was also the most highly induced gene in IL-13–treated cells (279-fold when compared with untreated cells).[4,27] Molecular analyses defined 2 STAT6 binding sites in the *CCL26* promoter that were necessary for the induction of *CCL26* by IL-13 and by IL-4.[30,31] Furthermore, several coactivators, including poly-ADP ribosyl polymerase 14 (PARP14), have been shown to act on the *CCL26* locus. PARP14 was identified as a specific coregulator of STAT6 signaling, and its overexpression in esophageal epithelial cells enhanced IL-13–induced *CCL26* expression in a STAT6-dependent manner.[32,33] Finally, exposure of esophageal epithelial cells to acidic pH enhances eotaxin-3 release, providing a potential mechanism by which proton pump inhibitor (PPI) therapies could have some anti-inflammatory effects in EoE.[16] A role for the eotaxins and their receptor CCR3 is supported by studies in mice that have shown attenuated eosinophil levels and/or tissue remodeling in eotaxin and/or CCR3-deficient mice.[4,34,35]

Periostin

Periostin (*POSTN*) is a matricellular protein capable of interacting with multiple extracellular matrix molecules and cell surface receptors such as type 1 collagen and

Notch1, respectively.[36] Periostin is directly involved in regulating multiple cellular processes, including cell migration and adhesion.[36] Its influence on metastasis, tissue remodeling, and wound healing has made it a highly studied molecule in the context of various human diseases, such as cancer, asthma, and atopic dermatitis.[37–39] A 47-fold induction of periostin mRNA was observed in EoE, making it the second most highly upregulated gene in the EoE transcriptome.[4] The periostin protein was also increased in EoE, primarily localized within the lamina propria, indicating fibroblasts as the main cellular source of periostin induction.[40] TGF-β and IL-13 induced greater levels of periostin expression in esophageal fibroblasts than in esophageal epithelial cells.[40] Using periostin-deficient mice, Blanchard and colleagues[40] showed that periostin promotes allergic inflammatory responses in the lung and esophagus, partly through enhancing eosinophil adhesion. In skin keratinocytes, periostin can induce the expression of TSLP.[37] These collective findings suggest a molecular loop among TGF-β, periostin, and TSLP, which act synergistically to drive the esophageal pathophysiology associated with EoE. Circulating periostin levels help identify patients with asthma who will experience response to biologic therapeutics, such as anti-IgE and anti–IL-13, and seem to identify eosinophilic asthmatic phenotypes, extending the significance of the eosinophil/periostin connection from EoE to other common atopic disorders.[38,41,42]

Desmoglein 1

Desmoglein 1 (DSG1) is a transmembrane molecule belonging to the family of desmosomal cadherins that has an essential role in maintaining epithelial integrity through calcium-dependent intercellular adhesion. The focus on DSG1 as an etiologic component in human disease stemmed from observations linking DSG1 alteration to various dermatologic disorders, in which epithelial integrity and barrier function are compromised.[43,44] In EoE, *DSG1* mRNA is specifically downregulated in the esophageal mucosa of patients with active disease.[27,45] This specific decrease in *DSG1* was shown to result from IL-13 stimulation of differentiated esophageal epithelial cells.[45] Functionally, *DSG1*-deficient esophageal epithelial cells exhibited greater cell dissociation, weaker adhesive properties, and reduced capacity to form an intact epithelial barrier.[45] Moreover, the loss of *DSG1* triggered epithelial gene expression changes reflective of those in EoE biopsies, including increased *POSTN* expression.[45]

A key contributory role for DSG1 dysregulation in the allergic disease process was independently demonstrated in genetic studies that identified loss-of-function mutations in *DSG1* in consanguineous individuals with severe atopic dermatitis, multiple allergies, and metabolic wasting (SAM) syndrome. All 3 patients with SAM who were analyzed had failure-to-thrive diagnoses and multiple food allergies; notably, one patient also had an EoE diagnosis (see **Table 1**).[46] Skin biopsies from patients with SAM showed reduced *DSG1* expression and acantholysis, whereas isolated keratinocytes showed increased expression of IL-5 and TSLP.[46] An intronic mutation in *DSG1* showed a suggestive association with EoE risk.[20] Given this potential association and the findings in SAM syndrome, further investigation into EoE risk variants in *DSG1* is warranted (**Fig. 1**).

EPIGENETICS

Epigenetics are the heritable phenotypic modifications that result from gene activation or repression through mechanisms that are independent of changes to the DNA sequence.[47] Capable of being influenced by environmental stimuli, the epigenome lies at the crossroads of gene-environment interactions, placing it at the forefront

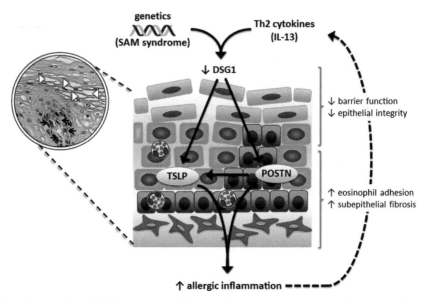

Fig. 1. Regulation of DSG1 promotes allergic inflammation. Decreased *DSG1* expression by Th2 cytokines (IL-13) or *DSG1* coding variants (as in SAM syndrome) alter the levels of functional DSG1, leading to impaired barrier function and reduced epithelial integrity. DSG1 deficiency also induces the expression of periostin (*POSTN*), which can lead to enhanced eosinophil adhesion and subepithelial fibrosis, and TSLP, either directly or indirectly through periostin, culminating in a proinflammatory cycle. The *arrowheads* signify dilated intracellular spaces.

for studying mechanisms underlying environmentally driven allergic inflammatory diseases. This article discusses in detail the current view of epigenetic regulation associated with EoE, which includes histone modification and DNA methylation, and posttranscriptional repression by microRNAs (miRNAs).

Histone Modification and DNA Methylation

Posttranslational modification of histone tails is an epigenetic mechanism that can alter the accessibility to gene promoters located proximally or distally to the modified histone. These reversible modifications, the most prominent of which include acetylation and methylation, are made by diverse families of modifying enzymes in monomeric or even multimeric fashion to exposed amino acid residues (typically lysine) of the histone tail.[48] The type of modification, the specific histone and position of the amino acid residue involved, and the degree to which the residue is modified can all influence the degree of gene activation or repression.[49] Much of what little is known about the involvement of epigenetics in EoE has been attained from biochemical studies of the promoter of the leading EoE candidate gene, *CCL26* (**Fig. 2**). The mapping of 2 STAT6 binding sites roughly established the promoter proximal regions required for IL-13–induced transcriptional activation of *CCL26*.[30] Further analysis demonstrated a requirement for 2 coactivators, activating transcription factor 2 (ATF2) and the histone acetyltransferase cyclic adenosine monophosphate (cAMP)–responsive element (CRE)–binding protein (CBP).[50] Chromatin immunoprecipitation assays indicated that STAT6, CBP, ATF2, and acetylated histone 3 bound within the same region of the *CCL26* promoter in esophageal epithelial cells after IL-13 treatment.[50] Thus, IL-13 induces the formation of a multiprotein complex on the

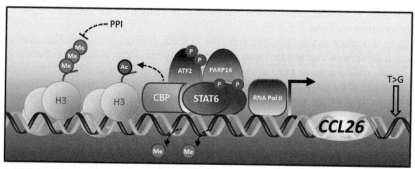

Fig. 2. Genetic and epigenetic regulation of the *CCL26* locus. *CCL26* expression is induced on phosphorylation (*P*) of STAT6 by Th2 cytokines (IL-13 and IL-4). Complete activation of the *CCL26* promoter by phosphorylated STAT6 is aided presumably by the opening of the *CCL26* promoter region by DNA demethylation, CBP-mediated acetylation (Ac) of histone 3 (H3), and interaction with cofactors such as CBP, phosphorylated ATF2, and PARP14. A genetic variant (T>G) in the 3′ untranslated region of *CCL26* is linked to EoE risk. Proton pump inhibitors (PPI) can silence *CCL26* expression by removing trimethylated (Me) H3 from the *CCL26* promoter region, potentially making the promoter inaccessible to phosphorylated STAT6 and RNA polymerase (Pol) II.

CCL26 promoter that includes CBP, leading to increases in acetylated histone 3 and opening of the *CCL26* promoter for additional transcriptional machinery. PPIs have been suggested to dampen the levels of trimethylated histone 3 lysine 4 (H3K4) and STAT6 bound to the *CCL26* promoter, resulting in decreased eotaxin-3 expression.[51] These findings could explain the emerging observation of PPI-responsive EoE, in which PPI therapy yields partial resolution of symptoms.[52]

In addition to the epigenetic regulation by histone acetylation, the *CCL26* promoter is also controlled by DNA methylation. DNA methylation occurs on cytosine nucleotides located within CpG (cytosine-guanine) dinucleotide motifs and, like other epigenetic marks, is dynamically regulated.[53] Two CpG sites in the *CCL26* promoter were identified as hypomethylated in esophageal epithelial cells derived from patients with EoE.[54] These data remarkably demonstrate the longevity of epigenetic marks in that they remain detectable even in cells cultured ex vivo through multiple rounds of cell division. The methylation status at 1 of the 2 CpG sites correlated with increased STAT6 binding to the *CCL26* promoter and induction of *CCL26* expression by IL-13.[54] Moreover, this CpG site flanks the CBP-binding sequence, and its methylation prohibited the binding of CBP to the *CCL26* promoter.[54] Collectively, these findings suggest that a coordinated interaction involving DNA demethylation followed by histone acetylation occurs at the *CCL26* promoter in response to IL-13.

MicroRNAs

miRNAs are short, noncoding RNAs that fine-tune the expression of target genes at the posttranscriptional level. miRNAs act to repress translation and/or induce mRNA degradation through binding complementary "seed" sequences in the 3′ untranslated region of target mRNAs, forming double-stranded RNA molecules that are digested within the RNA-induced silencing complex.[55] Much like their coding counterparts composing the EoE transcriptome, a select set of miRNAs has been shown to be dynamically altered in the esophageal mucosa of patients with EoE. The miRNA signature associated with EoE, which was distinct from both healthy controls and patients with chronic, noneosinophilic forms of esophagitis, included 21 upregulated and 11 downregulated miRNAs.[3]

Two of the most highly induced miRNAs in EoE, miR-21 and miR-223, also displayed the highest correlation with esophageal eosinophil levels in patients with EoE.[3] Both miRNAs have potentially significant functional implications in the pathophysiology of EoE. miR-21 is upregulated in multiple mouse models of allergic lung inflammation[56] and has been implicated in promoting eosinophil survival.[57] Induction of miR-223 in EoE showed significant correlations with the induction of the genes encoding Charcot-Leyden crystal protein (CLC), an eosinophil granule protein, and IL-5,[3] suggesting a role for miR-223 in eosinophil development. In vivo studies showed enhanced proliferation of eosinophil progenitors and a severe defect in eosinophil development from the bone marrow of miR-223–deficient mice.[58] However, how the localized increase of miR-223 in the esophageal mucosa affects terminally differentiated eosinophils within the Th2 microenvironment remains unknown.

Conversely, miR-375 is the most repressed miRNA in the EoE-associated signature. Mechanistically, IL-13 can downregulate miR-375 in cultured esophageal epithelial cells.[59] Exogenous expression of miR-375 in esophageal epithelial cells modulated the levels of several immunomodulatory genes at baseline and after IL-13 stimulation, indicating a unique role for miR-375 in the regulation of IL-13–induced transcriptional responses.[59] The interaction between epithelial-derived miR-375 and IL-13 has also been observed in the intestine with strikingly different results, wherein IL-13 treatment of intestinal epithelial cells enhanced miR-375 expression.[60] miR-375 was also shown to regulate goblet cell differentiation through targeting of Kruppel-like factor 5 (KLF5) and induce TSLP expression.[60] Taken together, these findings suggest that miRNA dysregulation affects multiple inflammatory processes connected to EoE.

The miRNA signature associated with EoE exhibited near-complete reversibility (27 of 32 dysregulated miRNAs, or 84%) during disease remission induced by swallowed fluticasone therapy.[3] Similar levels of normalization were observed in an independent, longitudinal EoE cohort analyzed both before and after steroid therapy, wherein only 32 of the 377 miRNAs analyzed, or fewer than 9%, remained dysregulated.[61] However, one miRNA, miR-675, was significantly elevated in patients experiencing EoE remission who were fluticasone-responsive compared with those who were unresponsive.[3] Several miRNAs, including miR-146a, miR-146b, and miR-223, were identified as dysregulated in plasma samples from patients with active EoE.[3] Together, these data implicate miRNAs as potential biomarkers for EoE diagnosis and steroid responsiveness.

SUMMARY

In summary, gene expression profiling of patient tissue and screening for disease risk variants have taken unbiased approaches to reveal many of the critical molecular pathways underlying EoE pathogenesis. Although these pathways continue to undergo rigorous investigation, new research into the epigenetic modification of immunoregulatory genes such as CCL26 and a dysregulated miRNA signature in EoE add additional layers to the molecular entities governing the transcriptome of the inflamed esophageal mucosa. In addition, there has been increasing recognition of EoE associated with several Mendelian disorders such as SAM syndrome (DSG1), connective tissue disorders (TGFBR1/2 mutations), and PTEN hamartoma tumor syndromes (see **Table 1**).[62] Although many challenges exist and much work remains, dissecting the genetic and epigenetic factors of EoE and related genetic disorders represents a promising area for translational research aimed at novel therapies, noninvasive diagnostics, and biomarkers for therapy response.

REFERENCES

1. Sherrill JD, Rothenberg ME. Genetic dissection of eosinophilic esophagitis provides insight into disease pathogenesis and treatment strategies. J Allergy Clin Immunol 2011;128:23–32.
2. Blanchard C, Wang N, Rothenberg ME. Eosinophilic esophagitis: pathogenesis, genetics, and therapy. J Allergy Clin Immunol 2006;118:1054–9.
3. Lu TX, Sherrill JD, Wen T, et al. MicroRNA signature in patients with eosinophilic esophagitis, reversibility with glucocorticoids, and assessment as disease biomarkers. J Allergy Clin Immunol 2012;129:1064–75.e1069.
4. Blanchard C, Wang N, Stringer KF, et al. Eotaxin-3 and a uniquely conserved gene-expression profile in eosinophilic esophagitis. J Clin Invest 2006;116: 536–47.
5. Bochner BS, Book W, Busse WW, et al. Workshop report from the National Institutes of Health Taskforce on the Research Needs of Eosinophil-Associated Diseases (TREAD). J Allergy Clin Immunol 2012;130:587–96.
6. Kagalwalla AF, Shah A, Li BU, et al. Identification of specific foods responsible for inflammation in children with eosinophilic esophagitis successfully treated with empiric elimination diet. J Pediatr Gastroenterol Nutr 2011;53:145–9.
7. Jensen ET, Kappelman MD, Kim H, et al. Early life exposures as risk factors for pediatric eosinophilic esophagitis. J Pediatr Gastroenterol Nutr 2013;57:67–71.
8. Almansa C, Krishna M, Buchner AM, et al. Seasonal distribution in newly diagnosed cases of eosinophilic esophagitis in adults. Am J Gastroenterol 2009;104: 828–33.
9. Spergel JM, Book WM, Mays E, et al. Variation in prevalence, diagnostic criteria, and initial management options for eosinophilic gastrointestinal diseases in the United States. J Pediatr Gastroenterol Nutr 2011;52:300–6.
10. Hurrell JM, Genta RM, Dellon ES. Prevalence of esophageal eosinophilia varies by climate zone in the United States. Am J Gastroenterol 2012;107:698–706.
11. Dellon ES, Peery AF, Shaheen NJ, et al. Inverse association of esophageal eosinophilia with Helicobacter pylori based on analysis of a US pathology database. Gastroenterology 2011;141:1586–92.
12. Rayapudi M, Mavi P, Zhu X, et al. Indoor insect allergens are potent inducers of experimental eosinophilic esophagitis in mice. J Leukoc Biol 2010;88: 337–46.
13. Pope SM, Fulkerson PC, Blanchard C, et al. Identification of a cooperative mechanism involving interleukin-13 and eotaxin-2 in experimental allergic lung inflammation. J Biol Chem 2005;280:13952–61.
14. Noti M, Wojno ED, Kim BS, et al. Thymic stromal lymphopoietin-elicited basophil responses promote eosinophilic esophagitis. Nat Med 2013;19:1005–13.
15. International HapMap Consortium. The International HapMap Project. Nature 2003;426:789–96.
16. Blanchard C, Stucke EM, Burwinkel K, et al. Coordinate interaction between IL-13 and epithelial differentiation cluster genes in eosinophilic esophagitis. J Immunol 2010;184:4033–41.
17. Aceves SS, Newbury RO, Chen D, et al. Resolution of remodeling in eosinophilic esophagitis correlates with epithelial response to topical corticosteroids. Allergy 2010;65:109–16.
18. Abonia JP, Wen T, Stucke EM, et al. High prevalence of eosinophilic esophagitis in patients with inherited connective tissue disorders. J Allergy Clin Immunol 2013;132:378–86.

19. Frischmeyer-Guerrerio PA, Guerrerio AL, Oswald G, et al. TGFbeta receptor mutations impose a strong predisposition for human allergic disease. Sci Transl Med 2013;5:195ra194.

20. Rothenberg ME, Spergel JM, Sherrill JD, et al. Common variants at 5q22 associate with pediatric eosinophilic esophagitis. Nat Genet 2010;42:289–91.

21. Ziegler SF. The role of thymic stromal lymphopoietin (TSLP) in allergic disorders. Curr Opin Immunol 2010;22:795–9.

22. Siracusa MC, Saenz SA, Tait Wojno ED, et al. Thymic stromal lymphopoietin-mediated extramedullary hematopoiesis promotes allergic inflammation. Immunity 2013;39:1158–70.

23. Sherrill JD, Gao PS, Stucke EM, et al. Variants of thymic stromal lymphopoietin and its receptor associate with eosinophilic esophagitis. J Allergy Clin Immunol 2010;126:160–5.e163.

24. Gudbjartsson DF, Bjornsdottir US, Halapi E, et al. Sequence variants affecting eosinophil numbers associate with asthma and myocardial infarction. Nat Genet 2009;41:342–7.

25. Collins MH, Blanchard C, Abonia JP, et al. Clinical, pathologic, and molecular characterization of familial eosinophilic esophagitis compared with sporadic cases. Clin Gastroenterol Hepatol 2008;6:621–9.

26. Wen T, Stucke EM, Grotjan TM, et al. Molecular diagnosis of eosinophilic esophagitis by gene expression profiling. Gastroenterology 2013;145:1289–99.

27. Blanchard C, Mingler MK, Vicario M, et al. IL-13 involvement in eosinophilic esophagitis: transcriptome analysis and reversibility with glucocorticoids. J Allergy Clin Immunol 2007;120:1292–300.

28. Lucendo AJ, De Rezende L, Comas C, et al. Treatment with topical steroids downregulates IL-5, eotaxin-1/CCL11, and eotaxin-3/CCL26 gene expression in eosinophilic esophagitis. Am J Gastroenterol 2008;103:2184–93.

29. Bhattacharya B, Carlsten J, Sabo E, et al. Increased expression of eotaxin-3 distinguishes between eosinophilic esophagitis and gastroesophageal reflux disease. Hum Pathol 2007;38:1744–53.

30. Blanchard C, Durual S, Estienne M, et al. Eotaxin-3/CCL26 gene expression in intestinal epithelial cells is up-regulated by interleukin-4 and interleukin-13 via the signal transducer and activator of transcription 6. Int J Biochem Cell Biol 2005;37:2559–73.

31. Hoeck J, Woisetschlager M. Activation of eotaxin-3/CCLI26 gene expression in human dermal fibroblasts is mediated by STAT6. J Immunol 2001;167:3216–22.

32. Goenka S, Boothby M. Selective potentiation of Stat-dependent gene expression by collaborator of Stat6 (CoaSt6), a transcriptional cofactor. Proc Natl Acad Sci U S A 2006;103:4210–5.

33. Krishnamurthy P, Sherrill JD, Parashette K, et al. Correlation of increased PARP14 and CCL26 expression in biopsies from children with eosinophilic esophagitis. J Allergy Clin Immunol 2014;133:577–80.

34. Mishra A, Hogan SP, Brandt EB, et al. An etiological role for aeroallergens and eosinophils in experimental esophagitis. J Clin Invest 2001;107:83–90.

35. Mishra A, Rothenberg ME. Intratracheal IL-13 induces eosinophilic esophagitis by an IL-5, eotaxin-1, and STAT6-dependent mechanism. Gastroenterology 2003;125:1419–27.

36. Kudo A. Periostin in fibrillogenesis for tissue regeneration: periostin actions inside and outside the cell. Cell Mol Life Sci 2011;68:3201–7.

37. Masuoka M, Shiraishi H, Ohta S, et al. Periostin promotes chronic allergic inflammation in response to Th2 cytokines. J Clin Invest 2012;122:2590–600.

38. Jia G, Erickson RW, Choy DF, et al. Periostin is a systemic biomarker of eosino-philic airway inflammation in asthmatic patients. J Allergy Clin Immunol 2012; 130:647–54.e610.

39. Wong GS, Lee JS, Park YY, et al. Periostin cooperates with mutant p53 to mediate invasion through the induction of STAT1 signaling in the esophageal tu-mor microenvironment. Oncogenesis 2013;2:e59.

40. Blanchard C, Mingler MK, McBride M, et al. Periostin facilitates eosinophil tissue infiltration in allergic lung and esophageal responses. Mucosal Immunol 2008;1: 289–96.

41. Corren J, Lemanske RF, Hanania NA, et al. Lebrikizumab treatment in adults with asthma. N Engl J Med 2011;365:1088–98.

42. Hanania NA, Wenzel S, Rosen K, et al. Exploring the effects of omalizumab in allergic asthma: an analysis of biomarkers in the EXTRA study. Am J Respir Crit Care Med 2013;187:804–11.

43. Chavanas S, Bodemer C, Rochat A, et al. Mutations in SPINK5, encoding a serine protease inhibitor, cause Netherton syndrome. Nat Genet 2000;25:141–2.

44. Amagai M, Matsuyoshi N, Wang ZH, et al. Toxin in bullous impetigo and staph-ylococcal scalded-skin syndrome targets desmoglein 1. Nat Med 2000;6: 1275–7.

45. Sherrill JD, Kc K, Wu D, et al. Desmoglein-1 regulates esophageal epithelial bar-rier function and immune responses in eosinophilic esophagitis. Mucosal Immu-nol 2013. [Epub ahead of print].

46. Samuelov L, Sarig O, Harmon RM, et al. Desmoglein 1 deficiency results in se-vere dermatitis, multiple allergies and metabolic wasting. Nat Genet 2013;45: 1244–8.

47. Bonasio R, Tu S, Reinberg D. Molecular signals of epigenetic states. Science 2010;330:612–6.

48. Kouzarides T. Chromatin modifications and their function. Cell 2007;128: 693–705.

49. Bernstein BE, Kamal M, Lindblad-Toh K, et al. Genomic maps and comparative analysis of histone modifications in human and mouse. Cell 2005;120:169–81.

50. Lim EJ, Lu TX, Blanchard C, et al. Epigenetic regulation of the IL-13-induced hu-man eotaxin-3 gene by CREB-binding protein-mediated histone 3 acetylation. J Biol Chem 2011;286:13193–204.

51. Zhang X, Cheng E, Huo X, et al. Omeprazole blocks STAT6 binding to the eotaxin-3 promoter in eosinophilic esophagitis cells. PLoS One 2012;7:e50037.

52. Dohil R, Newbury RO, Aceves S. Transient PPI responsive esophageal eosino-philia may be a clinical sub-phenotype of pediatric eosinophilic esophagitis. Dig Dis Sci 2012;57:1413–9.

53. Jones PA. Functions of DNA methylation: islands, start sites, gene bodies and beyond. Nat Rev Genet 2012;13:484–92.

54. Lim E, Rothenberg ME. Demethylation of the human Eotaxin-3 gene promoter leads to the elevated expression of Eotaxin-3. J Immunol 2014;192(1):466–74.

55. Behm-Ansmant I, Rehwinkel J, Izaurralde E. MicroRNAs silence gene expres-sion by repressing protein expression and/or by promoting mRNA decay. Cold Spring Harb Symp Quant Biol 2006;71:523–30.

56. Lu TX, Munitz A, Rothenberg ME. MicroRNA-21 is up-regulated in allergic airway inflammation and regulates IL-12p35 expression. J Immunol 2009;182: 4994–5002.

57. Lu TX, Lim EJ, Itskovich S, et al. Targeted ablation of miR-21 decreases murine eosinophil progenitor cell growth. PLoS One 2013;8:e59397.

58. Lu TX, Lim EJ, Besse JA, et al. MiR-223 deficiency increases eosinophil progenitor proliferation. J Immunol 2013;190:1576–82.

59. Lu TX, Lim EJ, Wen T, et al. MiR-375 is downregulated in epithelial cells after IL-13 stimulation and regulates an IL-13-induced epithelial transcriptome. Mucosal Immunol 2012;5:388–96.

60. Biton M, Levin A, Slyper M, et al. Epithelial microRNAs regulate gut mucosal immunity via epithelium-T cell crosstalk. Nat Immunol 2011;12:239–46.

61. Lu S, Mukkada VA, Mangray S, et al. MicroRNA profiling in mucosal biopsies of eosinophilic esophagitis patients pre and post treatment with steroids and relationship with mRNA targets. PLoS One 2012;7:e40676.

62. Henderson CJ, Ngeow J, Collins MH, et al. Increased prevalence of eosinophilic gastrointestinal disorders (EGID) in pediatric PTEN hamartoma tumor syndromes (PHTS). J Pediatr Gastroenterol Nutr 2013. [Epub ahead of print].

Allergic Mechanisms in Eosinophilic Esophagitis

Joshua B. Wechsler, MD[a], Paul J. Bryce, PhD[b],*

KEYWORDS

- Eosinophilic esophagitis • Allergic mechanism • Atopic • Antigen sensitization
- T-helper lymphocyte type 2 immunity • Pathogenesis

KEY POINTS

- Eosinophilic esophagitis shares a clinical link with other atopic diseases and is caused by immune dysregulation secondary to allergic sensitization to dietary or aeroallergens.
- Allergic sensitization, which may occur via multiple routes, drives the formation of allergen-specific IgE and T cells, which seem to participate in the esophageal hypersensitivity response.
- Loss of tolerance is likely critical to pathogenesis, and may be secondary to regulatory T-cell imbalance.
- Eosinophilic esophagitis is dominated by T-helper lymphocyte type 2–mediated eosinophil-predominant inflammation, with key contributions from mast cells, basophils, epithelial cells, and dendritic cells.

INTRODUCTION

Chronic tissue infiltration of eosinophils is the hallmark of allergic inflammatory diseases, which include asthma, atopic dermatitis, and eosinophilic gastrointestinal diseases (EGIDs). Eosinophilic esophagitis (EoE), a type of EGID, is characterized by eosinophil-predominant inflammation isolated to the esophagus, the only organ in the gastrointestinal (GI) tract that is homeostatically devoid of eosinophils. There is significant evidence of a role for allergic mechanisms as the driving force in EoE. The foundation for this understanding began almost 20 years ago, when Kelly and colleagues[1] reported that children with EoE resolved inflammation and clinical symptoms on amino acid–based diets. EoE is strongly linked to atopic disease and most often occurs comorbidly with asthma, eczema, allergic rhinitis, and anaphylactic food allergy, and a strong family history of such disorders is equally as common.[2,3] The tissue

[a] Division of Gastroenterology, Hepatology and Nutrition, Department of Pediatrics, Ann & Robert H. Lurie Children's Hospital of Chicago, 225 East Chicago Avenue, Chicago, IL 60611, USA; [b] Division of Allergy-Immunology, Department of Medicine, Feinberg School of Medicine, Northwestern University, 240 East Huron Street, M315, Chicago, IL 60611, USA
* Corresponding author.
E-mail address: p-bryce@northwestern.edu

Gastroenterol Clin N Am 43 (2014) 281–296
http://dx.doi.org/10.1016/j.gtc.2014.02.006
0889-8553/14/$ – see front matter © 2014 Elsevier Inc. All rights reserved.

inflammatory response in EoE is similar to other allergic inflammatory disorders and is characterized by a dysregulated immune response, with both IgE-mediated and non–IgE-mediated T-helper cell type 2 (Th2) responses. Cross-sensitization to aeroallergens seems to be common, and recent literature has begun to define antigen presentation, as well as the role of mast cells and basophils. In this review, our understanding of the allergic mechanisms involved in the pathogenesis of EoE are examined, based on clinical and translational studies in humans as well as experimental models in genetically modified animals.

CLINICAL ASSOCIATIONS OF EoE WITH ALLERGIC DISEASES

Despite being frequently managed by gastroenterology specialists, there are several unique features of EoE that reflect the allergic nature of this disorder. During the last few decades, the prevalence of allergic diseases has been increasing fast: in Westernized countries, more than a quarter of the population has allergic eczema, allergic rhinitis, or food allergy.[4] Paralleling this trend, epidemiologic studies show an increase in the number of children and adults with EoE.[5,6] In 2006, the prevalence of pediatric EoE in Australia was estimated to have increased 18-fold over the previous 10 years, and a US study reported a 35-fold increase over a similar time period.[7,8] This increasing prevalence is supported by an increasing incidence; population-based data from Olmsted County, MN show that the incidence of EoE increased from 0.35 to 9.45 per 100,000 persons from 1991 to 1995 to 2001 to 2005.[9] Similarly, a population-based study of pediatric and adult patients with EoE in Switzerland reported increased incidence from 2 to 6 per 100,000 persons from 1989 to 2004,[10] and findings from the Netherlands reported an increased incidence from 0.01 per 100,000 in 1996 to 1.31 per 100,000 in 2010.[5] This worldwide increase in EoE mirrors the trends in atopic diseases, although whether this is caused by a true increase in disease incidence, increased disease recognition, or improved access to endoscopy remains unclear.[11]

Beyond these parallels in disease incidence, several clinical studies have reported significant comorbidity of EoE with other atopic diseases. Although the prevalence of comorbid atopic disease varies between these studies, perhaps because of regional population differences, they show that most (50%–80%) patients with EoE also have atopy and other allergic diseases, including rhinitis, asthma, and eczema.[12] Although these allergic diseases can commonly be seen to follow the atopic march, whereby early in life, appearance of eczema and food allergy are observed and predispose for rhinitis and asthma several years later. EoE has a profoundly broad age range of onset and so seems to not adhere to this established concept. However, the strong clinical links between EoE and other well-described allergic diseases seem to imply shared pathogenic mechanisms.

HYPERSENSITIVITY IN EoE: IMMEDIATE OR DELAYED?

According to the National Institute of Allergy and Infectious Diseases–convened Guidelines for the Diagnosis and Management of Food Allergy in the United States,[13] food allergy was broadly defined as an abnormal immunologic hypersensitivity response to specific food proteins that leads to adverse clinical reactions. Within this definition, EoE is clearly an example of food antigen–driven hypersensitivity. However, hypersensitivity reactions can be further classified based on the mechanisms of antigen recognition: IgE (immediate type) or the T-cell receptor (delayed type).

In immediate-type IgE-mediated hypersensitivity, typically associated with anaphylaxis or urticaria, cross-linking of IgE and its receptor by antigen leads to the rapid release of preformed mediators from mast cells and basophils. Histamine is a key molecule in this process, and histamine receptors are important in regulating the physiologic responses.[14] This early antigen-specific rapid response is followed by the subsequent de novo synthesis and release of lipid mediators, cytokines, and chemokines, which can drive a late phase response in some individuals, with infiltration of inflammatory cells, including eosinophils.

Most patients with EoE have compelling evidence of IgE-mediated hypersensitivity to foods, as determined by increased food-specific IgE or abnormal skin prick test (SPT), despite food-induced anaphylaxis occurring in only around 15% of these patients.[2,15,16] Mechanistically, it has been shown that IgE-bearing mast cells are increased in the esophageal mucosa of patients with EoE, particularly those who are atopic.[17,18] Thus, it may be that the immediate hypersensitivity response in EoE occurs in a localized fashion exclusively in the esophagus, similar to what is seen in oral allergy syndrome. Although the involvement of IgE-mediated activation of mast cells in responses in the esophagus of patients with EoE remains to be defined, the early phase reaction could enhance blood flow and muscle contractility via release of histamine,[19,20] whereas the late phase reaction could contribute to the recruitment of eosinophils, similar to processes that have been noted in allergen-induced eosinophil recruitment in atopic dermatitis.[21]

Although the role of IgE-mediated hypersensitivity remains unclear, non–IgE-mediated reactions are increasingly understood to participate in EoE. These delayed-type reactions, often referred to as T-cell–mediated hypersensitivity, are characterized by the activation of antigen-specific T cells and subsequent recruitment of inflammatory cells. Delayed-type hypersensitivity (DTH) associated with allergic inflammatory disease is classically characterized by a Th2-predominant immune response, with increased interleukin 4 (IL-4), IL-5, and IL-13 levels, along with eosinophilic inflammation.[22] In clinical diagnosis, patch testing, whereby antigen is applied to the skin so as to elicit a DTH-associated response, has been shown to significantly improve predictive values over SPT alone, highlighting the likely contribution of this arm of the immune response in responses of patients with EoE.[23] The IgE-mediated and T-cell–mediated arms may intersect, because IgE has been shown to enhance DTH responses in mice.[24]

ALLERGIC SENSITIZATION
Dependent on IgE or T Cells?

The loss of tolerance and subsequent sensitization to antigen are critical events in the initiation of allergic conditions, involving coordinated involvement of antigen-presenting cells (APCs), T cells, and B cells, to prime the adaptive immune system for subsequent responses to antigen exposures. In particular, allergic sensitization associates with the generation of allergen-specific Th2 cells, which proliferate and differentiate into antigen-specific effector and memory T cells. In addition, these Th2 cells play a critical role in B-cell production of allergen-specific IgE, through their ability to generate IL-4.

In EoE, allergic sensitization is clearly evident: regardless of atopic status, patients with EoE have increased density of B cells and expression of IgE in the esophagus along with evidence of local class switching.[25] Specific IgEs for foods that trigger active disease are commonly detected in patients with EoE in the absence of anaphylaxis, although they may be present at low levels, perhaps reflecting local production.[26] Peripheral blood mononuclear cells from patients with EoE show allergen-specific cytokine responses that correlate with this increase in specific IgE (although some patients have allergen-specific cytokine responses without increased specific IgE levels, consistent with non-IgE–mediated allergic sensitization).[27] In addition, mouse models of EoE-like disease, whereby sensitization is elicited via cutaneous or respiratory allergen exposure, show increased antigen-specific IgE levels, and a clear dependency on T cells but are still able to traffic eosinophils to the esophagus in the absence of either B cells or IgE.[28,29] Thus, allergic sensitization in EoE drives the formation of allergen-specific IgE and T cells; however, they potentially have independent roles in the underlying disease pathogenesis.

Tolerance

In animal models, allergic sensitization commonly occurs to an antigen for which the animal is naive; however, in EoE, in which the mean age at diagnosis is 33.5 years, sensitization often occurs to antigens already in the diet or environment that have been tolerated.[30] This finding suggests that loss of tolerance may be critical to facilitate the subsequent immune sensitization. Several early-life risk factors have been found for EoE, including antibiotic use in infancy, cesarean delivery, preterm birth, and lack of breastfeeding,[31] all of which have been suggested by other studies to alter the development of tolerance. One critical cell type that seems to play a role in the maintenance of tolerance is the regulatory T (Treg) cell, characterized by expression of Foxp3. In EoE, an imbalance between effector and Treg cells was shown by Stuck and colleagues,[32] who found the proportion of Foxp3$^+$CD3$^+$ T cells was 50% reduced in EoE compared with healthy controls. Using an intranasal aeroallergen-induced murine model of EoE, Zhu and colleagues[33] found a similar alteration in the frequency of CD4$^+$ T-cell subsets in the esophagus of allergen-challenged mice compared with saline-challenged mice. Not surprisingly, it was FOXP3$^+$ cells that were critically reduced among these cell populations. Although these studies suggest that there may be a relative lack of Treg-type T cells at the site of inflammation, it remains to be determined whether this alteration in Treg cells has simply a sustaining effect in EoE or whether Treg imbalances are critical to promoting allergic sensitization.

Route of Sensitization

An interesting question that remains in EoE is the site at which allergic sensitization occurs. Clinical studies of early-life risk factors have not supported a specific route of sensitization in EoE. However, a variety of animal models of allergic disease have shown that allergic sensitization can occur via the skin, airway, or gut.[28,34,35] Experimental animal models of EoE suggest that sensitization may not require esophageal allergen exposure. Akei and colleagues[36] found that epicutaneous antigen sensitization in the form of repeated allergen administration to the shaved back of mice followed by an intranasal allergen challenge facilitated an EoE-like disease that was IL-5 dependent and, to a lesser extent, IL-4 and IL-13 dependent. More recently, Noti and colleagues[28] found that sensitization to egg or peanut protein could occur during skin inflammation or injury (tape stripping) in a thymic stromal lymphopoietin (TSLP)-dependent, basophil-dependent, and IgE-independent manner. Sensitization also seems to be effective via the lungs, because repeated exposure to aeroallergens via intranasal administration increased antigen-specific IgG1 levels and was sufficient to induce eosinophilic inflammation in the esophagus.[35] Neither intragastric nor oral administration of aeroallergens was sufficient to induce EoE-like disease. It is likely, therefore, that antigen sensitization can occur at several sites, including lung and skin, and likely depends on a variety of host and environmental factors, but further studies are required to determine what is clinically relevant in EoE.

Aeroallergens

Many patients with EoE show evidence of polysensitization, not just to multiple foods but also to environmental aeroallergens.[37] Although the functional role of allergic sensitization to aeroallergens is not entirely clear, there is evidence both in animal models and clinically that it may participate in driving elements of the EoE disease. Several studies have described seasonal variation in a subset of patients in whom disease worsening occurred during pollen season, regardless of therapy.[38,39] It remains unclear whether swallowed aeroallergen directly promotes active disease or inhaled aeroallergen exacerbates concomitant airway disease, as could be interpreted from the murine studies with intranasal aeroallergen. Primary allergic sensitization to aeroallergens may also contribute to food sensitization as a result of cross-reactivity or cross-sensitization. Detection of this phenomenon has become possible with the use of protein microarrays, which allow for simultaneous assessment of specific IgE antibodies against multiple recombinant or purified natural allergen components, so-called component-resolved diagnostics. Using this technique, Simon and colleagues[40] found IgE antibodies against food-specific allergen components were rare in Swiss patients with EoE and cross-reactive responses were common. These investigators noted that the dominant pattern of cross-reactivity was to profilins, pathogenesis-related (PR)-10 and lipid transfer proteins. These findings were validated by a group in the Netherlands, who also found that most food sensitizations in patients with EoE are a result of cross-sensitization to PR-10 proteins present in birch pollen.[41] These proteins can pass through the esophagus intact, but are degraded in the stomach, which could limit inflammation to the esophagus. Thus, sensitization to aeroallergens, which can occur via the skin or airway, may be a significant factor in the development of EoE and explain some of the comorbidity with atopic disease.

ANTIGEN PRESENTATION IN THE ESOPHAGUS

Antigen presentation plays a crucial role in initiating a highly specific immune response to a foreign protein. APCs engulf, process, and show peptides coupled to major histocompatibility complex (MHC) class II peptides on their cell membrane. Cell surface costimulatory molecules also help determine whether presented antigen provokes an immunogenic or tolerogenic T-lymphocyte response. In EoE, the mechanistic understanding of this process is limited, but it seems that both professional APCs such as dendritic cells (DCs) and nonprofessional APCs such as epithelial cells play a role.

The primary professional APC in the esophagus seems to be the Langerhans cell, a type of DC found in all squamous epithelia,[42] particularly the epidermis. Langerhans cells of the esophagus are structurally similar to those in the skin and are located along the papillae of the lamina propria and in the suprabasal region.[43] These myeloid DCs, identified by the surface marker CD1a, are increased in density in children with EoE compared with controls and are reduced after treatment.[44] However, there are contradictory data from a study in adults with EoE, which found no differences in CD1a density before/after treatment or with controls.[45] This finding may be because of histopathologic variability or may represent a key etiologic difference between children and adults with EoE. In addition, Langerhans cells of the upper GI tract express the high-affinity IgE receptor, FcϵRI,[46] for which expression increases in active EoE.[47] IgE signaling on APCs has been proposed to enhance antigen uptake and enhance the development and activation of allergen-specific T cells.[48] Although the role of Langerhans cells in EoE is unclear, they are critical to the pathogenesis of atopic diseases such as eczema, and their proximity to T cells in the esophagus suggests a possible interaction and pathologic function.

Under pathologic conditions, epithelial cells at mucosal surfaces act as nonprofessional APCs and can regulate immune responses at the site of exposure. Antigen presentation by small bowel epithelium is well established and likely plays a role in food hypersensitivity.[49,50] Mulder and colleagues[51] found that basal epithelial cells in EoE biopsies express the MHC class II protein HLA-DR. Using the human esophageal epithelial HET-1A cell line, which maintains characteristics of basal esophageal epithelium, these investigators showed the ability of these cells to engulf, process, and present antigen in an interferon γ (IFN-γ)-dependent manner, as well as stimulate T-helper cell activation. IFN-γ, which is increased in biopsy tissue of patients with EoE, enhanced expression of MHC class II, whereas IL-4 enhanced costimulatory molecule expression. Thus, although the esophageal epithelium is unlikely to play a role in the early initiation of an immune response, given the dependence on cytokine priming, it may play a role in perpetuating EoE-associated inflammation.

Controversially, recent literature has suggested that eosinophils may also function as APCs at the site of inflammation.[52] In asthmatics, eosinophils seem to express the MHC class II protein, HLA-DR, dependent on stimulation by granulocyte-macrophage colony-stimulating factor, as well as costimulatory molecules CD40, CD80, and CD86, and can traffic to regional lymph nodes after exposure to antigen, bringing them close to T cells for presentation.[53,54] Likewise, in EoE, tissue eosinophils have been shown to express increased HLA-DR,[55] as well as CD40 and CD80,[56] supporting the potential capacity for antigen presentation. However, the evidence to support the ability of eosinophils to engulf and process protein antigens seems lacking and limits their ability to function in similar ways to professional APCs, such as DCs. One postulated mechanism, whereby MHC II loading occurs from exogenous peptides generated from the protease-rich milieu in EoE, remains to be fully established. In addition, the nature of the interaction between T cells and antigen-presenting eosinophils is not well understood; thus, the extent to which eosinophils act as APCs to initiate or even sustain the inflammatory process is unclear.

T-LYMPHOCYTE IMMUNE RESPONSES

Murine studies on mice lacking various components of the adaptive immune system have established a critical role for T cells in EoE.[29] Similar to other atopic diseases, such as allergic asthma and eczema, tissue inflammation in EoE is characterized by a Th2-type inflammatory response. This finding was initially described by Straumann and colleagues[57] in 2001, who observed increased T cells and IgE+ mast cells in esophageal biopsies of patients with EoE associated with IL-5 expression in the infiltrating inflammatory cells. Since that initial study, several reports have confirmed these findings and described increased levels of IL-4 and IL-13 in biopsy samples.[25,58,59] Peripheral blood mononuclear cells from patients with EoE also produce IL-5 and IL-13 in response to specific allergen stimulation,[27] and murine models of EoE have provided additional support that a Th2-mediated response is required for pathogenicity.[29,36,60] Blanchard and colleagues[59] examined a large cohort of patients with EoE and found enhanced expression of both IL-4 and IL-5 in atopic individuals with EoE compared with nonatopic individuals. In addition, the study noted concerted expression of IL-5 and IL-13, suggesting that a common cell type is responsible for their production.

Although much of the focus has been on the Th2 cell in EoE, Th1-associated cytokines are also an important part of the inflammatory response, and likely play a critical role in pathogenesis. This category includes tumor necrosis factor, which is expressed by esophageal epithelial cells,[57] and is involved in remodeling,[61] and IFN-γ, which is expressed by T cells after stimulation with IL-15[62] and is involved in priming the epithelium for antigen presentation.[51]

IL-4

Critical to the initiation of a Th2 response, IL-4 promotes differentiation of naive T-helper cells into Th2 cells as well as B-cell class switching to produce IgE. Although the initial source of IL-4 in atopic disease is not entirely clear, recent work has proposed that TSLP-elicited basophils may be important.[28,63,64] In the esophagus, IL-4 not only sustains the Th2 response but also contributes directly to recruitment of eosinophils by stimulating eotaxin production in esophageal epithelial cells.[65] Th2 cells are considered to be an important source of IL-4 in EoE, which is enhanced by IL-15 stimulation.[62] Countering this concept, IL-4 expression levels correlate poorly with the other Th2-associated cytokines, IL-5 and IL-13,[59] and suggest that other cells may be relevant sources.

IL-5

Of the Th2 cytokines, IL-5 is the most well studied in EoE and seems to be central to the disease. In the GI tract, IL-5$^+$ allergen-specific T-cell responses differentiate EGIDs from IgE-mediated immediate hypersensitivity, characterized by IL-5$^-$ Th2 responses.[66] IL-5 is produced primarily by Th2 cells, although additional sources include mast cells and eosinophils. It acts on the bone marrow to stimulate eosinophil proliferation and differentiation and regulates survival and activation of eosinophils.[67] Mice lacking IL-5 fail to recruit eosinophils to the esophagus in intranasal aeroallergen-induced EoE, whereas mice transgenic for IL-5 under the control of the T-cell–specific CD2 promoter (CD2-IL5) develop chronic esophageal eosinophilia and mastocytosis.[68,69] Trafficking of eosinophils by IL-5 likely occurs by priming of eosinophil responses to chemokines such as eotaxins (CCL11, CCL24, and CCL26), or by upregulating homing receptors.[60] IL-5 also has a role in tissue remodeling, because mice with CD2-IL-5–mediated esophageal eosinophilia have increased collagen accumulation in the lamina propria and extended stromal papillae, whereas IL-5–deficient mice do not in similar model studies.[60,69] Although clinical and murine studies has shown a central role for IL-5 in the allergic mechanisms of EoE, and there is variable downregulation of IL-5 expression after treatment with fluticasone,[70] anti-IL-5 biological therapy has shown limited clinical efficacy,[71] suggesting that, although IL-5 plays an important role in EoE disease, blocking IL-5 may not be sufficient to prevent the immunopathology of EoE in humans.

IL-13

IL-13 is a pleotropic cytokine that exerts pathologic effects when excessively produced by activating local tissue inflammatory responses; its cellular sources include Th2 cells and activated eosinophils.[27,57,72] In EoE, active inflammation is self-perpetuating, because infiltrating eosinophils secrete IL-13, which acts to enhance further recruitment of eosinophils to the esophagus by inducing STAT6-dependent eotaxin expression in the epithelium.[73–75] The critical interaction between IL-13 and the esophageal epithelium in driving EoE was highlighted by Blanchard and colleagues,[58] who found a significant overlap between the transcriptome of primary esophageal epithelial cells treated with IL-13 and total RNA from biopsies of patients with EoE, which was reversible with steroid therapy. IL-13 also recruits eosinophils by promoting fibroblasts to produce periostin, which increases eosinophil adhesion to fibronectin.[76] Intratracheal IL-13 was sufficient to induce experimental EoE in mice in an eotaxin/IL-5/STAT-6–dependent manner[73] but was not required, because intranasal aeroallergen-induced EoE had only mildly reduced esophageal eosinophilia in IL-13–deficient mice,[36,77] which may be caused by exaggerated Th17 responses.[78] IL-13 also plays key roles in barrier function, by downregulating genes involved in the epithelial cell differentiation, such as desmoglein-1, filaggrin, and involucrin,[75,79] and eosinophil-independent tissue remodeling by promoting collagen deposition, angiogenesis, and epithelial hyperplasia.[80] IL-13 is a prominent T-cell mediator in EoE pathogenesis with broad function and may be predicted as a likely factor that prevented efficacy from targeted IL-5 therapy. Ongoing clinical trials with anti-IL-13 will serve to better understand its role in pathogenesis and relevance as a therapeutic target.

B LYMPHOCYTES AND IGE

Formation of antigen-specific IgE is a principal effector function of Th2 cells, which promote class switching in B cells by stimulation with IL-4. IgE can bind to its high-affinity receptor, FcεRI, on the surface of mast cells and basophils, where subsequent engagement with polyvalent antigen triggers hypersensitivity responses, as described earlier. This process is central to the pathogenesis of many atopic disorders, including anaphylaxis, allergic bronchospasm, and urticaria. In addition, there are several antigen-independent immune functions of IgE, which include enhancement of mast cell survival, maintenance of mast cell location, and DC migration.[81] Clinical studies have documented the presence of allergen-specific IgE in patients with EoE, and SPT is commonly abnormal, providing evidence of immediate hypersensitivity to a variety of foods, and specific IgE has been suggested to contribute to symptoms.[40] A clinical study of omalizumab,[82] a monoclonal antibody directed against IgE, in the treatment of EoE found clinical but not histologic or endoscopic improvement. This finding may have pathogenic implications, because it suggests that some acute symptoms in EoE may be associated with IgE-mediated activation of mast cells or basophils.[18] However, many patients have no evidence of food-specific IgE, or abnormal SPT, and as described earlier, experimental studies in mice have shown that eosinophil recruitment is IgE independent, indicating a critical need for more translational and murine studies to fully understand the contribution of IgE to disease pathogenesis.

EOSINOPHILS

Both acute and chronic allergic reactions are associated with tissue eosinophilia. Antigen-driven recruitment of eosinophils occurs through critical mediators like IL-5 and the eotaxin family of chemokines, as well as lipid mediators like prostaglandin D2 (PGD2). At the site of inflammation, eosinophils become activated where they modulate immune responses and can damage the surrounding tissue.[83] Activation promotes secretion of various mediators that have been linked to EoE, including cytokines such as IL-4, IL-5, IL-13, and transforming growth factor β (TGF-β), chemokines such as CCL5/RANTES and CCL11/eotaxin-1, and lipid mediators such as leukotriene C_4.[59,84] These molecules have profound effects on the inflammatory response, which include upregulation of adhesion molecules, enhanced cellular trafficking and activation, and regulation of vascular permeability and muscle contraction. In addition, eosinophils secrete toxic granule protein that damages gut epithelium, including eosinophil peroxidase, eosinophil cationic protein, eosinophil-derived neurotoxin, and major basic protein, all of which have been shown to be increased in EoE tissues.[85]

The regulation over eosinophil recruitment to the esophagus seems similar to other atopic inflammatory diseases and is largely associated with the chemotactic effects of the eotaxin proteins, which are critical for maintenance of tissue eosinophilia. In EoE, eotaxin-3 (CCL26) was shown to be the most highly expressed gene in the esophagus, and expression levels strongly correlated with disease severity.[86] Eotaxin-deficient mice have been described as having markedly impaired esophageal eosinophilia,[87] even when overexpression of IL-5 is genetically introduced.[60] The relative increase in esophageal eosinophils in these IL-5 transgenic/eotaxin-deficient mice, when compared with control mice, suggest that additional chemotactic factors participate. These factors may include histamine, generated from mast cells or basophils, because thioperamide, a nonselective blocker of the histamine 3 and 4 receptor, inhibited eosinophil infiltration to the esophagus in an allergen-inhalation model of EoE in guinea pigs.[88] In addition, PGD2, a prostanoid largely produced by mast cells, is sufficient to drive eosinophils to the esophagus because injection of a PGD2 agonist into the esophagus led to rapid recruitment of eosinophils in guinea pigs, and pretreatment with a selective antagonist limited this experimental EoE-like disease.[89] Also, in adults with corticosteroid-resistant EoE, treatment of 8 weeks with OC000459, a selective antagonist of CRTH2, the receptor for PGD2, led to reduced tissue eosinophilia and clinical symptoms.[90]

The eosinophil is critical to many aspects of the histopathology of EoE. Mice deficient in the eosinophil lineage have a significant reduction in basal layer and lamina propria collagen thickness and fail to develop esophageal strictures as detected by barium esophagram.[68,69] These mice still maintain evidence of esophageal motility dysfunction, suggesting that this aspect of the disease is eosinophil independent.[68] In oral ovalbumin-induced EoE in mice, antibody targeting of Siglec-F, the mouse homolog of Siglec-8, which is highly expressed on eosinophils, and which mediates their apoptosis and clearance, reduced esophageal eosinophilia associated with reduced angiogenesis, basal zone hyperplasia, and fibronectin deposition.[91] These studies implicate the eosinophil as a critical damage-inducing mediator of EoE.

MAST CELLS

Despite being derived from the same $CD34^+$ progenitor cell type as eosinophils, mast cells are normally resident in the mucosa and submucosa of the esophagus. Their best-characterized function involves cross-linking of IgE, which binds to the high-affinity receptor, FcεRI, and becomes activated after engagement with antigen. Similar to eosinophils, mast cells store and produce an abundant number of inflammatory mediators that might participate in the pathogenesis of EoE. These mediators include TGF-β1, Th2 cytokines IL-4, IL-5, and IL-13, as well as eotaxins, histamine, leukotrienes, lipid mediators, and proteases, which can collectively contribute to fibrosis, tissue inflammation, or recruitment and activation of eosinophils.[92]

Mast cells are considered to be a major player in allergic disease, although the nature of their role in EoE pathogenesis remains unclear. Numerous studies have observed an increase in mast cell density in biopsies from patients with EoE,[18,57,86] and this correlates with both eosinophil density and basal zone hyperplasia and is responsive to swallowed steroids.[45] Mast cell activation occurs locally in EoE, because ultrastructural changes in cytoplasmic granules are detectable by electron microscopy,[18] and genes such as carboxypeptidase A3, tryptase, and histamine decarboxylase are increased in esophageal tissue, and normalize with therapy.[93] In the smooth muscle of patients with EoE, mast cell numbers are increased and express TGF-β1, which is capable of enhancing muscle contraction, suggesting a potential role in symptoms.[84] Atopic patients with EoE can be distinguished from nonatopic patients by the presence of IgE on esophageal mast cells, suggesting that mast cell activation may occur by alternative mechanisms in nonatopic patients.[17]

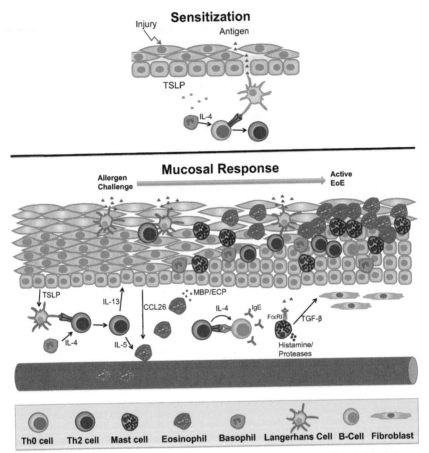

Fig. 1. Proposed allergic mechanisms involved in the pathogenesis of EoE. (*Top*) Proposed mechanism of allergic sensitization in EoE. In the presence of epithelial injury, TSLP production is elicited from epithelium. This process primes basophils to produce IL-4, which promotes allergic sensitization after antigen presentation to a naive T cell, which generates antigen-specific Th2 cells. (*Bottom*) Proposed mucosal response in EoE. Subsequent antigen challenge leads to recruitment and expansion of Th2 cells, which secrete IL-5 and IL-13, both critical in the recruitment of eosinophils and remodeling of the esophagus. Th2 cells locally promote class switching of B cells to produce antigen-specific IgE, which binds to the surface of mast cells. Activation of mast cells leads to the release of proinflammatory mediators such as TGF-β, which promotes remodeling and enhances muscle cell contractility. CCL26, Eotaxin-3; MPB, major basic protein; ECP, eosinophil cationic protein.

Mechanistically, the role of mast cells in EoE has been studied in mice and, similar to humans, there is an increase in density paralleling the increase in eosinophils.[68,77,87,94,95] In the intranasal aeroallergen-induced model of EoE, the increase in esophageal mast cells was time and challenge dependent. Although mast cell–deficient mice had reduced muscle cell hyperplasia and hypertrophy in this model, consistent with a role in remodeling, there was no effect on eosinophil recruitment.[95] Likewise, eosinophils are not required to recruit mast cells to the esophagus, but IL-5 seems to participate in recruiting mast cells, because CD2-IL5 transgenic/eosinophil-deficient mice had similar increased esophageal mast cell density to controls.[68]

This finding was supported clinically by subanalysis of a trial of mepolizumab in children, which also found reduced esophageal mast cells in treated patients.[96] Thus, it seems that mast cells have a multifunctional role in EoE, contributing to symptoms, remodeling, and tissue inflammation.

BASOPHILS

Despite an abundance of work defining the role of basophils in allergic inflammation, there have been limited studies investigating their pathogenic function in EoE. Recently, their potential involvement was shown using a novel murine model of EoE, whereby mice were sensitized to food antigen via the skin and EoE-like disease was initiated by repeated oral challenge with antigen.[28] In this model, antigen-specific IgE was detectable, but the mice developed EoE-like inflammation that was IgE independent. Instead, the investigators showed that EoE responses were associated with a significant expansion of basophils, driven by exposure to epithelial-derived TSLP, along with a Th2 response that was dominated by IL-4. These investigators established that depletion of basophils or deficiency of TSLP signaling resulted in loss of responses and included translational studies also showing increased TSLP and basophils in biopsies of patients with EoE. This new model provides unique insight into the mechanism by which IgE-independent allergic sensitization to antigen can facilitate eosinophil recruitment to the esophagus driven by basophils.

SUMMARY

EoE is a chronic inflammatory disease isolated to the esophagus that affects both children and adults. Animal models as well as studies in patients have helped to uncover various aspects of its pathogenesis, although many questions remain. EoE seems to share a significant clinical link with other atopic diseases, and there is strong evidence that it is caused by immune dysregulation secondary to allergic sensitization to dietary or aeroallergens. Although the role of IgE remains unclear, EoE is dominated by T-lymphocyte–mediated disease, with significant participation from mast cells, basophils, epithelial cells, and DCs, summarized in **Fig. 1**. What remains poorly understood is how the disease develops, and although there is some literature to suggest a role for loss of tolerance, further translational research is necessary to better characterize this aspect of the disease. As the complex immune mechanisms that govern EoE are uncovered, novel diagnostic and treatment options will move from bench to bedside.

REFERENCES

1. Kelly KJ, Lazenby AJ, Rowe PC, et al. Eosinophilic esophagitis attributed to gastroesophageal reflux: improvement with an amino acid-based formula. Gastroenterology 1995;109(5):1503–12.
2. Assa'ad AH, Putnam PE, Collins MH, et al. Pediatric patients with eosinophilic esophagitis: an 8-year follow-up. J Allergy Clin Immunol 2007;119(3):731–8.
3. Simon D, Marti H, Heer P, et al. Eosinophilic esophagitis is frequently associated with IgE-mediated allergic airway diseases. J Allergy Clin Immunol 2005;115(5): 1090–2.
4. Kiyohara C, Tanaka K, Miyake Y. Genetic susceptibility to atopic dermatitis. Allergol Int 2008;57(1):39–56.
5. van Rhijn BD, Verheij J, Smout AJ, et al. Rapidly increasing incidence of eosinophilic esophagitis in a large cohort. Neurogastroenterol Motil 2013;25(1): 47–52.e5.

6. Soon IS, Butzner JD, Kaplan GG, et al. Incidence and prevalence of eosinophilic esophagitis in children. J Pediatr Gastroenterol Nutr 2013;57(1):72–80.

7. Cherian S, Smith NM, Forbes DA. Rapidly increasing prevalence of eosinophilic oesophagitis in Western Australia. Arch Dis Child 2006;91(12):1000–4.

8. Liacouras CA, Spergel JM, Ruchelli E, et al. Eosinophilic esophagitis: a 10-year experience in 381 children. Clin Gastroenterol Hepatol 2005;3(12):1198–206.

9. Prasad GA, Alexander JA, Schleck CD, et al. Epidemiology of eosinophilic esophagitis over three decades in Olmsted County, Minnesota. Clin Gastroenterol Hepatol 2009;7(10):1055–61.

10. Straumann A, Simon HU. Eosinophilic esophagitis: escalating epidemiology? J Allergy Clin Immunol 2005;115(2):418–9.

11. Syed AA, Andrews CN, Shaffer E, et al. The rising incidence of eosinophilic oesophagitis is associated with increasing biopsy rates: a population-based study. Aliment Pharmacol Ther 2012;36(10):950–8.

12. Jyonouchi S, Brown-Whitehorn TA, Spergel JM. Association of eosinophilic gastrointestinal disorders with other atopic disorders. Immunol Allergy Clin North Am 2009;29(1):85–97, x.

13. Boyce JA, Assa'ad A, Burks AW, et al. Guidelines for the diagnosis and management of food allergy in the United States: report of the NIAID-sponsored expert panel. J Allergy Clin Immunol 2010;126(6 Suppl):S1–58.

14. Wechsler JB, Schroeder HA, Byrne AJ, et al. Anaphylactic responses to histamine in mice utilize both histamine receptors 1 and 2. Allergy 2013;68(10): 1338–40.

15. Spergel JM, Andrews T, Brown-Whitehorn TF, et al. Treatment of eosinophilic esophagitis with specific food elimination diet directed by a combination of skin prick and patch tests. Ann Allergy Asthma Immunol 2005;95(4):336–43.

16. Spergel JM. Eosinophilic esophagitis in adults and children: evidence for a food allergy component in many patients. Curr Opin Allergy Clin Immunol 2007;7(3): 274–8.

17. Mulder DJ, Mak N, Hurlbut DJ, et al. Atopic and non-atopic eosinophilic oesophagitis are distinguished by immunoglobulin E-bearing intraepithelial mast cells. Histopathology 2012;61(5):810–22.

18. Kirsch R, Bokhary R, Marcon MA, et al. Activated mucosal mast cells differentiate eosinophilic (allergic) esophagitis from gastroesophageal reflux disease. J Pediatr Gastroenterol Nutr 2007;44(1):20–6.

19. Feldman MJ, Morris GP, Dinda PK, et al. Mast cells mediate acid-induced augmentation of opossum esophageal blood flow via histamine and nitric oxide. Gastroenterology 1996;110(1):121–8.

20. Percy WH, Warren JM, Brunz JT. Characteristics of the muscularis mucosae in the acid-secreting region of the rabbit stomach. Am J Phys 1999;276(5 Pt 1): G1213–20.

21. Barata LT, Ying S, Meng Q, et al. IL-4- and IL-5-positive T lymphocytes, eosinophils, and mast cells in allergen-induced late-phase cutaneous reactions in atopic subjects. J Allergy Clin Immunol 1998;101(2 Pt 1):222–30.

22. Uzzaman A, Cho SH. Classification of hypersensitivity reactions. Allergy Asthma Proc 2012;33(Suppl 1):S96–9.

23. Spergel JM, Brown-Whitehorn T, Beausoleil JL, et al. Predictive values for skin prick test and atopy patch test for eosinophilic esophagitis. J Allergy Clin Immunol 2007;119(2):509–11.

24. Bryce PJ, Miller ML, Miyajima I, et al. Immune sensitization in the skin is enhanced by antigen-independent effects of IgE. Immunity 2004;20(4):381–92.

25. Vicario M, Blanchard C, Stringer KF, et al. Local B cells and IgE production in the oesophageal mucosa in eosinophilic oesophagitis. Gut 2010;59(1):12–20.
26. Erwin PC, Greene SB, Mays GP, et al. The association of changes in local health department resources with changes in state-level health outcomes. Am J Public Health 2011;101(4):609–15.
27. Yamazaki K, Murray JA, Arora AS, et al. Allergen-specific in vitro cytokine production in adult patients with eosinophilic esophagitis. Dig Dis Sci 2006; 51(11):1934–41.
28. Noti M, Wojno ED, Kim BS, et al. Thymic stromal lymphopoietin-elicited basophil responses promote eosinophilic esophagitis. Nat Med 2013;19(8):1005–13.
29. Mishra A, Schlotman J, Wang M, et al. Critical role for adaptive T cell immunity in experimental eosinophilic esophagitis in mice. J Leukoc Biol 2007;81(4):916–24.
30. Dellon ES, Jensen ET, Martin CF, et al. Prevalence of eosinophilic esophagitis in the United States. Clin Gastroenterol Hepatol 2013. [Epub ahead of print].
31. Jensen ET, Kappelman MD, Kim H, et al. Early life exposures as risk factors for pediatric eosinophilic esophagitis. J Pediatr Gastroenterol Nutr 2013;57(1): 67–71.
32. Stuck MC, Straumann A, Simon HU. Relative lack of T regulatory cells in adult eosinophilic esophagitis–no normalization after corticosteroid therapy. Allergy 2011;66(5):705–7.
33. Zhu X, Wang M, Crump CH, et al. An imbalance of esophageal effector and regulatory T cell subsets in experimental eosinophilic esophagitis in mice. Am J Physiol Gastrointest Liver Physiol 2009;297(3):G550–8.
34. Ganeshan K, Neilsen CV, Hadsaitong A, et al. Impairing oral tolerance promotes allergy and anaphylaxis: a new murine food allergy model. J Allergy Clin Immunol 2009;123(1):231–8.e4.
35. Rayapudi M, Mavi P, Zhu X, et al. Indoor insect allergens are potent inducers of experimental eosinophilic esophagitis in mice. J Leukoc Biol 2010;88(2):337–46.
36. Akei HS, Mishra A, Blanchard C, et al. Epicutaneous antigen exposure primes for experimental eosinophilic esophagitis in mice. Gastroenterology 2005; 129(3):985–94.
37. Slack MA, Erwin EA, Cho CB, et al. Food and aeroallergen sensitization in adult eosinophilic esophagitis. Ann Allergy Asthma Immunol 2013;111(4):304–5.
38. Spergel JM, Brown-Whitehorn TF, Beausoleil JL, et al. 14 years of eosinophilic esophagitis: clinical features and prognosis. J Pediatr Gastroenterol Nutr 2009;48(1):30–6.
39. Wang FY, Gupta SK, Fitzgerald JF. Is there a seasonal variation in the incidence or intensity of allergic eosinophilic esophagitis in newly diagnosed children? J Clin Gastroenterol 2007;41(5):451–3.
40. Simon D, Straumann A, Dahinden C, et al. Frequent sensitization to Candida albicans and profilins in adult eosinophilic esophagitis. Allergy 2013;68(7):945–8.
41. van Rhijn BD, van Ree R, Versteeg SA, et al. Birch pollen sensitization with cross-reactivity to food allergens predominates in adults with eosinophilic esophagitis. Allergy 2013;68(11):1475–81.
42. de Fraissinette A, Schmitt D, Thivolet J. Langerhans cells of human mucosa. J Dermatol 1989;16(4):255–62.
43. Terris B, Potet F. Structure and role of Langerhans' cells in the human oesophageal epithelium. Digestion 1995;56(Suppl 1):9–14.
44. Teitelbaum JE, Fox VL, Twarog FJ, et al. Eosinophilic esophagitis in children: immunopathological analysis and response to fluticasone propionate. Gastroenterology 2002;122(5):1216–25.

45. Lucendo AJ, Navarro M, Comas C, et al. Immunophenotypic characterization and quantification of the epithelial inflammatory infiltrate in eosinophilic esophagitis through stereology: an analysis of the cellular mechanisms of the disease and the immunologic capacity of the esophagus. Am J Surg Pathol 2007; 31(4):598–606.

46. Bannert C, Bidmon-Fliegenschnee B, Stary G, et al. Fc-epsilon-RI, the high affinity IgE-receptor, is robustly expressed in the upper gastrointestinal tract and modulated by mucosal inflammation. PLoS One 2012;7(7):e42066.

47. Yen EH, Hornick JL, Dehlink E, et al. Comparative analysis of FcepsilonRI expression patterns in patients with eosinophilic and reflux esophagitis. J Pediatr Gastroenterol Nutr 2010;51(5):584–92.

48. Bieber T. The pro- and anti-inflammatory properties of human antigen-presenting cells expressing the high affinity receptor for IgE (Fc epsilon RI). Immunobiology 2007;212(6):499–503.

49. Buning J, von Smolinski D, Tafazzoli K, et al. Multivesicular bodies in intestinal epithelial cells: responsible for MHC class II-restricted antigen processing and origin of exosomes. Immunology 2008;125(4):510–21.

50. Heyman M. Symposium on 'dietary influences on mucosal immunity'. How dietary antigens access the mucosal immune system. Proc Nutr Soc 2001;60(4): 419–26.

51. Mulder DJ, Pooni A, Mak N, et al. Antigen presentation and MHC class II expression by human esophageal epithelial cells: role in eosinophilic esophagitis. Am J Pathol 2011;178(2):744–53.

52. Akuthota P, Wang H, Weller PF. Eosinophils as antigen-presenting cells in allergic upper airway disease. Curr Opin Allergy Clin Immunol 2010;10(1):14–9.

53. Shi HZ, Humbles A, Gerard C, et al. Lymph node trafficking and antigen presentation by endobronchial eosinophils. J Clin Invest 2000;105(7):945–53.

54. Wang HB, Ghiran I, Matthaei K, et al. Airway eosinophils: allergic inflammation recruited professional antigen-presenting cells. J Immunol 2007;179(11): 7585–92.

55. Patel AJ, Fuentebella J, Gernez Y, et al. Increased HLA-DR expression on tissue eosinophils in eosinophilic esophagitis. J Pediatr Gastroenterol Nutr 2010;51(3): 290–4.

56. Le-Carlson M, Seki S, Abarbanel D, et al. Markers of antigen presentation and activation on eosinophils and T cells in the esophageal tissue of patients with eosinophilic esophagitis. J Pediatr Gastroenterol Nutr 2013;56(3): 257–62.

57. Straumann A, Bauer M, Fischer B, et al. Idiopathic eosinophilic esophagitis is associated with a T(H)2-type allergic inflammatory response. J Allergy Clin Immunol 2001;108(6):954–61.

58. Blanchard C, Mingler MK, Vicario M, et al. IL-13 involvement in eosinophilic esophagitis: transcriptome analysis and reversibility with glucocorticoids. J Allergy Clin Immunol 2007;120(6):1292–300.

59. Blanchard C, Stucke EM, Rodriguez-Jimenez B, et al. A striking local esophageal cytokine expression profile in eosinophilic esophagitis. J Allergy Clin Immunol 2011;127(1):208–17, 217.e1–7.

60. Mishra A, Hogan SP, Brandt EB, et al. IL-5 promotes eosinophil trafficking to the esophagus. J Immunol 2002;168(5):2464–9.

61. Persad R, Huynh HQ, Hao L, et al. Angiogenic remodeling in pediatric EoE is associated with increased levels of VEGF-A, angiogenin, IL-8, and activation of the TNF-alpha-NFkappaB pathway. J Pediatr Gastroenterol Nutr 2012;55(3):251–60.

62. Zhu X, Wang M, Mavi P, et al. Interleukin-15 expression is increased in human eosinophilic esophagitis and mediates pathogenesis in mice. Gastroenterology 2010;139(1):182–93.e7.

63. Siracusa MC, Saenz SA, Hill DA, et al. TSLP promotes interleukin-3-independent basophil haematopoiesis and type 2 inflammation. Nature 2011;477(7363): 229–33.

64. Giacomin PR, Siracusa MC, Walsh KP, et al. Thymic stromal lymphopoietin-dependent basophils promote Th2 cytokine responses following intestinal helminth infection. J Immunol 2012;189(9):4371–8.

65. Cheng E, Zhang X, Huo X, et al. Omeprazole blocks eotaxin-3 expression by oesophageal squamous cells from patients with eosinophilic oesophagitis and GORD. Gut 2013;62(6):824–32.

66. Prussin C, Lee J, Foster B. Eosinophilic gastrointestinal disease and peanut allergy are alternatively associated with IL-5+ and IL-5(-) T(H)2 responses. J Allergy Clin Immunol 2009;124(6):1326–32.e6.

67. O'Byrne PM, Inman MD, Parameswaran K. The trials and tribulations of IL-5, eosinophils, and allergic asthma. J Allergy Clin Immunol 2001; 108(4):503–8.

68. Mavi P, Rajavelu P, Rayapudi M, et al. Esophageal functional impairments in experimental eosinophilic esophagitis. Am J Physiol Gastrointest Liver Physiol 2012;302(11):G1347–55.

69. Mishra A, Wang M, Pemmaraju VR, et al. Esophageal remodeling develops as a consequence of tissue specific IL-5-induced eosinophilia. Gastroenterology 2008;134(1):204–14.

70. Lucendo AJ, De Rezende L, Comas C, et al. Treatment with topical steroids downregulates IL-5, eotaxin-1/CCL11, and eotaxin-3/CCL26 gene expression in eosinophilic esophagitis. Am J Gastroenterol 2008;103(9):2184–93.

71. Reddy V, Ghaffari G. Eosinophilic esophagitis: review of nonsurgical treatment modalities. Allergy Asthma Proc 2013;34(5):421–6.

72. Straumann A, Kristl J, Conus S, et al. Cytokine expression in healthy and inflamed mucosa: probing the role of eosinophils in the digestive tract. Inflamm Bowel Dis 2005;11(8):720–6.

73. Mishra A, Rothenberg ME. Intratracheal IL-13 induces eosinophilic esophagitis by an IL-5, eotaxin-1, and STAT6-dependent mechanism. Gastroenterology 2003;125(5):1419–27.

74. Blanchard C, Durual S, Estienne M, et al. Eotaxin-3/CCL26 gene expression in intestinal epithelial cells is up-regulated by interleukin-4 and interleukin-13 via the signal transducer and activator of transcription 6. Int J Biochem Cell Biol 2005;37(12):2559–73.

75. Blanchard C, Stucke EM, Burwinkel K, et al. Coordinate interaction between IL-13 and epithelial differentiation cluster genes in eosinophilic esophagitis. J Immunol 2010;184(7):4033–41.

76. Blanchard C, Mingler MK, McBride M, et al. Periostin facilitates eosinophil tissue infiltration in allergic lung and esophageal responses. Mucosal Immunol 2008; 1(4):289–96.

77. Niranjan R, Rayapudi M, Mishra A, et al. Pathogenesis of allergen-induced eosinophilic esophagitis is independent of interleukin (IL)-13. Immunol Cell Biol 2013;91(6):408–15.

78. He R, Kim HY, Yoon J, et al. Exaggerated IL-17 response to epicutaneous sensitization mediates airway inflammation in the absence of IL-4 and IL-13. J Allergy Clin Immunol 2009;124(4):761–70.e1.

79. Sherrill JD, Kc K, Wu D, et al. Desmoglein-1 regulates esophageal epithelial barrier function and immune responses in eosinophilic esophagitis. Mucosal Immunol 2013. [Epub ahead of print].

80. Zuo L, Fulkerson PC, Finkelman FD, et al. IL-13 induces esophageal remodeling and gene expression by an eosinophil-independent, IL-13R alpha 2-inhibited pathway. J Immunol 2010;185(1):660–9.

81. Bryce PJ, Oettgen HC. Antigen-independent effects of immunoglobulin E. Curr Allergy Asthma Rep 2005;5(3):186–90.

82. Rocha R, Vitor AB, Trindade E, et al. Omalizumab in the treatment of eosinophilic esophagitis and food allergy. Eur J Pediatr 2011;170(11):1471–4.

83. Hogan SP, Rosenberg HF, Moqbel R, et al. Eosinophils: biological properties and role in health and disease. Clin Exp Allergy 2008;38(5):709–50.

84. Aceves SS, Chen D, Newbury RO, et al. Mast cells infiltrate the esophageal smooth muscle in patients with eosinophilic esophagitis, express TGF-beta1, and increase esophageal smooth muscle contraction. J Allergy Clin Immunol 2010;126(6):1198–204.e4.

85. Furuta GT, Kagalwalla AF, Lee JJ, et al. The oesophageal string test: a novel, minimally invasive method measures mucosal inflammation in eosinophilic oesophagitis. Gut 2013;62(10):1395–405.

86. Blanchard C, Wang N, Stringer KF, et al. Eotaxin-3 and a uniquely conserved gene-expression profile in eosinophilic esophagitis. J Clin Invest 2006;116(2):536–47.

87. Rajavelu P, Rayapudi M, Moffitt M, et al. Significance of para-esophageal lymph nodes in food or aeroallergen-induced iNKT cell-mediated experimental eosinophilic esophagitis. Am J Physiol Gastrointest Liver Physiol 2012;302(7):G645–54.

88. Yu S, Stahl E, Li Q, et al. Antigen inhalation induces mast cells and eosinophils infiltration in the guinea pig esophageal epithelium involving histamine-mediated pathway. Life Sci 2008;82(5–6):324–30.

89. Zhang S, Wu X, Yu S. Prostaglandin D2 receptor d-type prostanoid receptor 2 mediates eosinophil trafficking into the esophagus. Dis Esophagus 2013. [Epub ahead of print].

90. Straumann A, Hoesli S, Bussmann C, et al. Anti-eosinophil activity and clinical efficacy of the CRTH2 antagonist OC000459 in eosinophilic esophagitis. Allergy 2013;68(3):375–85.

91. Rubinstein E, Cho JY, Rosenthal P, et al. Siglec-F inhibition reduces esophageal eosinophilia and angiogenesis in a mouse model of eosinophilic esophagitis. J Pediatr Gastroenterol Nutr 2011;53(4):409–16.

92. Shakoory B, Fitzgerald SM, Lee SA, et al. The role of human mast cell-derived cytokines in eosinophil biology. J Interferon Cytokine Res 2004;24(5):271–81.

93. Hsu Blatman KS, Gonsalves N, Hirano I, et al. Expression of mast cell-associated genes is upregulated in adult eosinophilic esophagitis and responds to steroid or dietary therapy. J Allergy Clin Immunol 2011;127(5):1307–8.e3.

94. Cho JY, Rosenthal P, Miller M, et al. Targeting AMCase reduces esophageal eosinophilic inflammation and remodeling in a mouse model of egg induced eosinophilic esophagitis. Int Immunopharmacol 2013;18(1):35–42.

95. Niranjan R, Mavi P, Rayapudi M, et al. Pathogenic role of mast cells in experimental eosinophilic esophagitis. Am J Physiol Gastrointest Liver Physiol 2013;304(12):G1087–94.

96. Otani IM, Anilkumar AA, Newbury RO, et al. Anti-IL-5 therapy reduces mast cell and IL-9 cell numbers in pediatric patients with eosinophilic esophagitis. J Allergy Clin Immunol 2013;131(6):1576–82.

Clinical Implications and Pathogenesis of Esophageal Remodeling in Eosinophilic Esophagitis

Ikuo Hirano, MD[a], Seema S. Aceves, MD, PhD[b],*

KEYWORDS

- Eosinophilic esophagitis • Remodeling • Fibrosis • Gastroesophageal reflux disease
- Dysphagia • Endoscopy • Esophagitis

KEY POINTS

- Remodeling changes in eosinophilic esophagitis include epithelial basal zone hyperplasia, lamina propria fibrosis, expansion of the muscularis propria, and increased vascularity.
- Esophageal inflammation in eosinophilic esophagitis drives the remodeling process with mediators that include IL-5, IL-13, TGFβ1, mast cells, fibroblasts, and eosinophils.
- Recent studies have provided increasing evidence that the primary symptoms of esophageal dysfunction in children and adults as well as clinical complications of eosinophilic esophagitis are consequences of esophageal remodeling and fibrostenosis.
- Esophageal remodeling in eosinophilic esophagitis can be demonstrated using widely available tests, such as histopathology, barium esophagram, upper endoscopy, and endoscopic ultrasonography.
- Clinical trials need to account for the presence and reversibility of esophageal remodeling to fully elucidate the potential benefits and limitations of therapeutic interventions.

INTRODUCTION

Since the initial case descriptions 2 decades ago, eosinophilic esophagitis (EoE) has emerged as an important clinical entity with steadily rising prevalence.[1] In children, EoE is an increasingly recognized etiology for feeding disorders and manifests with poor weight gain, anorexia, vomiting, regurgitation, abdominal pain, and dysphagia. In adult patients, EoE is one of the most common causes of dysphagia. An increasing

[a] Division of Gastroenterology, Northwestern University Feinberg School of Medicine, 676 North Saint Clair, Suite 1400, Chicago, IL 60611, USA; [b] Division of Allergy and Immunology, Departments of Pediatrics and Medicine, University of California, San Diego, Rady Children's Hospital, San Diego, 9500 Gilman Drive, MC-0760, La Jolla, CA 92093-0760, USA
* Corresponding author. 9500 Gilman Drive, MC-0760, La Jolla, CA 92093-0760.
E-mail address: saceves@ucsd.edu

Gastroenterol Clin N Am 43 (2014) 297–316
http://dx.doi.org/10.1016/j.gtc.2014.02.015
0889-8553/14/$ – see front matter © 2014 Elsevier Inc. All rights reserved.

gastro.theclinics.com

number of studies have shown that the primary symptoms in children and adults, as well as clinical complications of EoE, are consequences of esophageal remodeling and fibrostenosis. This article focuses on the current understanding of the pathogenesis, clinical detection, and therapeutic implications of esophageal remodeling in EoE.

DEFINITION OF ESOPHAGEAL REMODELING

The concept of eosinophil-associated tissue remodeling stems from diseases such as the hypereosinophilic syndrome and asthma. Remodeling can be defined as tissue changes in target organs that result in end organ dysfunction. Remodeling is associated with histologic alterations, such as fibrosis and angiogenesis, which are caused by changes in cellular function, phenotype, and products. Remodeling itself may not be a pathogenic process, as it could be considered to represent a protective mechanism akin to wound healing. However, when remodeling is not controlled, presumably due to unbridled inflammation, there are negative consequences for organ function. Indeed, the natural history of untreated EoE is to progress to stricture formation, at least in adults.[2,3]

In EoE, remodeling changes are seen histologically in both the epithelium and subepithelium (**Fig. 1**). Epithelial changes include basal zone hyperplasia and increased length of the vascular papillae. The papillae are intrusions of the subepithelium into the epithelial space and, as such, are likely a further reflection of subepithelial expansion. Subepithelial changes include lamina propria fibrosis with increased collagen deposition and thickness and increased vascularity with vascular activation. Muscularis remodeling changes include smooth muscle hypertrophy and hyperplasia. Together these tissue changes are the likely mechanisms for the esophageal

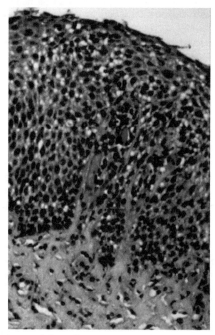

Fig. 1. Histopathology of remodeling changes in EoE. The squamous epithelium shows basal zone hyperplasia and LP shows increased collagen density in EoE. (original magnification ×400)

dysfunction that characterizes EoE and underlies the clinical complications of dysphagia, strictures, food impactions, esophageal rigidity, and dysmotility. Ultimately it is the potential control of the clinical consequences of remodeling that motivates practitioners to treat EoE. In this vain, the assumption is that control of inflammation is equated to control of remodeling. However, this has yet to be systematically proven.

Although it is recommended that there is recurrent tissue procurement for EoE management, this is not the case in other eosinophil-associated diseases. This paucity of repeatedly acquired human tissue has limited our understanding of the true clinical implications of tissue remodeling. For this reason, EoE provides a unique opportunity to understand the clinical complications, natural history, and reversibility of eosinophil-associated tissue remodeling. This is further underscored by the fact that young children have recurrent tissue assessments, allowing us to investigate the long-term effects of tissue architectural changes on esophageal function and EoE progression. If EoE is akin to asthma, a person's fibrotic phenotype may be defined very early in life.

For the purposes of this review, tissue remodeling as it relates to EoE is considered to be composed of epithelial changes, including basal cell hyperplasia and epithelial mesenchymal transition, subepithelial changes of fibrosis and angiogenesis, and smooth muscle hypertrophy. We provide a summary of the current molecular and clinical data that support the hypothesis that esophageal tissue remodeling (1) is driven by EoE-associated esophageal inflammation, and (2) is the underlying etiology for major EoE clinical symptoms and complications.

PATHOGENESIS OF ESOPHAGEAL REMODELING IN EoE

Inflammatory mediators and cells clearly play a role in driving esophageal remodeling (**Table 1, Fig. 2**). Animal models demonstrate that mice lacking eosinophils or the eosinophilopoetic cytokine interleukin (IL)-5, have significantly less collagen deposition and fibronectin expression than their wild-type littermates.[4,5] In addition, mice that have decreased esophageal eosinophils also have decreased basal zone hyperplasia.[5] Importantly, a lack of eosinophils, even in the presence of IL-5 overexpression, leads to decreases in stricture formation. In contrast, there is no effect of eosinophil loss on esophageal dysmotility.[6] Overexpression of IL-13 causes esophageal stricture that is not reversible by the subsequent removal of IL-13.[6] This underscores a number of important concepts. First, there is a dependence on eosinophilic inflammation to drive strictures. Second, interleukins in the absence of subsets of cellular inflammation can have distinct effects. Third, various esophageal remodeling features can be uncoupled and can use distinct mechanistic pathways (see **Fig. 2**).

Esophageal eosinophils in EoE produce the profibrotic factor, transforming growth factor beta-1 (TGFβ1), which can increase the production of collagen, fibronectin, and other extracellular matrix proteins.[7–9] TGFβ1 mRNA and protein levels are elevated in the epithelium and subepithelium of pediatric and adult subjects with EoE when compared with control subjects. In addition to TGFβ1, other profibrotic molecules, including CC chemokine ligand 18 (CCL-18) and fibroblast growth factor 9 (FGF-9) are increased in subjects with EoE, suggesting that there are also TGFβ1 independent pathways to fibrosis.[10,11] Increased numbers of lamina propria (LP) cells that express phosphorylated Smad2/3, part of the canonical TGFβ1 transcription factor complex, are also found in the LP of pediatric subjects with EoE. Profibrotic factors, such as FGF-9 and TGFβ1, also can have effects on the function of epithelial cells, including proliferation and epithelial mesenchymal transformation.[11,12]

Mast cells are important in EoE pathogenesis. Indeed, the numbers of mast cells infiltrating the deeper esophageal layers, such as the muscularis mucosa, can exceed

Table 1
Mediators of esophageal remodeling in eosinophilic esophagitis

Mediator	Remodeling Effects	Evidence
IL-5	Increased collagen	Animal models
	Increased smooth muscle contraction force	Animal models
	Increased epithelial TGFβ1	Human anti–IL-5 trials
	Increased tenascin C	Human anti–IL-5 trials
IL-13	Increased collagen deposition	Animal models
	Increased esophageal thickness	
	Stricture formation	
Periostin	Increased periostin deposition in lamina propria	Human in vitro studies
	Increased eosinophil trafficking	
Siglec-8	Increased fibronectin	Animal models
	Increased angiogenesis	
Smad3	Increased fibronectin	Animal models
	Increased angiogenesis	
TGFβ1	Increased fibrosis	Human in vitro studies
	Smooth muscle cell contraction	
TSLP	Increased food impactions	Animal models
Eosinophils	Increased fibrosis	Animal models
	Strictures	
	Increased tenascin	Human anti–IL-5 studies
	Increased epithelial TGFβ1	
Mast cells	Smooth muscle hypertrophy and hyperplasia	Animal studies
Basophils	Increased food impactions	Animal studies

Abbreviations: IL, interleukin; TGFβ1, transforming growth factor beta 1; TSLP, thymic stromal lymphopoietin.

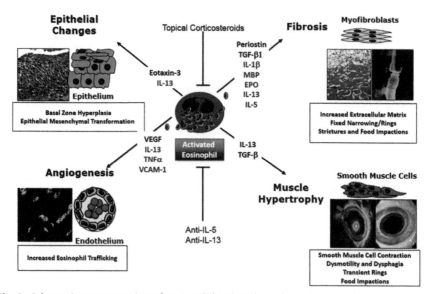

Fig. 2. Schematic representation of eosinophil-induced esophageal remodeling, key interleukins, and cytokines and its clinical consequences. *Red arrow* indicates the thickened esophageal wall. (*Adapted from* Aceves SS, Ackerman SJ. Relationships between eosinophilic inflammation, tissue remodeling, and fibrosis in eosinophilic esophagitis. Immunol Allergy Clin North Am 2009;29(1):197–211, xiii–xiv; with permission.)

the numbers of eosinophils.[13] Both eosinophils and mast cells also provide a source of TGFβ1 in EoE and a distinct mast cell transcript signature is present in both pediatric and adult subjects with EoE.[13–15] Mast cells are found in couplets with eosinophils in the esophagus of subjects with EoE and eosinophils produce the mast cell survival and recruitment factor, IL-9, suggesting that there is an intricate balance between eosinophilia and mastocytosis in EoE.[16] Animal studies have shown that mast cells and eosinophils travel together in EoE models. There is a decrease in smooth muscle hypertrophy and proliferation in mast cell–deficient mice.[17] As such, it is likely that mast cells not only promote fibrosis but also alter smooth muscle function during the process of esophageal remodeling.

IL-13 is a master regulator in EoE, functioning to increase both IL-5 and eotaxin-3 in the esophagus.[18,19] Pulmonary overexpression of IL-13 using a Clara cell promoter demonstrates increased fibrosis and esophageal circumference.[20] The effects of IL-13 can be independent of eosinophils and can promote the formation of irreversible strictures.[6,20] Both IL-13 and TGFβ1 increase the levels of periostin, an extracellular matrix protein that promotes the migration and adherence of eosinophils, thus propagating inflammation in EoE.[21]

Subepithelial angiogenesis is present in EoE.[5,7,22] Consistent with this, there are elevated levels of proangiogenic factors, including vascular endothelial growth factor (VEGF) and angiotensin in the esophagus of pediatric subjects with EoE.[22] Increased vascularity provides elevated numbers of conduits for the transport of inflammatory cells into the esophagus. Elevated levels of vascular activation factors described in EoE, such as vascular cell adhesion molecule 1, allow vessels to have increased tethering and transmigration of inflammatory cells.[7,22] Indeed, mice deficient in eosinophils have diminished levels of angiogenesis.[5]

Human studies using endoscopic ultrasound demonstrate increased esophageal thickness through all the esophageal layers, including the concentric and longitudinal muscle layers, in pediatric and adult subjects with EoE.[9,23] Subsets of subjects with EoE have altered esophageal motility on manometric studies that assess concentric muscle function and studies that analyze both concentric and longitudinal muscle layers demonstrate significant changes in the coordination between these smooth muscle layers.[24–27] Functionally, TGFβ1 can cause direct contraction of primary esophageal smooth muscle cells in culture, suggesting that inflammatory cell–derived growth factors can alter esophageal muscle cell function.[13,28] In addition, transgenic mice that overexpress IL-5 have increased longitudinal and circular smooth muscle contraction force.[6] Interestingly, these IL-5 transgenic mice that lack eosinophils continue to have increased contraction force, demonstrating that although strictures depend on the presence of eosinophils, dysmotility uses other inflammatory cells and/or factors.[6] Human data demonstrate that there is transmural inflammation with both eosinophilia and mastocytosis of the muscularis propria.[29,30] It is likely that the presence of such inflammatory cells and their chemical mediators would have functional consequences in EoE. Consistent with this concept, mice deficient in thymic stromal lymphopoietin (TSLP) or basophils are protected from food impactions in an experimental EoE model, demonstrating that TSLP and basophils play significant roles in esophageal dysfunction.[31]

RELATIONSHIP OF ESOPHAGEAL REMODELING WITH CLINICAL MANIFESTATIONS AND COMPLICATIONS

The clinical presentations of EoE reflect esophageal dysfunction. These functional changes in the esophagus likely reflect esophageal remodeling. In adults, EoE is dominated by symptoms of dysphagia and food impaction, whereas in children symptoms more commonly mimic gastroesophageal reflux disease (GERD) with dysphagia and food impactions becoming more prominent in adolescence. In adult subjects, there are 2 determinants for esophageal food impaction risk: (1) a reduction in luminal diameter and (2) limitation in esophageal mural distensibility. These features can occur concurrently or separately. Esophageal strictures, defined as a reduction of normal caliber, can be identified in 30% to 80% of adults with EoE, whereas decreased distensibility is reported in more than 70% of adults with EoE. It is important to note that the rates of esophageal mural rigidity have not been defined in pediatric EoE and, as such, the disease duration of EoE that causes decreased esophageal compliance in children is not clear. Certainly, esophageal strictures are uncommonly identified in children (<5% of subjects with EoE), even though food impactions occur in up to 30% of subjects. In adults, strictures defined as a reduction in luminal diameter to less than 10 mm have been reported in 38%.[2] The strictures can involve any portion of the esophagus, with many patients demonstrating diffusely compromised esophageal diameter, a condition termed "narrow or small-caliber" esophagus.[32] It is possible that lower-grade esophageal stenosis is underreported in the literature because of a lack of sensitivity for such luminal narrowing using the currently available endoscopic and radiographic techniques. Duration of untreated disease has been associated with increased risk of esophageal stricture, supporting the concept of progressive esophageal remodeling in EoE that may explain phenotypic differences between children and adults (**Fig. 3**).[2,33,34]

Both food impactions and strictures have significant complications. For example, food impactions that require emergency room visits and urgent endoscopic extraction is reported in 30% to 55% of adult cohorts with complications that include chest pain, as well as the risks of aspiration, esophageal tears, and esophageal perforation.[1] Esophageal perforation is also a recognized complication of endoscopic extraction of food impactions, particularly when food extraction is performed using rigid

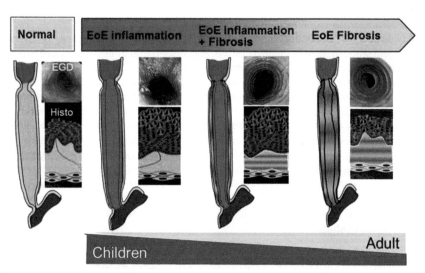

Fig. 3. Conceptual model of the consequences of esophageal remodeling. Esophageal remodeling over time leads to increasing subepithelial fibrosis that is associated with progressive esophageal structuring and narrow-caliber esophagus. This model may explain phenotypic differences between pediatric and adult presentations of eosinophilic esophagitis.

endoscopy. Furthermore, several reports of esophageal perforation related to esophageal dilation of strictures have led to reluctance in performing this therapy in EoE.[35]

Additional potential complications of EoE as they relate to esophageal remodeling include impaired quality of life and risk of nutritional deficiency because of dietary restriction. Most aspects of diminished quality of life in adults with EoE are related to the need for dietary modification and social embarrassment, as well as anxiety created by choking episodes.[36] Nutritional concerns in EoE can be related to food aversion that may be secondary to the inflammatory response to specific food antigens. In adults, decreased esophageal mural compliance and distensibility may limit the tolerability of specific foods due to texture, most commonly meat.[26,37]

CLINICAL METHODS TO ASSESS REMODELING IN EoE
Barium Radiography

A variety of methods have been used in clinical practice and investigative studies to demonstrate the remodeling consequences of EoE (**Table 2**). One of the oldest methods to evaluate the structure of the gastrointestinal tract is barium radiography. Early case series demonstrated the association of marked restriction of the esophageal luminal caliber with EoE, characterized as a narrow caliber or small-caliber esophagus.[32] **Fig. 4** illustrates the diffuse nature of this finding. The multiple, ringlike stenoses spanning lengths of the esophagus were initially confused with congenital esophageal stenosis but were subsequently recognized to be a characteristic feature of EoE.[38] Most recently, Alexander characterized restriction of the esophageal diameter in a cohort of adults with EoE, demonstrating a reduction in both the maximum and minimum diameters compared with controls.[39] Radiologic assessment of esophageal remodeling is clinically feasible but does not assess for variations in diameter as a function of intraluminal distension forces. A small volume of barium with low intrabolus distension pressure will have a tendency to provide falsely low estimates of the diameter of an esophageal stricture, as the stiffness of the esophageal wall limits the ability of the wall to expand. Limited studies have used cross-sectional imaging modalities, such as computed tomography or magnetic resonance imaging, to characterize the intramural effects of EoE (**Fig. 5**).[40]

Endoscopy

Endoscopically detected esophageal features of EoE include longitudinal furrows, white exudates (plaques), edema (loss of vascular markings), rings (trachealization), and strictures. Prospective studies in EoE have identified endoscopic abnormalities in 93% of patients with EoE.[41] Endoscopic findings in patients with EoE have been shown to vary by age. Younger patients are more likely to have findings of exudates, furrows, edema, or a normal-appearing esophagus, whereas adult patients are more likely to have strictures, rings, narrow-caliber esophagus, and crepe-paper mucosa.[33,42] Fibrostenotic features, including strictures and lumen-compromising rings, are commonly identified in adults with EoE but only among a minority of pediatric patients with EoE (**Fig. 6**). The extensive lacerations of the esophageal wall following esophageal dilation provide evidence of the longitudinal extent of the reduced esophageal elasticity in adults with EoE (see **Fig. 6**).[43] Pediatric studies demonstrate that features of exudates, furrows, and loss of vascular markings correlate with histologic epithelial features that include eosinophilic inflammation, whereas only loss of vascular markings and furrows correlate with LP features of fibrosis.[44] In alignment with the concept that pediatric disease is more inflammatory and potentially less fibrotic in nature, endoscopy in pediatric EoE is commonly characterized by

Table 2
Clinical methods to detect esophageal remodeling in eosinophilic esophagitis

Method	Findings	Advantages	Disadvantages
Barium esophagram	Esophageal rings, strictures, narrow caliber esophagus	Availability, ease of testing, cost	Radiation exposure, 2-dimensional imaging, measures diameter but not distensibility or compliance
Upper endoscopy	Esophageal rings, strictures, narrow-caliber esophagus	Availability, routine use in management of EoE, capability of therapeutic dilation, validated classification, biopsy evaluation of histologic remodeling	Cost, limited accuracy in determination of stricture diameter
Esophageal manometry	Esophageal motor dysfunction including peristaltic integrity, esophageal pressurization, and esophagogastric junction function	Availability, cost, potential physiologic biomarker of esophageal remodeling	Patient tolerance, limited sensitivity and specificity of identified abnormalities, limited to measurement of circular and not longitudinal smooth muscle function
Esophageal biopsy	Lamina propria fibrosis, basal zone hyperplasia, rete peg elongation	Availability, routine use in management of EoE	Limited sensitivity for evaluable lamina propria, validation of methodology used for procurement and analysis needed, potential for sampling variability
Endoscopic ultrasonography	Increased thickness of mucosa, submucosa, muscularis propria	Availability, assessment of esophageal intramural remodeling	Cost, endoscope diameter may exceed esophageal diameter, validation of methodology needed, nonfunctional/nonquantifiable output
Functional luminal imaging	Reduction in esophageal distensibility and compliance	Objective quantification of organ-level esophageal remodeling consequences with demonstrated correlation with clinical outcomes	Limited availability, utility in pediatric patients unknown
Tissue biomarkers	TGFβ1, periostin, tenacin C, fibronectin	Potential increased sensitivity for remodeling, potential predictor of targeted therapies, may correlate with TGFβ1 genotypes/pharmacogenomics responses	Validation of methodology needed

Abbreviations: EoE, eosinophilic esophagitis; TGFβ1, transforming growth factor beta 1.

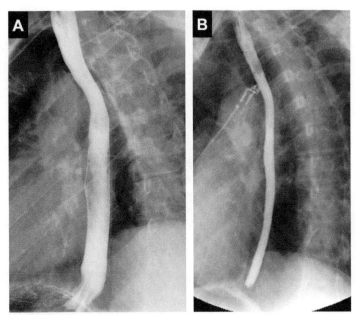

Fig. 4. Radiologic imaging in EoE. Barium esophagram in EoE. (*A*) A normal-caliber esophagus in a patient with GERD. (*B*) More than 50% reduction in luminal diameter of the entire esophagus in an adult with EoE, a manifestation referred to as a narrow or small-caliber esophagus.

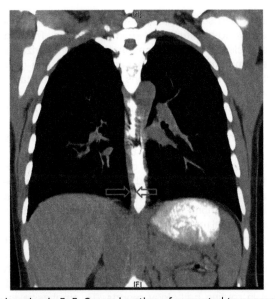

Fig. 5. Radiologic imaging in EoE. Coronal section of computed tomographic imaging illustrating the marked expansion of the esophageal wall in an adult with EoE. The imaging was obtained during ingestion of radiopaque contrast that clearly demarcates the inner lumen of the esophagus. The red arrows demarcate the mural thickness.

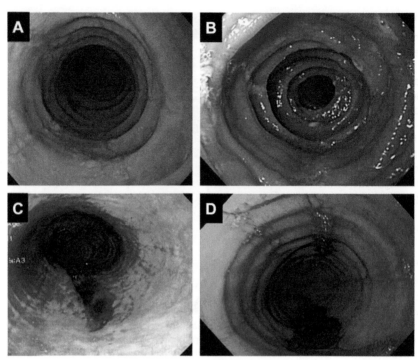

Fig. 6. Endoscopic imaging of 4 adult patients with EoE. (*A, B*) Remodeling changes of esophageal rings and stricture. (*C, D*) Esophageal mural tears that occurred following esophageal dilation, likely indicative of diffuse loss of esophageal elasticity.

inflammatory features with severe mucosal exudates. The presence of furrows and edema has been shown to be similar between age groups. The endoscopic findings correlate with typical clinical presentations that are characterized by anorexia/early satiety, GERD-like symptoms, and dysphagia in children and dysphagia with food impaction in adults.[45,46] These observations support an important distinction in the prevalence of fibrostenotic consequences of esophageal eosinophilia in different age groups and the concept of progressive remodeling with duration of disease (see **Fig. 3**).

A classification and grading system to assess the endoscopic findings in EoE has been proposed.[47] The acronym for the Endoscopic REFerence Scoring system, EREFS, designates the 5 major features of EoE (edema, rings, exudates, furrows, and stricture). This instrument was created to standardize and grade the endoscopic assessment performed by gastroenterologists. Although most features have good interobserver agreement among gastroenterologists, some of the endoscopic features that reflect esophageal remodeling were eliminated because of lack of sensitivity or problems with definition of terminology. Specifically, EREFS does not include either narrow-caliber esophagus or crepe-paper esophagus, which may be more specific signs of EoE remodeling likely related to the loss of tissue elasticity.[43] EREFS is an important tool that accounts for aspects of esophageal remodeling that are not currently captured in routine pathology reports. To emphasize the significance of endoscopically detected remodeling, the occurrence of food impaction, a clinically relevant symptom outcome of EoE, has recently been shown to be associated with the assessment of ring severity using the EREFS system.[46]

Endoscopic and Endoluminal Ultrasonography

Endoscopic ultrasonography depiction of expansion of the muscularis propria was described in an early case report of an elderly patient with eosinophilic esophagitis.[40] A small pediatric case series demonstrated significant increases in thickness of the combined mucosal-submucosa as well as muscularis propria in children with EoE.[23] Most recently, Straumann and colleagues[48] used endoscopic ultrasonography in a controlled trial of topical budesonide and demonstrated significant remodeling effects in adults with EoE. Doubling of the thickness of the mucosa and a 50% increase in the thickness of the muscularis propria were found, with the most marked difference being a threefold increase in submucosal thickness. Consistent with the natural history of EoE being a chronic, progressive disease associated with submucosal remodeling, the magnitude of the relative increases in mural thickness demonstrated in adults is greater than found in children with EoE (see **Fig. 3**). This observation supports the concept that remodeling in EoE is an ongoing process, with progression based on duration of disease.

Esophageal Manometry

The expansion of the muscularis propria on imaging, as well as reports of dysphagia in EoE in the absence of identified esophageal stricture, have led to the concept that esophageal motor function may be affected in EoE. Of note, the first 2 cases of "eosinophilic esophagitis" were reported in adults with major esophageal motility disorders; one having achalasia and the second having esophageal spasm.[49,50] Although these patients would be excluded from the current definition of EoE due to the presence of a major esophageal motility disorder and concomitant eosinophilic gastroenteritis,[1] the concept was introduced regarding potential for esophageal eosinophilia to result in esophageal motor dysfunction. A recent case report described an adult with more characteristic features of EoE with manometric findings consistent with achalasia.[51] The patient's dysphagia and manometry improved, but did not normalize, following treatment of systemic corticosteroids. Subsequent esophageal motility studies in adults with EoE have demonstrated hypertensive or weak peristaltic function in a subset of patients with EoE.[25,52] Nurko and colleagues[53] used prolonged ambulatory esophageal manometry to demonstrate a higher frequency of high-amplitude contractions and ineffective peristalsis in children with EoE compared with GERD or controls. Peristaltic dysfunction was observed during episodes of dysphagia, although cause and effect could not be differentiated, as the presence of a food bolus could itself secondarily alter esophageal motor function.

An investigation of adults using high-resolution esophageal manometry and Chicago classification systematically compared a cohort of 50 patients with EoE, 50 patients with GERD, and 50 healthy controls and demonstrated normal peristalsis in 64%, with 36% demonstrating nonspecific esophageal motor patterns dominated by weak and failed peristalsis.[24] Although such abnormalities could contribute to dysphagia, they are not accepted as major motility disorders because of limited direct correlation with symptoms. Furthermore, the frequency of these abnormal patterns was not significantly different from the motility abnormalities in the cohort of patients with GERD. A novel finding in this study was abnormal esophageal pressurization, characterized by pan esophageal pressurization in 16% and distal esophageal pressurization in 18%. Demonstration of this finding was accentuated by using a higher volume of swallowed boluses. Another study from Spain substantiated this observation through the demonstration of pan esophageal pressurization in 48% of patients with EoE and none of a control group.[54] The esophageal pressurization events in EoE may reflect reduced esophageal mural compliance secondary to the trans mural remodeling demonstrated on endoscopic ultrasonography imaging or alterations in motility that may occur secondary to EoE-associated inflammation and remodeling.

Conventional esophageal motility evaluates esophageal circular muscle function but does not assess longitudinal muscle contractions that are responsible for axial shortening of the esophagus. Using high-frequency ultrasonographic imaging, Korsapati and Mittal[27] assessed longitudinal muscle function in patients with EoE. Compared with healthy controls, patients with EoE showed significantly reduced longitudinal muscle peak thickness as well as duration of contraction. These results are consistent with selective longitudinal but not circular muscle dysfunction in EoE. However, an alternate explanation of the defect identified is that the longitudinal muscle function is intact but that transmural remodeling alterations in EoE mechanically restrict the ability of the esophagus to shorten. Regardless of the underlying cause, impaired esophageal shortening can be a mechanism that limits effective esophageal bolus transport and thereby contributes to dysphagia and food impactions.

In summary, the available studies evaluating esophageal motor function in EoE have demonstrated both hypercontractile and hypocontractile esophageal body functional abnormalities in subsets of children and adults that could impair esophageal bolus transport, especially when combined with structural defects. It should be acknowledged, however, that the manometric patterns identified are nonspecific and do not meet criteria for accepted, major esophageal motility disorders. Differences between motor patterns in children and adults are currently unclear but could potentially explain phenotypic distinctions in their clinical presentations. In most adults with EoE with normal peristalsis and lower esophageal sphincter relaxation, dysphagia is likely the result of reduced luminal caliber that is the consequence of decreased esophageal compliance and increased esophageal fibrosis/stiffness due to tissue remodeling. Increased esophageal pressurization events in adults with EoE may reflect the reduced ability of the esophagus to (1) adequately distend in response to an ingested bolus or (2) effectively clear the bolus due to defects in longitudinal muscle function or (3) a combination thereof. In children, esophageal motor defects may have a more substantial role in impairing bolus transit, a concept that needs further investigation. In addition to their possible clinical implications, functional deficits in EoE provide important insights regarding the pathophysiologic effects of esophageal eosinophilic inflammation.

Functional Luminal Imaging Probe

Fibrostenotic consequences of EoE can be visually estimated by endoscopy. However, the severity of esophageal rigidity cannot be quantified using standard endoscopy. As such, the novel and quantitative assessment of esophageal mural compliance at the whole-organ level using a functional luminal imaging probe (FLIP) is a better approach for assessing not only esophageal thickness but also the functional consequences of remodeling. The FLIP technology incorporates a multichannel electrical impedance catheter and manometric sensor surrounded by an infinitely compliant bag that is filled with an electrode conducting solution. As the bag is filled with the solution, the probe simultaneously ascertains the esophageal luminal diameter and pressure at multiple points along the catheter assembly. The resulting pressure-volume curves provide a detailed interrogation of the distensibility of the esophageal wall. An initial study of FLIP in patients with EoE demonstrated a significant reduction in distensibility in EoE compared with control subjects (**Fig. 7**).[37] A

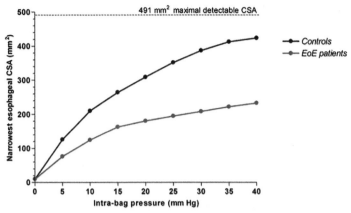

Fig. 7. Functional luminal imaging in EoE quantified remodeling effects of the esophagus. Esophageal distensibility plots in control subjects (*blue*) and EoE (*red*) demonstrating diminished distensibility for distension pressures higher than 5 mm Hg. The calculated value for constant cross-sectional area (CSA) in spite of increasing distension pressure is used to generate the distensibility plateau. (*Data from* Kwiatek MA, Hirano I, Kahrilas PJ, et al. Mechanical properties of the esophagus in eosinophilic esophagitis. Gastroenterology 2011;140(1):82–90.)

parameter called the distension plateau characterized the maximum ability of the esophagus to expand in spite of increasing intraluminal pressure at the point of minimal luminal diameter of the esophageal body. The distension plateau was reduced by 50% in EoE compared with controls.

Nicodème and colleagues[46] recently reported on the assessment of 70 patients with EoE who underwent endoscopy with esophageal biopsy and high-resolution impedance planimetry using a functional lumen-imaging probe. These patients were followed prospectively and rates of food impaction assessed. The study found that patients with a history of food impactions exhibited significantly lower esophageal distensibility, as measured by distensibility plateau values, than those with dysphagia alone. Decreased esophageal distensibility was found to be associated with an increased risk of food impaction and need for dilation during a 4- to 12-month follow-up period. The distensibility plateau was shown to be a more reliable predictor of food impaction risk than findings on endoscopy, although endoscopic estimations of strictures were not included in this comparison. Importantly, no correlation was found between epithelial eosinophil density and food impaction risk, need for dilation, or distensibility. The lack of correlation between esophageal distensibility and mucosal eosinophil density provides a number of potential insights into EoE disease mechanisms. Although epithelial eosinophilic inflammation is used to define one parameter of disease activity, it may not reflect the degree of submucosal disease activity. This is of particular relevance because the pathogenesis of remodeling lies largely below the mucosal surface. Mucosal eosinophilia is likely the harbinger of deeper tissue eosinophilia, as is seen in the LP and muscular layers in EoE. In turn, eosinophilia travels in conjunction with other inflammatory cells and mediators that drive fibrosis, angiogenesis, stenosis, and smooth muscle changes. As such, it appears that although fibrostenosis is an important determinant of clinically relevant symptoms and complications, the histologic finding of eosinophilic inflammation is likely to be the most relevant determinant for the future risk of fibrostenosis.

EFFECTIVENESS OF AVAILABLE THERAPIES FOR REMODELING IN EoE

EoE therapies are rapidly evolving as the mechanisms underlying the disease become better understood. Most drugs are in the early stages of development and none are currently approved by regulatory authorities for use in patients outside of clinical trials. Elimination diet therapy has demonstrated effectiveness similar to medical therapies in terms of resolution of mucosal eosinophilic inflammation. The primary end points used to judge the efficacy of therapies are symptoms and esophageal eosinophilic infiltration and to date have not been able to account for effects on esophageal remodeling.[34]

At this time, the most significant therapeutic efficacy on remodeling has been demonstrated with the use of topical, swallowed corticosteroids (**Table 3**). The benefits of these agents have been convincing in terms of resolving tissue inflammation.[9,55–57] Symptom benefits have been more difficult to demonstrate, likely because of limitations in available patient-reported outcome instruments, behavior modifications to compensate for symptoms, and the symptom-mucosal eosinophilia dissociation related to esophageal remodeling.[34,58] Available studies demonstrate heterogeneity regarding the ability to topical steroids to improve esophageal subepithelial fibrosis in EoE. It is likely that the ability to improve fibrotic changes depends on the degree of fibrosis, the duration of the disease, and the age of the subject with EoE. Aceves and colleagues[59] first described significant reduction in severity of fibrosis by using topical budesonide in children with EoE. This observation was confirmed by 2 subsequent pediatric series that used diet, topical fluticasone, or both, as well as in one adult study using topical budesonide.[9,60,61] It is important to note that in all of these studies, fibrosis improvement paralleled epithelial inflammatory improvement. In those patients who either did not improve with therapy or who were receiving placebo, both inflammation and fibrosis persisted.[9,59] Improvement of fibrostenosis with steroids has been less consistent in adult studies of EoE. A significant improvement in esophageal fibrosis using a histopathologic fibrosis score was demonstrated in a randomized controlled trial of adults following 15 days of topical budesonide by Straumann and colleagues.[9] In contrast, fibrosis score was reduced but did not reach

Table 3		
Eosinophilic esophagitis therapies and effect on esophageal remodeling		
Therapy	**Effectiveness**	**Population**
Topical corticosteroids	Decreased LP fibrosis in subsets of subjects	Adult and pediatric
	Decreased vascular activation in subset	Pediatric
	Decreased TGFβ1 in subset	Adult and pediatric
	Decreased pSmad2/3 in subset	Pediatric
Elimination diet	Decreased fibrosis	Pediatric
Elemental diet	Decreased thickening, plaques, no change in rings or strictures	Adult
Anti–IL-5	Decreased tenascin, decreased TGFβ1	Adult
Esophageal dilation	No change in inflammation or remodeling; does not address underlying disease etiology	Adult
Systemic steroids	No data	
Montelukast	No data	
Anti–IL-13	Results pending publication	Adult

Abbreviations: IL, interleukin; LP, lamina propria; TGFβ1, transforming growth factor beta 1.

statistical significance in an uncontrolled, prospective study following a year of topical fluticasone used in a nonconventional formulation.[9,10] In a follow-up, long-term maintenance, randomized controlled trial, Straumann and colleagues[48] demonstrated that neither epithelial eosinophilia nor histologic fibrosis control was well retained on low-dose budesonide (one-fourth of the initial 15-day treatment dose). In addition, although low-dose budesonide caused significant improvement in the mucosal thickness after 12 months of therapy, the submucosal and muscularis propria expansion on endoscopic ultrasonography were not significantly improved. Although both Aceves[56] (pediatric) and Straumann[9] (adult) have shown reduction in TGFβ1 expression after topical steroid therapy, a study of fluticasone demonstrated decreases only in CCL-18.[10] These differences in the results suggest several possibilities, such as an inability of topical corticosteroids to penetrate the deeper esophageal layers or phenotypic distinctions among subjects who have concordance versus discordance between epithelial inflammation and subepithelial fibrosis.

Given the conflicting data on improvement in histopathologic and biomarkers for remodeling, the variability of the clinical outcomes of controlled trials of topical steroids is not surprising. Prospective studies in adults with EoE with both topical steroids have demonstrated symptom improvement but persistence of endoscopically detected esophageal features of fibrostenosis, including rings and strictures.[9,33,62] In some contrast, Alexander and colleagues[39] found improvements in esophageal lumen diameter in the subset of subjects with more restricted pretreatment esophageal caliber following short-term topical budesonide. However, there were no significant improvements in luminal caliber on barium esophagram following 6 weeks of topical steroids among subjects who initially had a normal-caliber esophagus. Treatment of adults with elemental formula demonstrated improvements in endoscopic features that reflect inflammation (furrows, plaques) but not in the features of rings or strictures that likely reflect long-term tissue remodeling.[63] Together, the current therapeutic trials suggest that shorter-duration EoE and/or less severely remodeled esophagi may be more likely to demonstrate reversal of fibrosis.

Although corticosteroids are a frontline therapy for children and adults with EoE, there is a subset of patients with EoE patients who are steroid refractory.[64–66] In addition, given its chronic nature, EoE seems to require long-term topical corticosteroids or dietary management. As such, corticosteroid or elimination diet sparing agents and/or novel therapeutic strategies are of significant appeal in EoE.[66] To date, there have been 3 randomized studies in pediatric and adult EoE using anti–IL-5 and a single trial each in adults using anti–IL-13 and a CRTH2 antagonist. As such, these studies are still in their relative infancies. Studies using anti–IL-5 and CRTH2 antagonist have demonstrated statistically significant improvement with incomplete resolution of epithelial eosinophilia.[67–69] Symptoms were not significantly improved and the impacts on remodeling features were inconsistent with no significant changes in fibrosis in the pediatric anti–IL-5 study (one trial did not report results on fibrosis) but decreases in epithelial TGFβ1 and tenascin C in adult subjects.[68–70]

Animal models have provided preliminary preclinical data on potentially novel therapies that could improve EoE.[66] Treatment with anti–Siglec-F, the murine cognate for human Siglec-8,[71] causes decreased esophageal eosinophilia and concomitant decreases in remodeling.[5] Both angiogenesis and VEGF producing cells were decreased, as were basal zone hyperplasia and fibronectin expression. Smad3 is a member of the transcription factor complex downstream of canonical TGFβ1 signals. Mice deficient in Smad3, and therefore incapable of propagating TGFβ1 signals, have decreased fibrosis and angiogenesis with continued eosinophilia, demonstrating that antigen (ovalbumin)-induced esophageal remodeling can be diminished despite persistent eosinophilia in the face of absent TGFβ1 signals. As such, both anti–siglec-8 and anti-TGFβ1 therapies could be important for treating esophageal remodeling.[72] Current clinical trials using anti–IL-13 have been completed in adults with EoE but have not yet been published. Given its role in inducing fibrosis, strictures, and increased esophageal thickness in preclinical murine models, anti–IL-13 antibodies may represent an important therapeutic avenue in EoE.

The most rapidly effective treatment for symptomatic strictures in adults with EoE is esophageal dilation with either through-the-scope balloon or wire-guided bougie systems.[35] Dilation leads to mechanical disruption of fibrostenotic strictures. Relief of dysphagia is immediate and associated with significant patient-reported satisfaction.[73] Dilation, however, does not address the underlying inflammatory process responsible for the development of the stenosis. Although relief of dysphagia can continue for more than a year following esophageal dilation even in the absence of anti-inflammatory therapy, EoE is a chronic disease and symptomatic recurrence is expected in most patients.[2,74] As such, a reduction in esophageal inflammation and/or remodeling, rather than symptom relief, may be an appropriate primary end point of the therapeutics currently in development. Conceptually, inflammatory control will reduce the risk of ongoing esophageal remodeling and thereby prevent disease progression. Although this paradigm is yet unproven, the current emphasis on symptom outcomes only partially recognizes the contribution of remodeling effects and potentially deemphasizes the importance of anti-inflammatory benefits. Utilization of the most accurate therapeutic end points that acknowledge the fundamental importance of esophageal remodeling is essential to avoid overlooking valuable treatments for this important and growing disease.

In conclusion, remodeling changes are responsible for the major clinical symptoms and complications of EoE. Ongoing studies are investigating the mechanisms behind the chronic inflammation that drives the remodeling process. A variety of existing and novel biomarkers and tests provide important information on remodeling activity in patients with EoE. Clinical trials need to account for the presence and reversibility of esophageal remodeling to fully elucidate the potential benefits and limitations of therapeutic interventions.

REFERENCES

1. Liacouras CA, Furuta GT, Hirano I, et al. Eosinophilic esophagitis: updated consensus recommendations for children and adults. J Allergy Clin Immunol 2011;128(1):3–20.e6 [quiz: 21–2].
2. Schoepfer AM, Safroneeva E, Bussmann C, et al. Delay in diagnosis of eosinophilic esophagitis increases risk for stricture formation, in a time-dependent manner. Gastroenterology 2013;145(6):1230–6.e1–2.
3. Dellon ES, Gonsalves N, Hirano I, et al. ACG clinical guideline: evidenced based approach to the diagnosis and management of esophageal eosinophilia and eosinophilic esophagitis (EoE). Am J Gastroenterol 2013;108(5):679–92 [quiz: 693].
4. Mishra A, Wang M, Pemmaraju VR, et al. Esophageal remodeling develops as a consequence of tissue specific IL-5-induced eosinophilia. Gastroenterology 2008;134(1):204–14.
5. Rubinstein E, Cho JY, Rosenthal P, et al. Siglec-F inhibition reduces esophageal eosinophilia and angiogenesis in a mouse model of eosinophilic esophagitis. J Pediatr Gastroenterol Nutr 2011;53(4):409–16.

6. Mavi P, Rajavelu P, Rayapudi M, et al. Esophageal functional impairments in experimental eosinophilic esophagitis. Am J Physiol Gastrointest Liver Physiol 2012;302(11):G1347–55.
7. Aceves SS, Newbury RO, Dohil R, et al. Esophageal remodeling in pediatric eosinophilic esophagitis. J Allergy Clin Immunol 2007;119(1):206–12.
8. Mishra A. Mechanism of eosinophilic esophagitis. Immunol Allergy Clin North Am 2009;29(1):29–40, viii.
9. Straumann A, Conus S, Degen L, et al. Budesonide is effective in adolescent and adult patients with active eosinophilic esophagitis. Gastroenterology 2010;139(5):1526–37, 1537.e1.
10. Lucendo AJ, Arias A, De Rezende LC, et al. Subepithelial collagen deposition, profibrogenic cytokine gene expression, and changes after prolonged fluticasone propionate treatment in adult eosinophilic esophagitis: a prospective study. J Allergy Clin Immunol 2011;128(5):1037–46.
11. Mulder DJ, Pacheco I, Hurlbut DJ, et al. FGF9-induced proliferative response to eosinophilic inflammation in oesophagitis. Gut 2009;58(2):166–73.
12. Kagalwalla AF, Akhtar N, Woodruff SA, et al. Eosinophilic esophagitis: epithelial mesenchymal transition contributes to esophageal remodeling and reverses with treatment. J Allergy Clin Immunol 2012;129:1387–96.e7.
13. Aceves SS, Chen D, Newbury RO, et al. Mast cells infiltrate the esophageal smooth muscle in patients with eosinophilic esophagitis, express TGF-beta1, and increase esophageal smooth muscle contraction. J Allergy Clin Immunol 2010;126(6):1198–204.e4.
14. Abonia JP, Blanchard C, Butz BB, et al. Involvement of mast cells in eosinophilic esophagitis. J Allergy Clin Immunol 2010;126(1):140–9.
15. Hsu Blatman KS, Gonsalves N, Hirano I, et al. Expression of mast cell-associated genes is upregulated in adult eosinophilic esophagitis and responds to steroid or dietary therapy. J Allergy Clin Immunol 2011;127(5):1307–8.e3.
16. Otani IM, Anilkumar AA, Newbury RO, et al. Anti-IL-5 therapy reduces mast cell and IL-9 cell numbers in pediatric patients with eosinophilic esophagitis. J Allergy Clin Immunol 2013;131(6):1576–82.
17. Niranjan R, Mavi P, Rayapudi M, et al. Pathogenic role of mast cells in experimental eosinophilic esophagitis. Am J Physiol Gastrointest Liver Physiol 2013;304(12):G1087–94.
18. Blanchard C, Mingler MK, Vicario M, et al. IL-13 involvement in eosinophilic esophagitis: transcriptome analysis and reversibility with glucocorticoids. J Allergy Clin Immunol 2007;120(6):1292–300.
19. Blanchard C, Stucke EM, Burwinkel K, et al. Coordinate interaction between IL-13 and epithelial differentiation cluster genes in eosinophilic esophagitis. J Immunol 2010;184(7):4033–41.
20. Zuo L, Fulkerson PC, Finkelman FD, et al. IL-13 induces esophageal remodeling and gene expression by an eosinophil-independent, IL-13R alpha 2-inhibited pathway. J Immunol 2010;185(1):660–9.
21. Blanchard C, Mingler MK, McBride M, et al. Periostin facilitates eosinophil tissue infiltration in allergic lung and esophageal responses. Mucosal Immunol 2008;1(4):289–96.
22. Persad R, Huynh HQ, Hao L, et al. Angiogenic remodeling in pediatric EoE is associated with increased levels of VEGF-A, angiogenin, IL-8, and activation of the TNF-alpha-NFkappaB pathway. J Pediatr Gastroenterol Nutr 2012;55(3):251–60.
23. Fox VL, Nurko S, Teitelbaum JE, et al. High-resolution EUS in children with eosinophilic "allergic" esophagitis. Gastrointest Endosc 2003;57(1):30–6.

24. Roman S, Hirano I, Kwiatek MA, et al. Manometric features of eosinophilic esophagitis in esophageal pressure topography. Neurogastroenterol Motil 2011;23(3):208–14 e111.

25. Moawad FJ, Maydonovitch CL, Veerappan GR, et al. Esophageal motor disorders in adults with eosinophilic esophagitis. Dig Dis Sci 2011;56(5):1427–31.

26. Read AJ, Pandolfino JE. Biomechanics of esophageal function in eosinophilic esophagitis. J Neurogastroenterol Motil 2012;18(4):357–64.

27. Korsapati H, Babaei A, Bhargava V, et al. Dysfunction of the longitudinal muscles of the oesophagus in eosinophilic oesophagitis. Gut 2009;58(8):1056–62.

28. Abonia JP, Franciosi JP, Rothenberg ME. TGF-beta1: mediator of a feedback loop in eosinophilic esophagitis—or should we really say mastocytic esophagitis? J Allergy Clin Immunol 2010;126(6):1205–7.

29. Saffari H, Peterson KA, Fang JC, et al. Patchy eosinophil distributions in an esophagectomy specimen from a patient with eosinophilic esophagitis: implications for endoscopic biopsy. J Allergy Clin Immunol 2012;130(3):798–800.

30. Nicholson AG, Li D, Pastorino U, et al. Full thickness eosinophilia in oesophageal leiomyomatosis and idiopathic eosinophilic oesophagitis. A common allergic inflammatory profile? J Pathol 1997;183(2):233–6.

31. Noti M, Wojno ED, Kim BS, et al. Thymic stromal lymphopoietin-elicited basophil responses promote eosinophilic esophagitis. Nat Med 2013;19(8):1005–13.

32. Vasilopoulos S, Murphy P, Auerbach A, et al. The small-caliber esophagus: an unappreciated cause of dysphagia for solids in patients with eosinophilic esophagitis. Gastrointest Endosc 2002;55(1):99–106.

33. Straumann A, Schoepfer AM. Therapeutic concepts in adult and paediatric eosinophilic oesophagitis. Nat Rev Gastroenterol Hepatol 2012;9(12):697–704.

34. Hirano I. Therapeutic end points in eosinophilic esophagitis: is elimination of esophageal eosinophils enough? Clin Gastroenterol Hepatol 2012;10(7):750–2.

35. Hirano I. Dilation in eosinophilic esophagitis: to do or not to do? Gastrointest Endosc 2010;71(4):713–4.

36. Taft TH, Kern E, Keefer L, et al. Qualitative assessment of patient-reported outcomes in adults with eosinophilic esophagitis. J Clin Gastroenterol 2011;45(9):769–74.

37. Kwiatek MA, Hirano I, Kahrilas PJ, et al. Mechanical properties of the esophagus in eosinophilic esophagitis. Gastroenterology 2011;140(1):82–90.

38. Zimmerman SL, Levine MS, Rubesin SE, et al. Idiopathic eosinophilic esophagitis in adults: the ringed esophagus. Radiology 2005;236(1):159–65.

39. Lee J, Huprich J, Kujath C, et al. Esophageal diameter is decreased in some patients with eosinophilic esophagitis and might increase with topical corticosteroid therapy. Clin Gastroenterol Hepatol 2012;10(5):481–6.

40. Stevoff C, Rao S, Parsons W, et al. EUS and histopathologic correlates in eosinophilic esophagitis. Gastrointest Endosc 2001;54(3):373–7.

41. Kim HP, Vance RB, Shaheen NJ, et al. The prevalence and diagnostic utility of endoscopic features of eosinophilic esophagitis: a meta-analysis. Clin Gastroenterol Hepatol 2012;10(9):988–96.e5.

42. Straumann A, Aceves SS, Blanchard C, et al. Pediatric and adult eosinophilic esophagitis: similarities and differences. Allergy 2012;67(4):477–90.

43. Straumann A, Rossi L, Simon HU, et al. Fragility of the esophageal mucosa: a pathognomonic endoscopic sign of primary eosinophilic esophagitis? Gastrointest Endosc 2003;57(3):407–12.

44. Aceves SS, Ackerman SJ. Relationships between eosinophilic inflammation, tissue remodeling, and fibrosis in eosinophilic esophagitis. Immunol Allergy Clin North Am 2009;29(1):197–211, xiii–xiv.
45. Aceves SS, Newbury RO, Dohil MA, et al. A symptom scoring tool for identifying pediatric patients with eosinophilic esophagitis and correlating symptoms with inflammation. Ann Allergy Asthma Immunol 2009;103(5):401–6.
46. Nicodème F, Hirano I, Chen J, et al. Esophageal distensibility as a measure of disease severity in patients with eosinophilic esophagitis. Clin Gastroenterol Hepatol 2013;11(9):1101–7.e1.
47. Hirano I, Moy N, Heckman MG, et al. Endoscopic assessment of the oesophageal features of eosinophilic oesophagitis: validation of a novel classification and grading system. Gut 2013;62(4):489–95.
48. Straumann A, Conus S, Degen L, et al. Long-term budesonide maintenance treatment is partially effective for patients with eosinophilic esophagitis. Clin Gastroenterol Hepatol 2011;9(5):400–9.e1.
49. Dobbins JW, Sheahan DG, Behar J. Eosinophilic gastroenteritis with esophageal involvement. Gastroenterology 1977;72(6):1312–6.
50. Landres RT, Kuster GG, Strum WB. Eosinophilic esophagitis in a patient with vigorous achalasia. Gastroenterology 1978;74(6):1298–301.
51. Savarino E, Gemignani L, Zentilin P, et al. Achalasia with dense eosinophilic infiltrate responds to steroid therapy. Clin Gastroenterol Hepatol 2011;9(12):1104–6.
52. Lucendo AJ, Castillo P, Martin-Chavarri S, et al. Manometric findings in adult eosinophilic oesophagitis: a study of 12 cases. Eur J Gastroenterol Hepatol 2007;19(5):417–24.
53. Nurko S, Rosen R, Furuta GT. Esophageal dysmotility in children with eosinophilic esophagitis: a study using prolonged esophageal manometry. Am J Gastroenterol 2009;104(12):3050–7.
54. Martin Martin L, Santander C, Lopez Martin MC, et al. Esophageal motor abnormalities in eosinophilic esophagitis identified by high-resolution manometry. J Gastroenterol Hepatol 2011;26(9):1447–50.
55. Konikoff MR, Noel RJ, Blanchard C, et al. A randomized, double-blind, placebo-controlled trial of fluticasone propionate for pediatric eosinophilic esophagitis. Gastroenterology 2006;131(5):1381–91.
56. Dohil R, Newbury R, Fox L, et al. Oral viscous budesonide is effective in children with eosinophilic esophagitis in a randomized, placebo-controlled trial. Gastroenterology 2010;139(2):418–29.
57. Schroeder S, Fleischer DM, Masterson JC, et al. Successful treatment of eosinophilic esophagitis with ciclesonide. J Allergy Clin Immunol 2012;129(5):1419–21.
58. Rothenberg ME, Aceves S, Bonis PA, et al. Working with the US Food and Drug Administration: progress and timelines in understanding and treating patients with eosinophilic esophagitis. J Allergy Clin Immunol 2012;130(3):617–9.
59. Aceves SS, Newbury RO, Chen D, et al. Resolution of remodeling in eosinophilic esophagitis correlates with epithelial response to topical corticosteroids. Allergy 2010;65(1):109–16.
60. Abu-Sultaneh SM, Durst P, Maynard V, et al. Fluticasone and food allergen elimination reverse sub-epithelial fibrosis in children with eosinophilic esophagitis. Dig Dis Sci 2011;56(1):97–102.
61. Chehade M, Sampson HA, Morotti RA, et al. Esophageal subepithelial fibrosis in children with eosinophilic esophagitis. J Pediatr Gastroenterol Nutr 2007;45(3):319–28.

62. Alexander JA, Jung KW, Arora AS, et al. Swallowed fluticasone improves histologic but not symptomatic response of adults with eosinophilic esophagitis. Clin Gastroenterol Hepatol 2012;10(7):742–9.e1.

63. Peterson KA, Byrne KR, Vinson LA, et al. Elemental diet induces histologic response in adult eosinophilic esophagitis. Am J Gastroenterol 2013;108(5): 759–66.

64. Caldwell JM, Blanchard C, Collins MH, et al. Glucocorticoid-regulated genes in eosinophilic esophagitis: a role for FKBP51. J Allergy Clin Immunol 2010;125(4): 879–88.e8.

65. Wen T, Stucke EM, Grotjan TM, et al. Molecular diagnosis of eosinophilic esophagitis by gene expression profiling. Gastroenterology 2013;145(6):1289–99.

66. Kern E, Hirano I. Emerging drugs for eosinophilic esophagitis. Expert Opin Emerg Drugs 2013;18(3):353–64.

67. Straumann A, Hoesli S, Bussmann C, et al. Anti-eosinophil activity and clinical efficacy of the CRTH2 antagonist OC000459 in eosinophilic esophagitis. Allergy 2013;68(3):375–85.

68. Assa'ad AH, Gupta SK, Collins MH, et al. An antibody against IL-5 reduces numbers of esophageal intraepithelial eosinophils in children with eosinophilic esophagitis. Gastroenterology 2011;141(5):1593–604.

69. Spergel JM, Rothenberg ME, Collins MH, et al. Reslizumab in children and adolescents with eosinophilic esophagitis: results of a double-blind, randomized, placebo-controlled trial. J Allergy Clin Immunol 2012;129(2):456–63, 463.e1–3.

70. Straumann A, Conus S, Grzonka P, et al. Anti-interleukin-5 antibody treatment (mepolizumab) in active eosinophilic oesophagitis: a randomised, placebo-controlled, double-blind trial. Gut 2010;59(1):21–30.

71. Zimmermann N, McBride ML, Yamada Y, et al. Siglec-F antibody administration to mice selectively reduces blood and tissue eosinophils. Allergy 2008;63(9): 1156–63.

72. Kiwamoto T, Kawasaki N, Paulson JC, et al. Siglec-8 as a drugable target to treat eosinophil and mast cell-associated conditions. Pharmacol Ther 2012;135(3): 327–36.

73. Schoepfer AM, Gonsalves N, Bussmann C, et al. Esophageal dilation in eosinophilic esophagitis: effectiveness, safety, and impact on the underlying inflammation. Am J Gastroenterol 2010;105(5):1062–70.

74. Assa'ad AH, Putnam PE, Collins MH, et al. Pediatric patients with eosinophilic esophagitis: an 8-year follow-up. J Allergy Clin Immunol 2007;119(3):731–8.

Eosinophilic Gastroenteritis and Related Eosinophilic Disorders

Calman Prussin, MD

KEYWORDS

- Eosinophilic gastroenteritis • Eosinophilic gastritis • Eosinophilia • Food allergy
- EGID

KEY POINTS

- Eosinophilic gastroenteritis (EGE) is diagnosed by the presence of gastrointestinal symptoms, biopsies showing predominant eosinophilic infiltration, and the absence of allergic, parasitic, or other diseases that may cause eosinophilia.
- EGE is a rare disease affecting approximately 22 to 28 per 100,000 persons.
- Because EGE may vary by both the site of involvement (stomach, duodenum, jejunum) and the depth of involvement (mucosal, muscularis, or serosal disease), its manifestations are protean.
- Dietary therapy is effective in allergic EGE.
- Systemic and topical corticosteroids are effective treatments for EGE, but are limited by long-term corticosteroid side effects.

CLINICAL PRESENTATION OF EGE

Eosinophilic gastroenteritis (EGE) represents one member within the spectrum of diseases collectively referred to as eosinophilic gastrointestinal disorders (EGIDs), which includes eosinophilic esophagitis (EoE), gastritis, enteritis, and colitis. Although some patients present with EGID limited to the stomach (eosinophilic gastritis, EG) or duodenum (eosinophilic duodenitis), it is often simplest to refer to the combined entity of EGE. EoE as a clinical entity is effectively limited to "solitary EoE"; patients having coexistent EoE and EGE are a small minority. EoE and EGE are closely related disease entities, the relationship of which is discussed below. The diagnosis of EG is confirmed by a characteristic biopsy and/or eosinophilic ascitic fluid in the absence of other causes of gut eosinophilia.

The disease can affect patients of any age, but case series have noted a dominance of presentations starting in the third through fifth decade. As the prevalence of EoE has

Disclosures: The author has no competing financial interests.
Laboratory of Allergic Diseases, National Institute of Allergy and Infectious Diseases, National Institutes of Health, 10 Center Drive, MSC-1881, Bethesda, MD 20892-1881, USA
E-mail address: cprussin@niaid.nih.gov

Gastroenterol Clin N Am 43 (2014) 317–327
http://dx.doi.org/10.1016/j.gtc.2014.02.013
0889-8553/14/$ – see front matter Published by Elsevier Inc.

increased and there is an overall greater appreciation of EGID, it is likely that a second peak of incidence in the first decade of life will become better appreciated. As with EoE, there is a clear male predominance. An electronic survey sent to North American Allergists and Pediatric Gastroenterologists indicate prevalence for EGE of 22 to 28 per 100,000 persons.[1] Although no large longitudinal study has been performed, EGE is largely understood to be a chronic disease with few remissions after the first year.

The clinical features of EGE are protean and are related to the organs, tissue layers affected, and the intensity of eosinophilic inflammation.[2–6] Some patients present with dominant gastric or duodenal disease, whereas others have involvement of both organs. Dominant gastric disease often presents with nausea, vomiting, and early satiety. In contrast, dominant duodenal disease may present with malabsorption and protein-losing enteropathy. Both forms of EGE often have crampy abdominal pain and bloating as additional features. Because jejunal and ileal biopsies are not routinely obtained on endoscopy, it is not known how much these gut segments contribute to disease. Patients can variably present with either diarrhea or constipation.[7]

In addition to the varying distribution of eosinophils along the length of the gastrointestinal (GI) tract, multiple reports have cited EGE subtypes based on differing depth of eosinophilic infiltration.[3,8] The 3 well-described subtypes include dominant involvement of the mucosal, muscularis, and subserosal layers, respectively. Whether these actually represent different diseases or simply different presentations of the same disease is not known. The prevalence of each subtype is unknown because of reporting and referral biases. For example, surgical series report a predominance of muscularis disease with obstruction, whereas medical series primarily describe patients with mucosal involvement. Serosal disease is associated with eosinophilic ascites, but it is not known whether this reflects isolated serosal involvement or simply intense transmural eosinophilic inflammation.

In addition to the common presentations noted above, EGE can present with a variety of unusual manifestations. Patients may have gastric ulcer disease as a feature of their EGE.[9] Typically these ulcers do not respond well to proton pump inhibitor therapy, but do respond to either topical or systemic corticosteroids. There is a case report of ulcer disease responding to an elemental diet.[10]

In contrast to EoE, stricture formation is not a common feature of EGE. That said, a subset of perhaps 5% to 10% of EGE patients do have clinically significant strictures at some point. Such cases will typically present as an acute bowel obstruction with nausea, vomiting, crampy abdominal pain, and bloating.[11] Such bowel obstructions appear to be a combination of both mechanical obstruction due to stricture and functional obstruction due to inflammation, edema, and decreased GI motility. Most of the time these obstructions are reversible with corticosteroid treatment, suggesting that in many cases there is a functional component that can be reversed with treatment.[12] As such, clinically stable EGE patients presenting with bowel obstruction should generally first be treated with parenteral corticosteroid therapy, such as methyl prednisolone 1 to 2 mg/kg/d, and carefully observed.

EGE can occasionally involve the hepatobiliary tree. Pancreatitis is the best described hepatobiliary complication of EGE.[13] It is not clear if this is due to eosinophilic infiltration of the pancreas, gall bladder, or hepatobiliary ducts or to a secondary cause. In addition, EGE can rarely present with eosinophilic cholangitis.[14,15]

PATHOGENESIS OF EGE

The many similarities between EGE and EoE suggest they share a common pathogenesis. Shared features include tissue eosinophilic inflammation, coexisting allergic disease, peripheral eosinophilia, and polysensitization to food allergens. The most compelling clinical feature of EoE is its responsiveness to elemental and highly restricted diets.[16,17] Several case series suggest that at least a subpopulation of EGE is also responsive to elemental and 6-food elimination diets.[18,19] These findings underscore the concept that both EoE and EGE are food allergen–driven eosinophilic inflammatory bowel diseases.

In an early report, Jaffe and colleagues[20] noted increased interleukin (IL)-5 expression in peripheral blood mononuclear cells from EGE patients. Consistent with in vivo activation by food allergen, this IL-5 message was constitutively produced by CD4 T cells in the peripheral blood mononuclear cell. A role for IL-5 in driving the peripheral eosinophilia has been further established by the use of therapeutic monoclonal anti-IL-5, which potently decreases peripheral eosinophils in EGE.[21]

In the author's work, food allergen-specific CD4 T-cell responses in EGE, peanut allergies, and healthy control subjects were examined and differing Th2 responses in these eosinophilic versus anaphylactic forms of food allergy were found.[22] Notably, EGE is uniquely associated with an IL-5+ Th2 (IL-5+, IL-13+) response to foods; conversely, in peanut allergy, the Th2 response is almost entirely IL-5− (IL-5−, IL-13+). This IL-5+ Th2 response is highly correlated to peripheral blood eosinophil count, further establishing a link between this Th2 subpopulation and eosinophilia. In recent work these IL-5+ Th2 cells have been further characterized as highly differentiated Th2 cells that require multiple rounds of antigen exposure to attain the IL-5+ Th2 phenotype.[23] These data suggest that in EGE these pathogenic proeosinophilic IL-5+ Th2 cells are the product of multiple rounds of food allergen stimulation in vivo.

EGE and EoE are defined by their respective sites of clinical disease. Despite these differences, their similarities far outweigh the differences and suggest the pathogenesis of these 2 forms of EGID have common mechanisms. The differences in site of disease may be due to local effects that may favor esophageal versus gastric eosinophilic inflammation. For example, EoE may be influenced by high concentrations of swallowed aeroallergen impacting the esophagus, or by gastroesophageal reflux. Alternatively, there may be specific homing signals or receptors that favor esophageal versus gastric homing.

DIAGNOSIS OF EGE

Unlike EoE, there are no consensus guidelines for the diagnosis of EGE. The diagnosis is based on typical symptoms coupled with increased gastric or intestinal eosinophils, in the absence of other potential causes of GI eosinophilia. There is no consensus on the requisite number of eosinophils needed for the diagnosis. As detailed in the accompanying article, "Histopathologic Features," based on studies of healthy controls, peak eosinophil counts of 30 eos/hpf in the stomach and 50 eos/hpf (eosinophils per high powered field) in the duodenum have been proposed for the diagnosis of EG and duodenitis, respectively.[24,25] Additional features, such as epithelial eosinophils, intraglandular eosinophils, and eosinophils in the muscularis, also weight toward the diagnosis of EGE. The intensity of eosinophilic inflammation is quite variable within an affected organ and can reach almost confluent density in some cases (**Fig. 1**). Accordingly, endoscopic biopsies should be obtained from 5 to 6 sites per affected organ, in a similar manner to the consensus procedures in EoE.[26]

Given the association of EGE with allergic disease, in clinical studies of "allergic" EGE, additional criteria have been used, such as immunoglobulin E (IgE) sensitization to multiple food allergens and peripheral blood eosinophilia.[22] These added criteria identify a subpopulation of EGE patients with more homogeneous immunologic

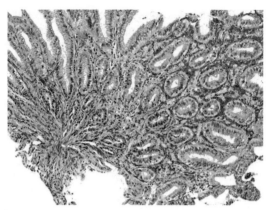

Fig. 1. Duodenal biopsy specimen showing intense areas of eosinophilic inflammation (hematoxylin-eosin, original magnification ×100).

findings and add to the specificity of diagnosis. However, such criteria should not be used as an absolute requirement for the diagnosis because there is a large fraction of EGE patients lacking these.

The gross endoscopic findings are often normal. Gastritis or ulcers may be present. The one observation that is relatively typical for EG is the presence of pseudopolyps.[10,27] These sessile lesions are not true polyps in that they are largely composed of dense collagen deposits with epithelium heaped on top. As such, they do not represent true polyps and do not contain hyperplastic glandular or epithelial components. Gastric pseudopolyps are the most common presentation (**Fig. 2**) and may occur in as many as 25% of EGE subjects (Calman Prussin, personal observation, 2014). Small bowel pseudopolyps may occur, but are less frequent (**Fig. 3**).

ESOPHAGEAL EOSINOPHILIA IN PATIENTS WITH EGE

As noted above, EoE and EGE share many clinical and pathogenic features. Thus, it is not surprising that a subgroup of patients have widespread EGID that includes their esophagus, stomach, and small bowel. In addition, on EGD, some patients with EoE will have increased numbers of gastric or duodenal eosinophils of unclear

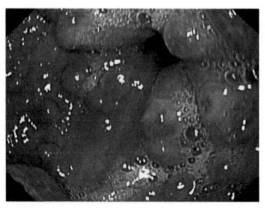

Fig. 2. Gastric pseudopolyps involving the gastric antrum and pyloris.

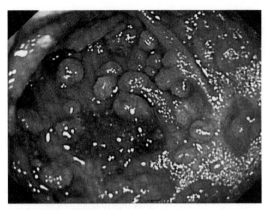

Fig. 3. Pseudopolyps within the terminal ileum.

significance. Gupta and colleagues found that 12% of pediatric EoE subjects had elevated gastric eosinophils, which they defined as greater than 10 eos/hpf. They noted no significant clinical differences between EoE patients with or without incidental gastric eosinophilia.[28] Conversely, in the author's adult EGE clinic, they noted ≈25% of EGE patients have greater than or equal to 15 eos/hpf in their esophagus (Prussin, personal observation). Notably, only about half of those EGE patients with increased esophageal eosinophils have dysphagia. This dysphagia often responds to swallowed topical corticosteroids.

EOSINOPHILIA IN PATIENTS WITH EGID

Patients with EGID frequently present with elevated blood eosinophilia. This elevation is particularly notable in EGE, in which most patients present with blood eosinophilia.[3,6] Blood eosinophilia can often be a source of concern because eosinophil counts are often elevated into the several thousand range. Indeed, many of the EGE patients in the author's clinic were initially referred for hypereosinophilic syndrome (HES), but after careful work-up it was apparent that despite very high blood eosinophils counts, their disease was limited to the GI tract and did not involve other end organs. The absolute eosinophil count (AEC), measured in eos/mm^3 or eos/μL, and not the percentage of eosinophils on the differential, is the metric used to follow eosinophilia.

Recently proposed diagnostic criteria for HES define it as blood eosinophilia of greater than 1500/mm^3 on at least 2 occasions or evidence of prominent tissue eosinophilia associated with symptoms and marked blood eosinophilia.[29] This definition further excludes "secondary causes of eosinophilia, such as parasitic or viral infections, allergic diseases, drug-induced or chemical-induced eosinophilia, hypoadrenalism, and neoplasms." Given that EGIDs are clearly allergic in cause, according to the new definition, EGID should not be considered a form of HES.

HES usually affects multiple organ systems, including the skin, lungs, GI tract, neurologic system, and heart.[30] Indeed, despite the frequency of high-grade eosinophilia in EGID, there is a conspicuous lack of reports in the literature of patients with stable allergic EGID of many years' duration at some later point transforming into an HES-like picture with skin ulcers, lung, heart, or neurologic involvement. That said, the GI tract is one of the more commonly affected organ systems in HES and clearly there are rare patients who clinically present as an overlap between HES and EGID.

To address potential HES in EGID patients with AEC greater than 1500 eos/mm^2, the following work-up is performed at initial presentation:

1. Drug history to examine for drug-induced eosinophilia
2. Travel history
3. Stool for ova and parasites
4. Strongyloides stercoralis serology
5. T-cell receptor clonality studies (to examine for a clonal T-cell population involved in lymphocytic HES)
6. FIP1-like 1/platelet-derived growth factor receptor αfusion gene studies (to examine for the most common cause of myeloid HES)
7. Cardiac echo (to rule out endomyocardial fibrosis)

In addition to HES, eosinophilic granulomatosis with polyangiitis (EGPA, formally known as Churg-Strauss syndrome) shares many features with EGID and can present with GI symptoms. GI symptoms associated with EGPA can include dysphagia, abdominal pain, vomiting, anorexia, and bloody diarrhea. EGPA should be considered in the differential in EGID patients with marked asthma, pulmonary symptoms, or nasal polyps. The lung disease in EGPA characteristically has migratory infiltrates seen on chest radiograph. Serum antineutrophil cytoplasmic antibodies should be examined. Ultimately, the diagnosis is best made by the demonstration of eosinophil-rich necrotizing granulomatous vasculitis in the lungs or other site of disease.

MANAGEMENT OF EGE

Because of the low prevalence of EGE, there are no placebo-controlled clinical trials examining therapeutic approaches. Although some patients may be optimally managed by the approaches noted below, most patients do not achieve complete remission of their EGE symptoms. As such, there is a great need for new approaches to the treatment of EGE.

Newly diagnosed patients are almost always responsive to systemic corticosteroid therapy. In patients who do not respond to corticosteroids, alternative diagnoses should be considered.[3] Doses of prednisone of 0.5 to 1 mg/kg typically induce a dramatic clinical improvement in 2 to 14 days. As such, short-term treatment with systemic corticosteroids is an excellent means to induce clinical remission.

Because of the long-term side effects of systemic corticosteroids, topical corticosteroids have been used in a similar manner to those in EoE. Early practitioners used oral beclomethasone, often diluted in corn oil. A major limitation of beclomethasone is its oral bioavailability of approximately 30% to 40%.[31] Given that beclomethasone has far greater oral bioavailability than other topical corticosteroids, it should not be used in the contemporary treatment of EGE.

In contrast to beclomethasone, budesonide has an oral bioavailability of about 10%.[32] Similar to its use in EoE, budesonide has been used for the treatment of EGE.[12,33–35] Unfortunately, all publications are single case reports and are subject to reporting bias.

In the United States and the European Union, the only commercial formulation of budesonide available in sufficient quantity to treat EGE is the controlled ileal release capsule preparation (Entocort EC). The controlled ileal release capsule provides optimal delivery to the terminal ileum, but provides minimal gastric delivery. Because most EGE patients have predominant gastric or duodenal disease, a solubilized modification of these capsules is used routinely to target topical activity to the upper GI tract. Such GI preparations of budesonide are not approved for use in pediatric patients, because their safety and efficacy has not been established in this population. Accordingly, any off-label use in pediatric patients should only be done after careful consideration of the risks, benefits, and alternatives.

For most symptomatic EGE patients therapy is initiated using prednisone at 0.4 to 0.8 mg/kg each morning to induce symptomatic remission. Simultaneously, solubilized budesonide is begun at 9 mg orally daily, taken at bedtime on an empty stomach. Patients are advised to open the budesonide capsules, crush the contents in a mortar and pestle, and dissolve it in 15 to 30 mL of water and juice. In this manner there is minimal additional dilution of the drug and its upper GI dwell time is maximized, thus maximizing topical activity. Once clinical symptoms are controlled, prednisone is tapered over the next 2 or more weeks. One to 2 months after the prednisone has been stopped, the budesonide dose is slowly tapered over an additional 2 to 4 months to the minimum required dose. For patients with substantial protein-losing enteropathy, in which jejunal or ileal disease is suspected, the intact controlled ileal capsule may be used.

Most adult patients get improvement of symptoms on 9 mg/d of budesonide. However, in many patients there are substantial systemic effects at that dose. A budesonide dose of 3 to 6 mg/d long term is preferable. Ultimately, corticosteroid therapy in EGE is an imperfect compromise between a dose that yields a tolerable level of systemic side effects and only partial treatment of symptoms. That said, at the present time there are few other feasible medical treatment options for most patients.

Fluticasone is a fluorinated corticosteroid that is widely used in EoE and is notable for having an exceedingly low oral bioavailability of less than or equal to 1%.[36] This low oral bioavailability makes it potentially an ideal drug for topical use in EGE. Unfortunately, fluticasone is only available in pulmonary and nasal inhalers, neither of which contain sufficient drug to treat EGE. Intriguingly, among pediatric EoE subjects with elevated gastric eosinophils who were treated with swallowed fluticasone, there was a significant decrease in gastric eosinophils,[28] which suggests that, particularly for gastric predominant EGE, higher doses of fluticasone are worthy of further study.

As in EoE, dietary therapy is an effective treatment in a large fraction of EGE patients. Chehade and colleagues[19] examined a cohort of 6 pediatric patients with allergic EGE and protein-losing enteropathy. All subjects responded to the elemental diet with a resolution of their clinical symptoms, hypoalbuminemia, and anemia in less than 4 weeks. When these same patients were managed with an eliminations diet, there was only limited success. Gonsalves and coworkers[18] published an abstract examining dietary therapy for 9 adults with EGE. Two subjects were treated with elemental diet and had resolution of both symptoms as well as tissue and blood eosinophilia. Seven subjects were treated with a 6-food elimination diet; of these, 4 of the 7 had resolution of both symptoms as well as tissue and blood eosinophilia. In sum, these data suggest that dietary approaches are generally effective, particularly in allergic EGE, and should be given greater consideration.

Because EGE is an allergic disease and is associated with IgE sensitization to multiple foods, an open-label clinical trial of the anti-IgE therapeutic monoclonal antibody was undertaken.[37] As expected, omalizumab effectively suppressed free IgE and IgE-dependent basophil responses. Although the primary endpoint of peripheral blood eosinophil count was significantly decreased during the 4-month trial, tissue eosinophilia and symptoms were only modestly affected. Coupled with similar negative reports of omalizumab in EoE, these data suggest that IgE blockade is not an effective treatment of EGID.[38–40]

Given the central role of IL-5 in eosinophil biology and the abundance of evidence that IL-5 plays a major role in EGID, therapeutic monoclonal antibodies against IL-5 have been used in EGID.[41] To this end, an open-label clinical trial of the anti-IL-5 therapeutic monoclonal antibody reslizumab (SCH55700) was undertaken in 4 subjects with EGE.[21] Reslizumab suppressed blood eosinophilia in a significant manner. However, tissue eosinophilia was only modestly suppressed and EGE symptoms were minimally affected. Additional work is needed to define the efficacy of such approaches better. The eosinophil-depleting anti-IL-5 receptor therapeutic monoclonal antibody benralizumab may allow this question to be addressed in a more substantial manner in the future.[42]

A variety of other drugs has been used to treat EGE and has been published in the literature, typically as case reports. Despite these generally positive reports, there are few controlled studies, nor is there a consensus among EGID specialists on the value of these drugs. Given the potential for reporting bias and nonreporting of negative data, until more definitive studies are done, these findings must be considered with some skepticism.

In several case reports montekukast has been described as an effective treatment of EGE in Refs.[43,44] Furthermore, a retrospective case series of pediatric EGID patients including both EGE and EoE, montelukast improved EGID symptoms.[45] In contrast, another report noted no benefit to treatment.[46] In a prospective study, 11 EoE subjects were induced into remission using swallowed fluticasone and then switched to montelukast for 3 months.[47] Montelukast did not maintain either symptomatic or histologic remission in this setting.

A variety of case reports have suggested sodium cromolyn is an effective treatment of EGE.[48–50] In contrast, another report notes its use was unsuccessful.[46] A clinical series of 14 EoE subjects treated with cromolyn at the University of Pennsylvania had no clinical or histologic improvement in their disease.[51]

Ketotifen is an H1 antihistamine that also has "mast cell stabilizing" activity. In the United States, it is only available in eye drops, but is available as a systemic drug in Canada and the European Union. An early clinical trial in EGE indicated efficacy and several positive case reports have been published through the years.[52,53] Suplatast is an anti-Th2 drug that inhibits the expression of Th2 cytokines, such as IL-5. Suplatast is not available in the United States and the European Union. Successful treatment of EGE with suplatast has been described in 2 single patient case reports, but the generalizability of these findings remains unclear.[54,55]

SUMMARY

EGE is a subset of EGID characterized by intense eosinophilic infiltration of the stomach and small bowel. Although the pathogenesis of EGE shares many features of EoE, the differing localization of eosinophilic inflammation in EGE results in a different constellation of disease. Corticosteroids remain the mainstay of treatment.

Unfortunately, in many patients low-dose topical corticosteroid therapy is not sufficiently effective to provide complete symptom relief. Thus, corticosteroid therapy in EGE is an imperfect compromise between a dose that yields a tolerable level of systemic side effects and only partial treatment of symptoms. Because EGE is a rare disease, relatively few clinical studies have been performed. As such, there is a large unmet need for new clinical therapeutic strategies.

REFERENCES

1. Spergel JM, Book WM, Mays E, et al. Variation in prevalence, diagnostic criteria, and initial management options for eosinophilic gastrointestinal diseases in the United States. J Pediatr Gastroenterol Nutr 2011;52(3):300–6.

2. Naylor AR. Eosinophilic gastroenteritis. Scott Med J 1990;35(6):163–5.
3. Talley NJ, Shorter RG, Phillips SF, et al. Eosinophilic gastroenteritis: a clinico-pathological study of patients with disease of the mucosa, muscle layer, and subserosal tissues. Gut 1990;31(1):54–8.
4. Kelly KJ. Eosinophilic gastroenteritis. J Pediatr Gastroenterol Nutr 2000; 30(Suppl):S28–35.
5. Khan S. Eosinophilic gastroenteritis. Best Pract Res Clin Gastroenterol 2005; 19(2):177–98.
6. Zhang L, Duan L, Ding S, et al. Eosinophilic gastroenteritis: clinical manifestations and morphological characteristics, a retrospective study of 42 patients. Scand J Gastroenterol 2011;46(9):1074–80.
7. Khan F, Chaudhry MA, Nusrat S, et al. Constipation–another manifestation of eosinophilic gastroenteritis. J Okla State Med Assoc 2012;105(4–5):134, 136.
8. Chang JY, Choung RS, Lee RM, et al. A shift in the clinical spectrum of eosinophilic gastroenteritis toward the mucosal disease type. Clin Gastroenterol Hepatol 2010;8(8):669–75 [quiz: e88].
9. Kristopaitis T, Neghme C, Yong SL, et al. Giant antral ulcer: a rare presentation of eosinophilic gastroenteritis–case report and review of the literature. Am J Gastroenterol 1997;92(7):1205–8.
10. Chehade M, Sicherer SH, Magid MS, et al. Multiple exudative ulcers and pseudopolyps in allergic eosinophilic gastroenteritis that responded to dietary therapy. J Pediatr Gastroenterol Nutr 2007;45(3):354–7.
11. Yun MY, Cho YU, Park IS, et al. Eosinophilic gastroenteritis presenting as small bowel obstruction: a case report and review of the literature. World J Gastroenterol 2007;13(11):1758–60.
12. Elsing C, Placke J, Gross-Weege W. Budesonide for the treatment of obstructive eosinophilic jejunitis. Z Gastroenterol 2007;45(2):187–9.
13. Lyngbaek S, Adamsen S, Aru A, et al. Recurrent acute pancreatitis due to eosinophilic gastroenteritis. Case report and literature review. JOP 2006;7(2):211–7.
14. Schoonbroodt D, Horsmans Y, Laka A, et al. Eosinophilic gastroenteritis presenting with colitis and cholangitis. Dig Dis Sci 1995;40(2):308–14.
15. Nashed C, Sakpal SV, Shusharina V, et al. Eosinophilic cholangitis and cholangiopathy: a sheep in wolves clothing. HPB Surg 2010;2010:906496.
16. Markowitz JE, Spergel JM, Ruchelli E, et al. Elemental diet is an effective treatment for eosinophilic esophagitis in children and adolescents. Am J Gastroenterol 2003;98(4):777–82.
17. Chehade M, Aceves SS. Food allergy and eosinophilic esophagitis. Curr Opin Allergy Clin Immunol 2010;10(3):231–7.
18. Gonsalves N, Doerfler B, Yang GY, et al. A prospective clinical trial of six food elimination diet or elemental diet in the treatment of adults with eosinophilic gastroenteritis. Gastroenterology 2009;136(5):A280.
19. Chehade M, Magid MS, Mofidi S, et al. Allergic eosinophilic gastroenteritis with protein-losing enteropathy: intestinal pathology, clinical course, and long-term follow-up. J Pediatr Gastroenterol Nutr 2006;42(5):516–21.
20. Jaffe JS, James SP, Mullins GE, et al. Evidence for an abnormal profile of interleukin-4 (IL-4), IL-5, and gamma-interferon (gamma-IFN) in peripheral blood T cells from patients with allergic eosinophilic gastroenteritis. J Clin Immunol 1994;14(5):299–309.
21. Kim YJ, Prussin C, Martin B, et al. Rebound eosinophilia after treatment of hypereosinophilic syndrome and eosinophilic gastroenteritis with monoclonal anti-IL-5 antibody SCH55700. J Allergy Clin Immunol 2004;114(6):1449–55.

22. Prussin C, Lee J, Foster B. Eosinophilic gastrointestinal disease and peanut allergy are alternatively associated with IL-5+ and IL-5(-) T(H)2 responses. J Allergy Clin Immunol 2009;124(6):1326–32.e6.
23. Upadhyaya B, Yin Y, Hill BJ, et al. Hierarchical IL-5 expression defines a subpopulation of highly differentiated human Th2 cells. J Immunol 2011;187(6): 3111–20.
24. Lwin T, Melton SD, Genta RM. Eosinophilic gastritis: histopathological characterization and quantification of the normal gastric eosinophil content. Mod Pathol 2011;24(4):556–63.
25. DeBrosse CW, Case JW, Putnam PE, et al. Quantity and distribution of eosinophils in the gastrointestinal tract of children. Pediatr Dev Pathol 2006;9(3):210–8.
26. Liacouras CA, Furuta GT, Hirano I, et al. Eosinophilic esophagitis: updated consensus recommendations for children and adults. J Allergy Clin Immunol 2011;128(1):3–20.e6 [quiz: 21–2].
27. Jimenez-Rivera C, Ngan B, Jackson R, et al. Gastric pseudopolyps in eosinophilic gastroenteritis. J Pediatr Gastroenterol Nutr 2005;40(1):83–6.
28. Ammoury RF, Rosenman MB, Roettcher D, et al. Incidental gastric eosinophils in patients with eosinophilic esophagitis: do they matter? J Pediatr Gastroenterol Nutr 2010;51(6):723–6.
29. Simon HU, Rothenberg ME, Bochner BS, et al. Refining the definition of hypereosinophilic syndrome. J Allergy Clin Immunol 2010;126(1):45–9.
30. Ogbogu PU, Bochner BS, Butterfield JH, et al. Hypereosinophilic syndrome: a multicenter, retrospective analysis of clinical characteristics and response to therapy. J Allergy Clin Immunol 2009;124(6):1319–25.e3.
31. Daley-Yates PT, Price AC, Sisson JR, et al. Beclomethasone dipropionate: absolute bioavailability, pharmacokinetics and metabolism following intravenous, oral, intranasal and inhaled administration in man. Br J Clin Pharmacol 2001; 51(5):400–9.
32. Friend DR. Review article: issues in oral administration of locally acting glucocorticosteroids for treatment of inflammatory bowel disease. Aliment Pharmacol Ther 1998;12(7):591–603.
33. Tan AC, Kruimel JW, Naber TH. Eosinophilic gastroenteritis treated with nonenteric-coated budesonide tablets. Eur J Gastroenterol Hepatol 2001;13(4):425–7.
34. Siewert E, Lammert F, Koppitz P, et al. Eosinophilic gastroenteritis with severe protein-losing enteropathy: successful treatment with budesonide. Dig Liver Dis 2006;38(1):55–9.
35. Lombardi C, Salmi A, Passalacqua G. An adult case of eosinophilic pyloric stenosis maintained on remission with oral budesonide. Eur Ann Allergy Clin Immunol 2011;43(1):29–30.
36. Hubner M, Hochhaus G, Derendorf H. Comparative pharmacology, bioavailability, pharmacokinetics, and pharmacodynamics of inhaled glucocorticosteroids. Immunol Allergy Clin North Am 2005;25(3):469–88.
37. Foroughi S, Foster B, Kim N, et al. Anti-IgE treatment of eosinophil-associated gastrointestinal disorders. J Allergy Clin Immunol 2007;120(3):594–601.
38. Fang JC, Hilden K, Gleich GJ, et al. A pilot study of the treatment of eosinophilic esophagitis with omalizumab. Gastroenterology 2011;140(Suppl 1):S235.
39. Rocha R, Vitor AB, Trindade E, et al. Omalizumab in the treatment of eosinophilic esophagitis and food allergy. Eur J Pediatr 2011;170(11):1471–4.
40. Loizou D, Louis-Jacques O, Enav B, et al. Elucidating mechanisms of allergic inflammation in eosinophilic esophagitis. J Allergy Clin Immunol 2013;131(2): Ab184.

41. Wechsler ME, Fulkerson PC, Bochner BS, et al. Novel targeted therapies for eosinophilic disorders. J Allergy Clin Immunol 2012;130(3):563–71.
42. Molfino NA, Gossage D, Kolbeck R, et al. Molecular and clinical rationale for therapeutic targeting of interleukin-5 and its receptor. Clin Exp Allergy 2012; 42(5):712–37.
43. Neustrom MR, Friesen C. Treatment of eosinophilic gastroenteritis with montelukast. J Allergy Clin Immunol 1999;104(2 Pt 1):506.
44. Schwartz DA, Pardi DS, Murray JA. Use of montelukast as steroid-sparing agent for recurrent eosinophilic gastroenteritis. Dig Dis Sci 2001;46(8):1787–90.
45. Vanderhoof JA, Young RJ, Hanner TL, et al. Montelukast: use in pediatric patients with eosinophilic gastrointestinal disease. J Pediatr Gastroenterol Nutr 2003;36(2):293–4.
46. Daikh BE, Ryan CK, Schwartz RH. Montelukast reduces peripheral blood eosinophilia but not tissue eosinophilia or symptoms in a patient with eosinophilic gastroenteritis and esophageal stricture. Ann Allergy Asthma Immunol 2003; 90(1):23–7.
47. Lucendo AJ, De Rezende LC, Jimenez-Contreras S, et al. Montelukast was inefficient in maintaining steroid-induced remission in adult eosinophilic esophagitis. Dig Dis Sci 2011;56(12):3551–8.
48. Van Dellen RG, Lewis JC. Oral administration of cromolyn in a patient with protein-losing enteropathy, food allergy, and eosinophilic gastroenteritis. Mayo Clin Proc 1994;69(5):441–4.
49. Perez-Millan A, Martin-Lorente JL, Lopez-Morante A, et al. Subserosal eosinophilic gastroenteritis treated efficaciously with sodium cromoglycate. Dig Dis Sci 1997;42(2):342–4.
50. Suzuki J, Kawasaki Y, Nozawa R, et al. Oral disodium cromoglycate and ketotifen for a patient with eosinophilic gastroenteritis, food allergy and protein-losing enteropathy. Asian Pac J Allergy Immunol 2003;21(3):193–7.
51. Liacouras CA, Spergel JM, Ruchelli E, et al. Eosinophilic esophagitis: a 10-year experience in 381 children. Clin Gastroenterol Hepatol 2005;3(12):1198–206.
52. Melamed I, Feanny SJ, Sherman PM, et al. Benefit of ketotifen in patients with eosinophilic gastroenteritis. Am J Med 1991;90(3):310–4.
53. Freeman HJ. Longstanding eosinophilic gastroenteritis of more than 20 years. Can J Gastroenterol 2009;23(9):632–4.
54. Shirai T, Hashimoto D, Suzuki K, et al. Successful treatment of eosinophilic gastroenteritis with suplatast tosilate. J Allergy Clin Immunol 2001;107(5):924–5.
55. Ishido K, Tanabe S, Higuchi K, et al. Eosinophilic gastroenteritis associated with giant folds. Dig Endosc 2010;22(4):312–5.

Eosinophilic Esophagitis
Overview of Clinical Management

Alain M. Schoepfer, MD[a], Ikuo Hirano, MD[b,*], David A. Katzka, MD[c]

KEYWORDS

- Eosinophilic esophagitis • Gastroesophageal reflux disease • Dysphagia
- Treatment end points • Patient-reported outcomes

KEY POINTS

- Recommended therapeutic end points in eosinophilic esophagitis (EoE) include symptoms (eg, dysphagia, chest pain), histologic activity, and endoscopic activity (especially strictures). Symptom assessment should examine meal modification and food-avoidance behaviors.
- Evidence is accumulating that maintenance therapy for EoE, by means of either swallowed topical corticosteroids or elimination diets, leads to a reduction of symptoms and esophageal remodeling processes that are associated with food bolus impactions.
- Esophageal dilation can offer long-lasting symptom improvement for EoE patients with esophageal remodeling not responsive to medical or diet therapy.

INTRODUCTION

This article covers several clinically relevant topics in the clinical management of eosinophilic esophagitis (EoE). First, which end points should be assessed in daily practice and in clinical trials are discussed. Second, the existing evidence to support maintenance treatment is highlighted, and the different therapeutic options discussed. Third, treatment options for patients refractory to standard therapies and for asymptomatic patients with esophageal eosinophilia are addressed. Finally, a therapeutic algorithm is presented.

Disclosures: A.M. Schoepfer received consulting fees and/or speaker fees and/or research grants from AstraZeneca, AG, Switzerland, Aptalis Pharma, Inc, Dr Falk Pharma, GmbH, Germany, Glaxo Smith Kline, AG, Nestlé S. A., Switzerland, and Novartis, AG, Switzerland. D.A. Katzka has no relevant financial, professional, or personal relationships to disclose. I. Hirano received consulting fees and/or speaker fees and/or research grants from Meritage Pharma, Inc, Aptalis Pharma, Inc, and Receptos, Inc.
[a] Division of Gastroenterology and Hepatology, Centre Hospitalier Universitaire Vaudois/CHUV, Rue de Bugnon 44, 07/2409, 1011 Lausanne, Switzerland; [b] Division of Gastroenterology, Esophageal Center, Northwestern University Feinberg School of Medicine, 676 North Saint Clair, Suite 1400, Chicago, IL 60611, USA; [c] Division of Gastroenterology and Hepatology, Mayo Clinic, 200 First Avenue, Southwest, Rochester, MN 55905, USA
* Corresponding author.
E-mail address: i-hirano@northwestern.edu

Gastroenterol Clin N Am 43 (2014) 329–344
http://dx.doi.org/10.1016/j.gtc.2014.02.014
0889-8553/14/$ – see front matter © 2014 Elsevier Inc. All rights reserved.
gastro.theclinics.com

END POINTS TO ASSESS TREATMENT EFFICACY
General Considerations

EoE has been defined as a clinicopathologic entity with symptoms of esophageal dysfunction and eosinophil-predominant esophageal inflammation.[1]

EoE activity can be assessed by patient-reported outcomes (PRO) in addition to biological markers, including endoscopic and histologic alterations as well as serologic biomarkers. One should discriminate between the use of outcomes in daily clinical practice and in clinical trials. For daily clinical practice the relevant outcomes are EoE-related symptoms, esophageal eosinophilia, and endoscopic features, especially the presence of esophageal strictures. In addition to these outcomes, quality of life and different biomarkers can become relevant in clinical trials.

Fig. 1 provides an overview of the different dimensions in which EoE activity can be measured. There is an ongoing debate as to whether EoE activity should be assessed based on PRO, biological components, or both dimensions. Which measures most accurately reflect disease activity depends on the impact of the disease's natural history on either PRO or biological markers. This concept is further illustrated by **Fig. 2**. In diseases such as migraine (PRO = headache; biological marker = abnormalities in functional magnetic resonance imaging [MRI]) or low back pain (PRO = pain; biological marker = MRI findings), activity assessment is mainly based on PRO measurement. At the other end of the spectrum there exist diseases in which patients may remain without any symptom for a long time but whereby appropriate biomarkers exist for activity assessment that are associated with distinct clinical outcomes, such as myocardial infarction in arterial hypertension (PRO = eg, quality of life; biological marker = blood pressure). In between these two poles there are diseases such as inflammatory bowel diseases (PRO = eg, bowel frequency, abdominal pain; biological marker = severity of endoscopically assessed inflammation) in which activity is determined by both PRO and biological markers.

Straumann and colleagues,[2] the first to publish on the natural history of 30 adult EoE patients, demonstrated that symptoms and eosinophil-predominant esophageal inflammation persisted over time. Several recent publications have demonstrated

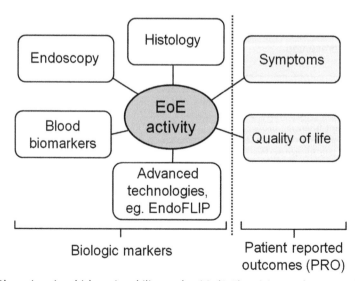

Fig. 1. Dimensions in which eosinophilic esophagitis (EoE) activity can be assessed.

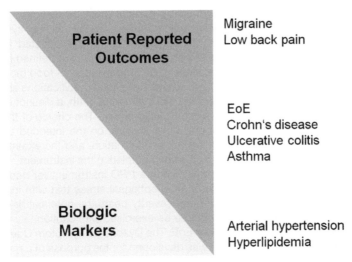

Migraine
Low back pain

EoE
Crohn's disease
Ulcerative colitis
Asthma

Arterial hypertension
Hyperlipidemia

Fig. 2. Patient-reported outcomes and biological markers in activity assessment of various diseases.

that long-standing eosinophil-predominant esophageal inflammation leads to deposition of subepithelial fibrous tissue, and that this remodeling process is associated with stricturing complications.[3-6] Current understanding suggests that symptom generation in EoE depends on active, eosinophil-predominant esophageal inflammation and associated esophageal remodeling processes. These observations support the recommendation that EoE activity assessment in daily practice and clinical trials should be performed using a combination of PRO and biological markers.[7]

There is currently no validated activity index to measure EoE activity in the different dimensions. Such an index is urgently needed to define end points for clinical trials, observational studies, and daily clinical practice. Several therapeutic trials have reported either a correlation or a dissociation between EoE-related symptoms and esophageal eosinophil counts, which might be related to the use of different, mostly nonvalidated instruments for symptom assessment.[8-11] The lack of a standardized, validated PRO instrument to assess EoE-associated symptom severity has several important implications. First, the results of different clinical trials are difficult to compare. Second, several therapeutic trials have documented heterogeneous associations between changes in PRO and biological markers. As such, the current situation poses a challenge for regulatory authorities to approve therapies for EoE management.[12-14] The US Food and Drug Administration (FDA) has identified the deficiency of clinically meaningful end points in EoE, calling for effective collaboration involving different interest groups (patients, physicians, researchers, pharmaceutical industry, and regulatory authorities).[13,14]

Current Status Regarding the Development of PRO Instruments

The development and validation of a PRO instrument to assess symptom severity in pediatric and adult EoE patients represents a challenge for several reasons. First, the leading EoE symptoms typically change in the pediatric population with ongoing age.[1,15] Second, again for pediatric patients, a cutoff age has to be chosen from which children are able to report on symptoms themselves; moreover, up to which age symptom reporting should be performed by parents must be decided. Third, the severity and frequency of dysphagia, which represents the leading symptom in adolescent and adult EoE patients, strongly depends on the ingested food consistencies; therefore, symptoms should be assessed according to defined food categories. Fourth, symptom severity may depend on food avoidance, food modification, or the time to ingest a standardized meal. These behavioral modifications should also be taken into account when developing a PRO instrument. Fifth, a distinct symptom-recall period has to be chosen for symptom assessment. The choice of the optimal symptom-recall period depends, among other factors, on the intended use of the PRO, the patient's ability to recall the required information, and the extent to which the patient is burdened by his or her EoE when completing the instrument.[16] All these factors should be considered when developing a PRO instrument for pediatric and adult EoE patients. The performance of an esophageal stress test with ingestion of a standardized meal to measure symptom severity bears the potential risk of acute food bolus impaction, and should therefore be exercised with caution.

Several PROs are being evaluated for EoE. The Dysphagia Symptom Questionnaire (DSQ) is a 3-item electronic PRO that was developed for the purpose of a pharmaceutical trial for EoE.[17] The DSQ is administered daily to assess the frequency and intensity of dysphagia caused by eating solid food.[17] The Eosinophilic Esophagitis Activity Index (EEsAI) study group is currently developing and validating a PRO instrument to assess EoE symptom severity. The EEsAI PRO instrument evaluates dysphagia severity according to 8 distinct food consistencies, and also takes into account behavioral adaptations such as food avoidance, food modification, and time to eat a regular meal (clinicaltrials.gov, NCT00939263). In 2011 Taft and colleagues[18] published a quality-of-life questionnaire for adult EoE patients. The Adult EoE Quality of Life (EoO-QOL-A) Questionnaire demonstrated good internal consistency and test-retest reliability.[18] Franciosi and colleagues[19] reported in 2011 on the qualitative methods of the Pediatric Eosinophilic Esophagitis Symptom Score (PEESS, version 2.0). The same group recently published a quality-of-life instrument for pediatric EoE patients.[20]

Overview of the Current Status Regarding the Development of Biological Measures

A classification and grading system for endoscopic assessment of esophageal features in EoE was recently published.[21] The EoE Endoscopic REFerence Score (EREFS) assesses 5 characteristic features of exudates, rings, edema (loss of vascular markings), furrows (longitudinal markings), and stricture. Definitions for endoscopic remission and mild, moderate, or severe endoscopic activity still need to be established.

The assessment of histologic activity is mainly based on the peak eosinophil count per high-power field (hpf) or the eosinophil load.[8–11] Additional histologic findings such as papillary elongation, basal layer hyperplasia, eosinophil degranulation, or subepithelial fibrosis have also been reported as parameters of histologic outcome. Dellon and colleagues[22] have shown that the number of reported peak eosinophil counts may not be necessarily comparable, as different microscope types with specific hpf sizes are being used. One way to overcome this issue would be the reporting of peak eosinophil counts standardized to mm^2. In analogy to the reporting of endoscopic severity, definitions regarding histologic remission and different semiquantitative degrees of histologic activity still need to be established.[7]

Furuta and colleagues[23] have recently evaluated the esophageal string test as a minimally invasive tool to assess the correlation between esophageal eosinophil counts and eosinophil granule proteins attached to the string. Excellent correlations were found between the level of eosinophil granule proteins extracted from the string and esophageal tissue eosinophilia.[23] Long-standing eosinophil-predominant inflammation leads to esophageal remodeling, resulting in stricture formation.[5,6] The Endo-FLIP, an impedance planimetry catheter–based device, measures esophageal compliance and distensibility and is thereby able to provide quantitative information on remodeling consequences in EoE.[24]

MAINTENANCE THERAPY

Only recently have studies begun to address the need and management options for long-term maintenance therapy in EoE. In examining the topic of maintenance therapy, limitations to existing assumptions should be acknowledged. (1) Although EoE is considered a chronic and lifelong disease, only 10 to 20 years of data exist, and spontaneous remission could occur. (2) The concept that untreated disease leads to a progressive fibrosis and stricture formation is largely based on retrospective data. (3) The current focus on control of esophageal eosinophilia as the end point of therapy ignores other potentially significant inflammatory pathways (eg, eosinophil degranulation proteins) and cells (eg, mast cells, basophils, lymphocytes).

Why is Maintenance Needed?

As in any chronic disease, the decision to use maintenance therapy balances the benefits of symptom control and prevention of disease progression with costs, side effects, and complications of long-term therapy. In the case of EoE, those in favor of observation and periodic treatment of symptom exacerbations might point out that many patients with EoE adapt to their disease, weight loss is uncommon, the disease remains isolated to the esophagus, and there are no neoplastic consequences.

On the other hand, EoE may be associated with morbidity. For example, food impaction is common, occurring in up to 35% of patients.[25–28] Patients with food impaction are indubitably at risk for perforation and aspiration. Furthermore, spontaneous perforation during food impaction (Boerhaave syndrome) has been reported.[26,29] Perforation may also occur with endoscopic bolus disimpaction and esophageal dilation. Although uncommonly requiring surgical repair, esophageal perforation results in chest pain, and careful inpatient observation is necessary.[30,31] The impact of EoE on the quality of life is now being examined.[32] Patients are commonly anxious or embarrassed by their slow eating and/or diet restrictions. As a result, important events such as business meals or social gatherings may be avoided. This scenario is particularly problematic among teenagers and young adults, a common demographic of the disease, of an age at which social stigmatisms are easily perceived.

The reason such complications ensue is the high rate of stricture formation. Indeed, once patients with EoE become or are diagnosed as young adults, the rate of esophageal stenosis reaches up to 40%.[33] In untreated patients, the natural history of persistent esophageal eosinophilia and increased collagen deposition supports the risk of progression.[2] In patients with initial successful treatment, disease regression is uncommon.[20,34] In a recent study from the Swiss EoE database, the duration of untreated disease (as measured through years of untreated symptoms) corresponded to the chance of stricture formation.[5] Specifically, after 30 years of untreated symptoms of EoE, 80% of patients had esophageal stricture formation.[5] Of note, these strictures were diagnosed with endoscopy. If one uses more sensitive tests to diagnose esophageal fibrosis, such as barium esophagography, endoscopic ultrasonography, or the EndoFLIP, the prevalence of strictures is even higher, including patients with a normal-appearing esophagus or alterations limited only to rings.[35–37] Studies with the EndoFLIP, a measurement of esophageal distensibility whereby patients may demonstrate a marked decrease in esophageal compliance presumably long before endoscopic strictures are evident, are particularly enlightening.[37]

There is also a good foundation of basic research that accounts for esophageal stricture formation in EoE. Specifically, careful analysis of tissue and inflammatory mediators in EoE has demonstrated the profibrotic process that results from the eosinophil-mediated inflammation in EoE.[38–41] For example, subepithelial collagen deposition is a common finding in these patients.[41] Moreover, many of the inflammatory mediators released from eosinophils are profibrotic. As a result, one of the main justifications for the use of maintenance therapy is to control esophageal inflammation and thereby prevent stricture formation.

Disease chronicity is a strong argument in favor of maintenance therapy. Prospective data demonstrate disease relapse in most, if not all patients, following cessation on initial therapy.[2,42] However, there are only limited data demonstrating that maintenance therapy prevents or reverses existing esophageal strictures.

What is the Goal of Maintenance Therapy?

The goal of maintenance therapy may focus on symptoms, control of histologic inflammation, or both. For symptom relief, periodic esophageal dilation may be as effective as swallowed fluticasone in reducing dysphagia.[43,44] Esophageal inflammation, however, is not lessened with dilation alone.[31] Thus, from a pathophysiologic point of view, the goal of maintenance medical therapy is to reduce esophageal eosinophilia and adverse consequences of esophageal remodeling. Unfortunately, as yet there are no data that can guide to what degree esophageal eosinophilia must be reduced, or even whether the eosinophil is the primary determinant of fibrotic change. More specifically, it is not known whether complete elimination of esophageal eosinophils is necessary or if fewer than 5, fewer than 10, or fewer than 15 eosinophils per hpf is sufficient. Indeed, in other chronic inflammatory diseases that lead to fibrosis, such as inflammatory bowel disease, investigators have long debated the appropriate end point of medical therapy, with more recent data suggesting that endoscopic demonstration of mucosal healing predicts sustained control of disease.[45] EoE is now approached in a similar manner, with the desired goal of sustained and complete elimination of eosinophilic inflammation.

Which Patients with EoE Should Be Considered for Maintenance Therapy?

Should all patients with EoE be treated with maintenance therapy? To some degree this depends on the safety and tolerability of the therapy. A patient whose esophageal inflammation remains under control with avoidance of a limited number of foods might continue with diet therapy indefinitely. On the other hand, for patients who use topical steroids, in whom the risk of long-term side effects is unclear, a more selective strategy may be appropriate. As a result, it may be important to identify subsets of EoE patients who are at greater risk of developing esophageal strictures or in whom clinically significant strictures already exist. Such patients might include those with repeated food impactions, those who relapse quickly with symptoms and/or esophageal eosinophilia off therapy, patients who cannot maintain their weight owing to severe diet restrictions, or those with narrow or small-caliber esophagus. It must be borne in mind that given the lack of data in this area, it is not known whether all or any of these specific subsets of EoE patients will respond to therapy. Patients with narrow-caliber esophagus or multiple severe atopic comorbidities may be less responsive to conventional therapies.[46]

What Potential Maintenance Treatments Exist and Are They Effective?

The potential treatments to maintain remission in EoE include steroids and elimination diet therapy. There are several reasons for which the use of steroids for maintenance therapy is an attractive option. First, there are clear data demonstrating excellent control of inflammatory change and reduction of tissue eosinophilia.[7] Second, studies in EoE have shown downregulation of genes associated with tissue remodeling following steroid therapy.[4,40,47,48] Furthermore, there are some clinical data suggesting an increase in stricture diameter with steroids based on endoscopic and/or radiologic assessment.[35,49] There are additional data demonstrating that steroids are effective in suppressing some of the key pathways and genes that mediate esophageal injury in EoE[50] and the abnormal transcriptome of EoE,[51,52] thus holding a mechanistic potential to reverse fibrosis.[4] In favor of diet therapy is the lack of concern for side effects as long as daily nutritional requirements are met. On the other hand, diet therapy poses greater challenges with identification of triggering food antigens and in lifelong avoidance of these antigens, particularly when multiple and/or common table foods are implicated.[33,53] This latter point is particularly relevant given the commonality of milk and wheat allergy identified in these patients. Elemental diets, though also effective,[54] are limited by tolerability and expense.

Another emerging issue in maintenance therapy is whether control of extraesophageal allergies positively affects esophageal disease. This contention is suggested in animal models by induction of esophageal eosinophilia through an initial priming mechanism of allergy in the lung or skin.[55] It is supported in humans by the finding of years of preceding airway allergies in most patients[56] as well as the inconsistent finding of flares of EoE during respiratory allergy seasons.[57] On identification of risk factors for EoE in patients with asthma, patients most typically have an allergic phenotype such as presence of allergic asthma and peripheral eosinophilia.[58] However, no controlled trials have been performed that demonstrate a beneficial effect of therapy directed toward extraesophageal allergic disease on EoE.

Data on Maintenance Therapy

Despite the theoretical benefits of maintenance steroid therapy, there is a distinct paucity of data available. In a randomized controlled trial conducted by Straumann and colleagues,[11] 28 patients were randomized to 0.25 mg of budesonide twice daily or placebo for 50 weeks. The favorable results from this trial demonstrated that budesonide reduced markers of inflammation, epithelial cell apoptosis, and remodeling events, without adverse side effects. Unfortunately, eosinophil count and symptoms significantly increased on both placebo and budesonide. A higher maintenance dosing of budesonide may have improved the therapeutic gain. These findings provide valuable data for defining an adequate maintenance dose, but further work needs to be performed to refine this approach.

Another looming issue on maintenance therapy is the potential long-term side effects of oral steroid therapies. In the Straumann trial, measurement of the effects of long-term budesonide on adrenal function are not discussed.[11] In a 3-month trial examining the use of swallowed topical steroids in children with EoE, there was no clear evidence of adrenal suppression.[59] Similarly, in another pediatric randomized study comparing prednisone with fluticasone, systemic effects such as Cushingoid features were only identified with systemic steroid administration.[60] When inhaled steroids are used for maintenance therapy in patients with asthma, both fluticasone and budesonide have been shown to slightly increase the risk for adrenal suppression.[61] One has to be careful in extrapolating the effects of steroid therapy in asthma to

EoE, as the distal esophagus venous network drains through the portal vein, exposing the drugs to hepatic first-pass metabolism. One also needs to consider that although it is assumed that little small-bowel or esophageal absorption occurs with the oral route of a topical steroid preparation, this is also not well studied.

Diet therapy has more robust and longer-term data on maintenance, albeit uncontrolled. In a series of 562 children studied for up to 14 years and treated mostly with diet, only 11 children remained in remission as defined by absence of esophageal eosinophilia.[57] On the other hand, improvement in symptoms and histology occurred in 98% of 381 patients studied long term and maintained on diet therapy, including 16% maintained on an elemental diet.[42] Lucendo and colleagues[33] reported that adult EoE patients on an empiric 6-food elimination diet had prolonged clinical and histopathologic remission for up to 3 years of follow-up.

Conclusions on Maintenance Therapy

Current data support the conceptual and clinical benefits of long-term maintenance therapy in EoE. At present, however, the appropriate patients to use maintenance therapy, the proper end point of therapy that will prevent and perhaps reverse complications of EoE, and the type of therapy that will provide the greatest benefit-to-risk ratio are unanswered questions. Nevertheless, it is reasonable to discuss the potential benefits of maintenance therapy in all patients with EoE, particularly those who have already evidenced disease complications. For those patients who have responded and are able to adhere to elimination diet therapy, maintenance is relatively straightforward. For those patients who have responded to short-term topical steroids, options include reduced-dose maintenance steroids, intermittent steroids, and clinical observation without therapy. Esophageal dilation, discussed next, may offer a long-term symptom improvement in selected patients.

ESOPHAGEAL DILATION

Esophageal dilation was one of the first therapies used to treat stricturing EoE.[62,63] Recent publications on the natural history of EoE have demonstrated that persisting eosinophil-predominant inflammation leads to the formation of esophageal strictures.[5,6] More than one-third of EoE patients suffer from one or several food bolus impactions necessitating endoscopic removal as an emergency procedure.[25,64] Esophageal dilation can be performed using either through-the-scope inflatable balloons or wire-guided Savary bougies. Strictures are readily recognized if a standard, diagnostic endoscope does not traverse the esophagus. It is not yet clear as to how accurate gastroenterologists are in detecting and reporting lower grades of esophageal strictures. It can be hypothesized that mild strictures or generalized esophageal narrowing will be underappreciated by the endoscopist.

A study by Schoepfer and colleagues[31] of 474 dilations in 207 EoE patients treated by esophageal dilation found that 67% of patients reported an improvement or absence of dysphagia following esophageal dilation. Patient acceptance for dilation was high.[31] Similarly, Dellon and colleagues[65] reported on a series of 36 EoE patients who were treated by a total of 70 dilations with a symptom response of 83%. A recently reported meta-analysis on 860 EoE patients, of whom 525 underwent at least 1 esophageal dilation and a total of 992 dilations, showed a clinical improvement in 75% of patients.[66]

Esophageal dilation may also be associated with several limitations, the first of which is the occurrence of postprocedural thoracic pain.[31] Postdilational pain may last for some days and responds favorably to analgesics.[31] Hospitalizations resulting from postprocedural pain are rare (about 1%).[66] A second limitation is that dilation does not influence the severity of eosinophil-predominant esophageal inflammation.[31] As a third limitation, dilation may be associated with esophageal perforation. Whereas earlier case series have reported a high complication rate,[67] subsequent studies consistently showed a lower perforation rate, approximating estimates of perforation risk for dilation for other benign esophageal disorders. Jung and colleagues[30] evaluated 293 dilations in 167 patients, and found a perforation rate of 1% (3 cases). In a series of 207 dilated patients (mean 2 dilations per patient), no case of esophageal perforation was documented.[31] A 2010 meta-analysis that included 468 patients having undergone 671 dilations found only 1 perforation (0.1%).[68] This result is comparable to that of the meta-analysis by Moawad and colleagues[66] reporting on 3 perforations during 992 dilations (0.3% perforation rate).

It is unknown as to which defined esophageal diameter should be targeted by dilation, but most patients show considerable symptomatic improvement when a diameter of 16 to 18 mm has been reached.[31] It has been recommended that the progression of dilation per session should be limited to 3 mm or less.[30] Mucosal tears or lacerations following dilation should not be regarded as a complication but rather as evidence of effective therapy.[68] Dilation-related esophageal bleedings that necessitate an endoscopic intervention do occur on rare occasion.[66]

PATIENTS REFRACTORY TO STANDARD THERAPIES

Patients with EoE with a limited or lack of response to initial diet or medical therapy include those with persistent symptoms, persistent esophageal inflammation, or both symptoms and inflammation. In addition, patients may demonstrate both symptoms and histologic response but have persistent esophageal luminal stenosis. As discussed earlier, the definition of symptom and histologic response has yet to be determined in either daily practice or clinical trials. With this caveat in mind, when both symptoms and inflammation persist, the initial therapy needs to be examined.

Patients not responding to topical steroids should be questioned as to adherence, dosing, and appropriate method of administration. Adherence to medications can be challenging for adolescent and adult patients, most of whom are unaccustomed to the use of medications on a long-term basis. Dose escalation of topical steroids is a consideration, as higher response rates have been reported in studies using fluticasone 880 μg twice daily compared with those using 440 μg twice daily.[8] Prospective studies comparing various dosing regimens are lacking, however. Anecdotal reports have noted patients failing to respond to swallowed fluticasone by inhaler administration who responded to liquid budesonide. This observation may be the result of inadvertent inhalation instead of swallowing of the aerosolized steroid. A randomized controlled trial compared swallowed budesonide administered via a nebulizer with a liquid suspension.[69] Although superiority was apparent with the liquid suspension, steroid formulations studied in clinical trials and used in clinical practice are delivered by metered dose inhalation, not nebulizers. Systemic steroids are often considered superior to topical steroids. A randomized trial, however, found similar efficacy in terms of the primary end point of a histopathology score for topical fluticasone compared with oral prednisone in a pediatric cohort.[60] The study did find that a secondary end point of histologic normalization was significantly greater with systemic steroids, supporting a potential role for systemic steroids in patients unresponsive to topical steroids.

Dietary therapy is an option for patients unresponsive to topical steroids, although there are only anecdotal reports regarding the effectiveness of this crossover strategy.

Several uncontrolled, retrospective studies indicate a greater response to elemental formula diets compared with empiric or allergy testing–directed elimination diet therapy. However, the tolerability and acceptability of elemental diets limits their widespread use. Other medical therapies including montelukast, cromolyn sodium, or antihistamines have shown limited benefits in a few small uncontrolled studies, and are considered second-line agents.[1] The effectiveness of therapies combining steroids, diet, montelukast, and antihistamines has not been reported.

Patients with resolution of eosinophilia but continued dysphagia with evidence of esophageal stenosis are candidates for esophageal dilation. The reversibility of esophageal remodeling in EoE with medical or diet therapies is discussed in an article elsewhere in this issue.[47–49] It should be noted that the reversal of esophageal submucosal fibrosis and remodeling in EoE may require prolonged therapy, whereas the epithelial inflammatory response may respond rapidly (within 2 weeks) with topical corticosteroid administration. Available studies have demonstrated modest improvement in esophageal lamina propria fibrosis and stricture in adults with EoE with short-term and intermediate-term (1 year) therapy with topical steroids.[11]

Novel biologic therapies have emerged for the treatment of EoE. Anti–immunoglobulin E, anti–interleukin (IL)-5, anti-IL-13, anti–tumor necrosis factor, and CRTH2-antagonist therapies have been reported in small studies.[70–72] Several of these studies included patients who were refractory or dependent on corticosteroid therapy. Significant histologic response was seen in pediatric studies of anti–IL-5 therapy, but symptom response was more difficult to demonstrate. Analogous to their use in inflammatory bowel disease, biologics therapy offers the potential of disease-modifying and steroid-sparing agents. More data on their use as monotherapy or in combination with existing therapies is needed.

TREATMENT OF ASYMPTOMATIC PATIENTS

Based on current consensus recommendations and clinical guidelines, patients with significant esophageal eosinophilia on biopsy but without symptoms would not meet the definition of EoE.[1] However, patients may have substantial esophageal luminal stenoses but do not report dysphagia, because of careful mastication, prolonged meal times, and/or food avoidance. The same situation may be encountered in patients initially diagnosed with EoE but achieving symptom but not histologic remission following medical or dietary therapy. At present, there is limited evidence to support additional treatment of such individuals. A more proactive approach might be considered in asymptomatic patients with esophageal eosinophilia and higher degrees of esophageal stenosis, and in treated patients without symptoms but with esophageal eosinophilia who have a history of disease complications such as food impaction or esophageal stricture. Given the uncertainties regarding the natural history of EoE, clinical follow-up for patients with esophageal eosinophilia even in the absence of symptoms is reasonable. Growing evidence supports the concept that untreated disease leads to higher degrees of esophageal stricture over time.[5]

THERAPEUTIC ALGORITHM

Given the many unknowns in EoE therapy and outcome assessment, it may seem venturesome to provide a therapy algorithm for clinical practice. Nevertheless, the authors provide here their approach in EoE patient management that is in line with recent clinical consensus recommendations and guidelines (**Fig. 3**).[1,7] Relevant end points

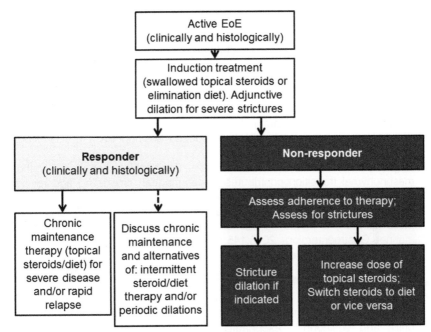

Fig. 3. Eosinophilic esophagitis (EoE) therapy algorithm.

for daily practice include EoE-related symptoms and esophageal eosinophilic inflammation. Patient history in adult EoE patients should not only include dysphagia and thoracic pain but also behavioral modifications such as food avoidance, food modification, and time taken to eat a regular meal. Dysphagia should be assessed according to distinct food consistencies, especially meat, rice, and bread. Endoscopic features, especially the presence of strictures, should be taken into account when establishing a therapy plan. Symptomatic EoE patients with esophageal eosinophilic inflammation should be treated either with swallowed topical corticosteroids or elimination diets. A reasonable clinical goal is to achieve an important reduction in EoE-related symptoms as well as esophageal eosinophilic inflammation. How much of residual esophageal eosinophilic inflammation can be tolerated is currently unknown. Evidence is increasing to support a maintenance therapy. In EoE patients in symptomatic remission, the authors recommend a yearly disease monitoring with symptom, endoscopic, and histologic assessments of sustained treatment response. In cases of persistent symptomatic esophageal strictures, esophageal dilation is an effective and safe approach.

SUMMARY

For clinical practice, therapeutic goals in EoE include relief of esophageal symptoms and improvement in eosinophilic inflammation and endoscopic features, particularly strictures. EoE activity indices that incorporate PROs are currently being validated and evaluated in the context of randomized, controlled clinical trials. Maintenance therapies are an important consideration for both pediatric and adult patients with EoE, especially in light of recent data reporting a substantial risk for esophageal stricture development in the setting of prolonged untreated disease.

REFERENCES

1. Liacouras CA, Furuta GT, Hirano I, et al. Eosinophilic esophagitis: updated consensus recommendations for children and adults. J Allergy Clin Immunol 2011;128:3–20.
2. Straumann A, Spichtin HP, Grize L, et al. Natural history of primary eosinophilic esophagitis: a follow-up of 30 adult patients for up to 11.5 years. Gastroenterology 2003;125:1660–9.
3. Mishra A, Wang M, Pemmaraju VR, et al. Esophageal remodeling develops as a consequence of tissue specific IL-5 induced eosinophilia. Gastroenterology 2008;134:204–14.
4. Kagalwalla AF, Akhtar N, Woodruff SA, et al. Eosinophilic esophagitis: epithelial mesenchymal transition contributes to esophageal remodeling and reverses with treatment. J Allergy Clin Immunol 2012;129:1387–96.
5. Schoepfer AM, Safroneeva E, Bussmann C, et al. Delay in diagnosis of eosinophilic esophagitis increases risk for stricture formation, in a time-dependent manner. Gastroenterology 2013;145:1230–6.
6. Dellon ES, Kim HP, Sperry SL, et al. A phenotypic analysis shows that eosinophilic esophagitis is a progressive fibrostenotic disease. Gastrointest Endosc 2013. [Epub ahead of print].
7. Dellon ES, Gonsalves N, Hirano I, et al. ACG clinical guideline: evidence based approach to the diagnosis and management of esophageal eosinophilia and eosinophilic esophagitis (EoE). Am J Gastroenterol 2013;108: 679–92.
8. Alexander JA, Jung KW, Arora AS, et al. Swallowed fluticasone improves histologic but not symptomatic response of adults with eosinophilic esophagitis. Clin Gastroenterol Hepatol 2012;10:742–9.
9. Pentiuk S, Putnam PE, Collins MH, et al. Dissociation between symptoms and histological severity in pediatric eosinophilic esophagitis. J Pediatr Gastroenterol Nutr 2009;48:152–60.
10. Straumann A, Conus S, Degen L, et al. Budesonide is effective in adolescent and adult patients with active eosinophilic esophagitis. Gastroenterology 2010;139:1526–37.
11. Straumann A, Conus S, Degen L, et al. Long-term budesonide maintenance treatment is partially effective for patients with eosinophilic esophagitis. Clin Gastroenterol Hepatol 2011;9:400–9.
12. US Food and Drug Administration. Patient-reported outcome measures: use in medical product development to support labeling claims. Available at: www.fda.gov/downloads/Drugs/Guidances/UCM193282.pdf. Accessed December 3, 2013.
13. Fiorentino R, Liu G, Pariser AR, et al. Cross-sector sponsorship of research in eosinophilic esophagitis: a collaborative model for rational drug development in rare diseases. J Allergy Clin Immunol 2012;130:613–6.
14. Rothenberg ME, Aceves S, Bonis PA, et al. Working with the US Food and Drug Administration: progress and timelines in understanding and treating patients with eosinophilic esophagitis. J Allergy Clin Immunol 2012;130:617–9.
15. Noel RJ, Putnam PE, Rothenberg ME. Eosinophilic esophagitis. N Engl J Med 2004;351:940–1.
16. Norquist JM, Girman C, Fehnel S, et al. Choice of recall period for patient-reported outcome (PRO) measures: criteria for consideration. Qual Life Res 2012;21:1013–20.

17. Dellon ES, Irani AM, Hill MR, et al. Development and field testing of a novel patient-reported outcome measure of dysphagia in patients with eosinophilic esophagitis. Aliment Pharmacol Ther 2013;38:634–42.
18. Taft TH, Kern E, Kwiatek MA, et al. The adult eosinophilic esophagitis quality of life questionnaire: a new measure of health-related quality of life. Aliment Pharmacol Ther 2011;34:790–8.
19. Franciosi JP, Hommel KA, DeBrosse CW, et al. Development of a validated patient-reported symptom metric for pediatric eosinophilic esophagitis: qualitative methods. BMC Gastroenterol 2011;11:126.
20. Franciosi JP, Hommel KA, Bendo CB, et al. PedsQL eosinophilic esophagitis module: feasibility, reliability, and validity. J Pediatr Gastroenterol Nutr 2013;57:57–66.
21. Hirano I, Moy N, Heckman MG, et al. Endoscopic assessment of the oesophageal features of eosinophilic oesophagitis: validation of a novel classification and grading system. Gut 2013;62:489–95.
22. Dellon ES, Aderoju A, Woosley JT, et al. Variability in diagnostic criteria for eosinophilic esophagitis: a systematic review. Am J Gastroenterol 2007;102:2300–13.
23. Furuta GT, Kagalwalla AF, Lee JJ, et al. The oesophageal string test: a novel, minimally invasive method measures mucosal inflammation in eosinophilic oesophagitis. Gut 2013;62:1395–405.
24. Kwiatek MA, Hirano I, Kahrilas PJ, et al. Mechanical properties of the esophagus in eosinophilic esophagitis. Gastroenterology 2011;140:82–90.
25. Straumann A, Bussmann C, Zuber M, et al. Eosinophilic esophagitis: analysis of food impaction and perforation in 251 adolescent and adult patients. Clin Gastroenterol Hepatol 2008;6:598–600.
26. Desai TK, Goldstein NS, Stecevic V, et al. Esophageal eosinophilia is common among adults with esophageal food impaction. Gastroenterology 2002;122:343.
27. Kerlin P, Jones D, Remedios M, et al. Prevalence of eosinophilic esophagitis in adults with food bolus obstruction of the esophagus. J Clin Gastroenterol 2007;41:356–61.
28. Prasad GA, Talley NJ, Romero Y, et al. Prevalence and predictive factors of eosinophilic esophagitis in patients presenting with dysphagia: a prospective study. Am J Gastroenterol 2007;102:2627–32.
29. Cohen MS, Kaufman A, Dimarino AJ, et al. Eosinophilic esophagitis presenting as spontaneous esophageal rupture (Boerhaave's syndrome). Clin Gastroenterol Hepatol 2007;5:A24.
30. Jung KW, Gundersen N, Kopacova J, et al. Occurrence and risk factors for complications after endoscopic dilation in eosinophilic esophagitis. Gastrointest Endosc 2011;73:15–21.
31. Schoepfer AM, Gonsalves N, Bussmann C, et al. Esophageal dilation in eosinophilic esophagitis: effectiveness, safety, and impact on the underlying inflammation. Am J Gastroenterol 2010;105:1062–70.
32. DeBrosse CW, Franciosi JP, King EC, et al. Long-term outcomes in pediatric-onset esophageal eosinophilia. J Allergy Clin Immunol 2011;128:132–8.
33. Lucendo AJ, Arias A, Gonzalez-Cervera J, et al. Empiric 6-food elimination diet induced and maintained prolonged remission in patients with adult eosinophilic esophagitis: a prospective study on the food cause of the disease. J Allergy Clin Immunol 2013;131:797–804.
34. Helou EF, Simonson J, Arora AS. Three-year follow-up of topical corticosteroid treatment for eosinophilic esophagitis in adults. Am J Gastroenterol 2008;103:2194–9.

35. Lee J, Huprich J, Kujath C, et al. Esophageal diameter is decreased in some patients with eosinophilic esophagitis and might increase with topical corticosteroid therapy. Clin Gastroenterol Hepatol 2012;10:481–6.

36. Fox VL, Nurko S, Teitelbaum JE, et al. High-resolution EUS in children with eosinophilic "allergic" esophagitis. Gastrointest Endosc 2003;57:30–6.

37. Roman S, Hirano I, Kwiatek MA, et al. Manometric features of eosinophilic esophagitis in esophageal pressure topography. Neurogastroenterol Motil 2011;23:208–14.

38. Aceves SS, Newbury RO, Dohil R, et al. Esophageal remodeling in pediatric eosinophilic esophagitis. J Allergy Clin Immunol 2007;119:206–12.

39. Aceves SS. Tissue remodeling in patients with eosinophilic esophagitis: what lies beneath the surface? J Allergy Clin Immunol 2011;128:1047–9.

40. Lucendo AJ, Arias A, De Rezende LC, et al. Subepithelial collagen deposition, profibrogenic cytokine gene expression, and changes after prolonged fluticasone propionate treatment in adult eosinophilic esophagitis: a prospective study. J Allergy Clin Immunol 2011;128:1037–46.

41. Lee S, de Boer WB, Naran A, et al. More than just counting eosinophils: proximal oesophageal involvement and subepithelial sclerosis are major diagnostic criteria for eosinophilic oesophagitis. J Clin Pathol 2010;63:644–7.

42. Liacouras CA, Spergel JM, Ruchelli E, et al. Eosinophilic esophagitis: a 10-year experience in 381 children. Clin Gastroenterol Hepatol 2005;3: 1198–206.

43. Bohm M, Richter JE, Kelsen S, et al. Esophageal dilation: simple and effective treatment for adults with eosinophilic esophagitis and esophageal rings and narrowing. Dis Esophagus 2010;23:377–85.

44. Bohm ME, Richter JE. Review article: oesophageal dilation in adults with eosinophilic oesophagitis. Aliment Pharmacol Ther 2011;33:748–57.

45. Schnitzler F, Fidder H, Ferrante M, et al. Mucosal healing predicts long-term outcome of maintenance therapy with infliximab in Crohn's disease. Inflamm Bowel Dis 2009;15:1295–301.

46. Noel RJ, Putnam PE, Collins MH, et al. Clinical and immunopathologic effects of swallowed fluticasone for eosinophilic esophagitis. Clin Gastroenterol Hepatol 2004;2:568–75.

47. Aceves SS, Newbury RO, Chen D, et al. Resolution of remodeling in eosinophilic esophagitis correlates with epithelial response to topical corticosteroids. Allergy 2010;65:109–16.

48. Caldwell JM, Blanchard C, Collins MH, et al. Glucocorticoid-regulated genes in eosinophilic esophagitis: a role for FKBP51. J Allergy Clin Immunol 2010;125: 879–88.

49. Lucendo AJ, Pascual-Turrion JM, Navarro M, et al. Endoscopic, bioptic, and manometric findings in eosinophilic esophagitis before and after steroid therapy: a case series. Endoscopy 2007;39:765–71.

50. Hsu Blatman KS, Gonsalves N, Hirano I, et al. Expression of mast cell-associated genes is upregulated in adult eosinophilic esophagitis and responds to steroid or dietary therapy. J Allergy Clin Immunol 2011;127:1307–8.

51. Lu TX, Lim EJ, Wen T, et al. MiR-375 is downregulated in epithelial cells after IL-13 stimulation and regulates an IL-13-induced epithelial transcriptome. Mucosal Immunol 2012;5:388–96.

52. Sherrill JD, Rothenberg ME. Genetic dissection of eosinophilic esophagitis provides insight into disease pathogenesis and treatment strategies. J Allergy Clin Immunol 2011;128:23–32 [quiz: 33–4].

53. Gonsalves N, Yang GY, Doerfler B, et al. Elimination diet effectively treats eosinophilic esophagitis in adults; food reintroduction identifies causative factors. Gastroenterology 2012;142:1451–9.e1 [quiz: e14–5].

54. Peterson K, Clayton F, Vinson LA, et al. Utility of an elemental diet in adult eosinophilic esophagitis. Gastroenterology 2011;140(Suppl 1):S180.

55. Rothenberg ME, Mishra A, Collins MH, et al. Pathogenesis and clinical features of eosinophilic esophagitis. J Allergy Clin Immunol 2001;108:891–4.

56. Simon D, Marti H, Heer P, et al. Eosinophilic esophagitis is frequently associated with IgE-mediated allergic airway diseases. J Allergy Clin Immunol 2005;115: 1090–2.

57. Spergel JM, Brown-Whitehorn TF, Beausoleil JL, et al. 14 years of eosinophilic esophagitis: clinical features and prognosis. J Pediatr Gastroenterol Nutr 2009;48:30–6.

58. Harer KN, Enders FT, Lim KG, et al. An allergic phenotype and the use of steroid inhalers predict eosinophilic oesophagitis in patients with asthma. Aliment Pharmacol Ther 2013;37:107–13.

59. Dohil R, Newbury R, Fox L, et al. Oral viscous budesonide is effective in children with eosinophilic esophagitis in a randomized, placebo-controlled trial. Gastroenterology 2010;139:418–29.

60. Schaefer ET, Fitzgerald JF, Molleston JP, et al. Comparison of oral prednisone and topical fluticasone in the treatment of eosinophilic esophagitis: a randomized trial in children. Clin Gastroenterol Hepatol 2008;6:165–73.

61. Clark DJ, Grove A, Cargill RI, et al. Comparative adrenal suppression with inhaled budesonide and fluticasone propionate in adult asthmatic patients. Thorax 1996;51:262–6.

62. Attwood SE, Smyrk TC, Demeester TR, et al. Esophageal eosinophilia with dysphagia, a distinct clinicopathologic syndrome. Dig Dis Sci 1993;38: 109–16.

63. Straumann A, Spichtin HP, Bernoulli R, et al. Idiopathic eosinophilic esophagitis: a frequently overlooked disease with typical clinical aspects and discrete endoscopic findings. Schweiz Med Wochenschr 1994;124:1419–29 [in German with English abstract].

64. Lucendo AJ, Friginal-Ruiz AB, Rodriguez B. Boerhaave's syndrome as the primary manifestation of adult eosinophilic esophagitis. Two case reports and a review of the literature. Dis Esophagus 2011;24:E11–5.

65. Dellon ES, Gibbs WS, Rubinas TC, et al. Esophageal dilation in eosinophilic esophagitis: safety and predictors of clinical response and complications. Gastrointest Endosc 2010;71:706–12.

66. Moawad FJ, Cheatham JG, DeZee KJ. Meta-Analysis: the safety and efficacy of dilation in eosinophilic esophagitis. Aliment Pharmacol Ther 2013;38:713–20.

67. Hirano I. Dilation in eosinophilic esophagitis: to do or not to do? Gastrointest Endosc 2010;71:713–4.

68. Jacobs JW Jr, Spechler SJ. A systematic review of the risk of perforation during esophageal dilation for patients with eosinophilic esophagitis. Dig Dis Sci 2010; 55:1512–5.

69. Dellon ES, Sheikh A, Speck O, et al. Viscous topical is more effective than nebulized steroid therapy for patients with eosinophilic esophagitis. Gastroenterology 2012;143:321–4.

70. Straumann A, Conus S, Grzonka P, et al. Anti-interleukin-5 antibody treatment (mepolizumab) in active eosinophilic esophagitis: a randomised, placebo-controlled, double-blind trial. Gut 2010;59:21–30.

71. Straumann A, Bussmann C, Conus S, et al. Anti-TNF-alpha (infliximab) therapy for severe adult eosinophilic esophagitis. J Allergy Clin Immunol 2008;122: 425–7.
72. Straumann A, Hoesli S, Bussmann C, et al. Anti-eosinophil activity and clinical efficacy of the CRTH2 antagonist OC000459 in eosinophilic esophagitis. Allergy 2013;68:375–85.

Steroids in Pediatric Eosinophilic Esophagitis

Emily M. Contreras, MD, Sandeep K. Gupta, MD*

KEYWORDS

- Children • Eosinophilic esophagitis • Steroids • Topical steroids • Fluticasone
- Budesonide • Ciclesonide

KEY POINTS

- Topical corticosteroids (CSs) (eg, swallowed fluticasone propionate [FP] and oral viscous budesonide [OVB]) are effective first-line therapies for pediatric eosinophilic esophagitis.
- Topical CSs have minimal known side effects when used for treatment of eosinophilic esophagitis.
- Systemic CSs have significant adverse effects and are now reserved for urgent situations where topical CSs are not effective or in patients who require rapid improvement in symptoms.

The goals for treatment of eosinophilic esophagitis (EoE) are improvements in symptoms and esophageal eosinophilic inflammation with the ideal endpoint complete resolution of the latter.[1] Once a diagnosis of proton pump inhibitor (PPI)-nonresponsive EoE is confirmed, treatment options include pharmacologic agents and/or dietary elimination. If pharmacologic therapy is chosen, topical CSs are effective and considered first line. Although these medications are currently not Food and Drug Administration approved for EoE, the 2 commonly used options are swallowed aerosolized FP and OVB. Systemic CSs (ie, prednisolone and methylprednisolone) may be useful if topical steroids are not effective or in patients who require rapid improvement in symptoms.

This article discusses the use of topical and systemic CSs for induction of remission and as maintenance treatment of pediatric EoE. The risks and benefits of these agents are outlined and some important and clinically relevant questions discussed.

Disclosures: E.M. Contreras has no disclosures; S.K. Gupta is a consultant for Meritage Pharmacia, QOL Medical, and Receptos Inc. He is in the speaker's bureau for both Abbott Nutrition and Nestle.

Division of Pediatric Gastroenterology, Hepatology, and Nutrition, Department of Pediatrics, Riley Hospital for Children, Indiana University School of Medicine, 705 Riley Hospital Drive, ROC 4210, Indianapolis, IN 46202, USA

* Corresponding author.

E-mail address: sgupta@iu.edu

Gastroenterol Clin N Am 43 (2014) 345–356

http://dx.doi.org/10.1016/j.gtc.2014.02.008

0889-8553/14/$ – see front matter © 2014 Elsevier Inc. All rights reserved.

gastro.theclinics.com

TOPICAL CORTICOSTEROIDS FOR INDUCTION

In 1998, Faubion and colleagues[2] described 4 children with eosinophilic inflammation isolated to the esophagus who improved clinically and histologically by swallowing aerosolized CSs (FP and beclomethasone) from an inhaler without use of a spacer. Over time, FP has become the topical CS used most often in EoE, although other agents are also used (discussed later). We will review prospective and randomized studies involving topical steroids used in pediatric eosinophilic esophagitis (**Table 1**). Adult studies are discussed elsewhere in this issue.

Fluticasone

In 2002, a prospective study using swallowed FP in children cited its ease of administration, low systemic absorption, and rapid first-pass metabolism by the liver to limit systemic side effects.[3] These children had symptoms of esophageal dysfunction (ie, chest pain, food impaction, dysphagia, feeding refusal, and vomiting), eosinophilic esophageal infiltration, normal 24-hour continuous monitoring of intraesophageal pH (pH probe), and lack of clinical response to an 8-week trial of PPI. FP dosing was age dependent, with a maximum of 880 μg/d divided twice daily. Four patients had no food allergens identified by history, radioimmunosorbent assay, or skin prick testing and were started directly on swallowed FP. Eleven patients were started on dietary restriction and nutritional counseling based on abnormal allergy testing or history; however, none of these patients had clinical improvement and 9 were subsequently treated with swallowed FP. All 13 patients who received FP had resolution of their presenting symptoms, and all 11 patients with post-treatment endoscopy showed improvement in histology with similar decreases in eosinophilia in proximal and distal esophageal biopsies.

A subsequent randomized, double-blind, placebo-controlled trial in children showed that 50% of FP-treated patients achieved complete histologic remission (≤1 eosinophil [EOS] per high-power field [HPF]) with a standard dose, regardless of patient age and/or size, of 880 μg/d divided twice daily.[4] Patient factors predictive of histologic resolution in this study included shorter stature and younger age. Unlike the previous study, proximal esophageal biopsies were more improved than those from the distal esophagus. Another randomized controlled trial comparing swallowed FP to oral prednisone (880–1760 μg/d based on age and 1 mg/kg/d to a maximum of 30 mg twice daily, respectively) showed complete histologic resolution in 50% of patients in FP group versus 81% in prednisone group at week 4; partial improvement in histologic grade was recorded in 94% of patients in both groups.[5] As expected, symptomatic improvement was seen more often compared with histologic reversal; 97.2% of FP patients and 100% of prednisone patients had resolution of presenting symptoms with therapy although symptoms recurred in approximately 45% of patients 12 weeks after treatment was stopped (**Fig. 1**A).

A recent prospective Italian study in children using a higher dose of FP (2250 μg/d) for 6 weeks reported higher likelihood (73.5%) in reaching post-treatment peak esophageal eosinophils of less than 6 eos/hpf and suggested that more severe esophageal inflammation (higher median peak eos/hpf, presence of eosinophilic abscesses, and peak mast cells/HPF) was associated with higher response rate to FP treatment.[6] Age and height did not affect response in this study.

Improvement in incidental gastric eosinophilic inflammation (≥10 eos/hpf) in patients otherwise similar to EoE patients was noted with FP.[7] Therefore, mild gastric eosinophilia should not exclude FP as a possible therapeutic option for esophageal eosinophilia.

The results of the first double-blind, randomized, placebo-controlled trial of FP (1760 μg/d) in children and adults are awaited.[8] Further studies are needed to determine ideal dosing regimen but current recommendations are listed in **Table 2**.

Budesonide

Budesonide is another topical steroid with proved efficacy for EoE. OVB was initially developed to help patients who were developmentally unable to perform the puff and swallow technique required for FP. The first studies to evaluate its efficacy mixed aqueous budesonide (0.5 mg/2 mL suspension, Budesonide Respules [Pulmicort], Astra-Zeneca, Wilmington, DE) with sucralose (see **Table 2** for recipe) to create a thickened slurry. A randomized, double-blind, placebo-controlled trial in children showed significant improvement in symptoms, endoscopic findings, and esophageal eosinophilia compared with placebo.[9] Patients less than 1.5 meters (5 feet) tall received 1 mg daily; patients greater than or equal to 5 feet tall received 2 mg daily for 3 months. Patients in both groups also received twice-daily lansoprazole (15 mg twice daily if less than 10 years old and 30 mg twice daily if greater than 10 years old). Peak eosinophil counts in the OVB group improved from 66.7 to 4.8 eos/hpf, with significant reductions in proximal, mid-, and distal esophageal eosinophilia.

No studies to date have compared FP and OVB in children.

Ciclesonide

Two small case series report a total of 8 children treated with ciclesonide, a topical CS also used in asthma, allergic rhinitis, and allergic conjunctivitis.[10,11] Six of the 8 patients showed histologic improvement; the 2 who did not respond had previous poor response to OVB as well. In asthma, inhaled ciclesonide seems to have similar effectiveness compared with inhaled FP and nebulized budesonide.[12] Larger randomized, drug-controlled studies are needed to see if this is the case in EoE.

TOPICAL CORTICOSTEROIDS FOR MAINTENANCE THERAPY

EoE is considered a chronic immune-mediated disease, yet long-term management has not been defined. Need for maintenance therapy is underscored by the observations that 45% of children had recurrence of symptoms within 12 weeks of discontinuing CS therapy[5] and esophageal eosinophilia recurred in a majority of patients[13] after 6 months off therapy (see **Fig. 1**). Straumann and colleagues[14] prospectively evaluated a maintenance regimen with swallowed nebulized budesonide (0.5 mg/d), in adolescents and adults after successful remission with 15 days of nebulized budesonide (2 mg/d). Patients placed on maintenance therapy of nebulized budesonide (0.5 mg/d) had increased eosinophil load compared with at remission/end of induction (31.8 to 0.4 eos/hpf, respectively). This increase was less pronounced when compared with patients placed on placebo after remission/end of induction (65.0 to 0.7 eos/hpf, respectively). Symptom scores were stable with maintenance therapy but increased with placebo. This study not only highlighted a shorter induction time of 15 days but also a newer mode of delivery (ie, via a nebulizer). Further studies with higher maintenance dose are needed to evaluate for efficacy and long-term adverse effects.

Maintenance therapy studies have not been done with FP or OVB or in children.

OTHER DELIVERY METHODS
Fluticasone

A tablet form (1.5 mg and 3 mg) of fluticasone is currently undergoing phase 1/2a trials in adolescents and adults.[15]

Table 1
Topical steroids in pediatric eosinophilic esophagitis, prospective and randomized controlled trials

Study	Type of Study	Control Group (n)	Histologic Criteria	Drug (n)	Dose (µg)	Length of Treatment	Primary Outcomes	Drug Efficacy[a] (%)	Control Group Response (%)	Other Outcomes	Adverse Events	Comments
Teitelbaum et al, 2002	Prospective	NA	>15 eos/hpf, superficial layering, and/or eosinophil microabscesses	FP (13)	2–4 yo: 88 BID 5–10 yo: 220 BID ≥11 yo: 440 BID	8 wk	Clinical improvement/ resolution of symptoms	100	NA	70% still had abnormal endoscopy (loss of vascular pattern, thickened longitudinal folds), but improved histology	18% With esophageal candidiasis, 9% (n = 1) symptomatic	8-wk PPI trial before diagnosis. Normal 24-h continuous pH monitoring; 9 of the patients who responded clinically to FP had failed allergy testing–based diet restriction.
Konikoff et al, 2006	Randomized, double-blind, placebo-controlled	Placebo (15)	>24 eos/hpf in any ×400 HPF and epithelial hyperplasia	FP (21)	440 BID	3 mo	Complete response: <1 eos/hpf Partial response: 1–24 eos/hpf	50 / 15	9 / 9	All FP responders: resolved distal furrowing, epithelial hyperplasia, and vomiting	Incidental esophageal candidiasis in 9% of FP pts (1/11)	Prior acid suppression therapy was not necessary for diagnosis. FP response higher in nonallergic individuals. FP response negatively correlates with patient age, height, and weight.
Schaefer et al, 2008	Randomized, comparator controlled	Prednisone 1 mg/kg/d (40)	≥15 eos/hpf with negative pH probe studies	FP (40)	1–10 yo: 220 QID 11–18 yo: 440 QID	4-wk Induction	Complete histologic resolution Improvement in biopsy grade (score based on basal cell zone % and # eos/hpf)	50 / 94	81 / 94	97% FP group had resolution of symptoms. 100% of prednisone group had resolution of symptoms.	Incidental esophageal candidiasis in 15% of FP patients; hyperphagia, weight gain in 40% of prednisone patients.	Symptom relapse in 44% of FP patients, 45% of prednisone 12 wk after treatment stopped.

Study	Design	Placebo (9)	Peak eos/hpf	Drug (n) dose	Dose	Duration	Primary Outcomes		Adverse Events	Comments
Dohil et al, 2010	Randomized, double-blind, placebo-controlled	Placebo (9)	≥20	OVB (15)	<5 ft Tall: 1000/d; ≥5 ft Tall: 2000/d	3 mo	Responders: <6 eos/hpf — 87, 0; Partial responders: 7–19 eos/hpf — 6.7, 11; Nonresponders ≥20 eos/hpf — 6.7, 89	Endoscopy score improved more in OVB vs placebo. Symptom score improved in OVB but not placebo group.	Oral candidiasis that responded to nystatin. Serum cortisol unchanged	All patients received PPI during drug period. <10 yo: Lansoprazole 15 mg BID; ≥10 yo: lansoprazole 30 mg BID. Placebo and PPI did not improve eosinophilia at any level.
Boldorini et al, 2013	Prospective	NA	>15 eos/hpf	FP (34) 750 TID		6 wk	Responders: ≤6 eos/hpf — 74, NA; Borderline: 7–20 eos/hpf — 0; Nonresponders: >20 eos/hpf — 26	All children had symptomatic improvement irrespective of histologic results. Responders had more severe inflammation (higher median peak eos/hpf, higher likelihood of eosinophilic microabscesses, and peak mast cells/HPF).	No adverse events seen	All children were nonresponders to PPI or 24-h pH monitoring was negative for gastroesophageal reflux. 4 Children had celiac disease, 3 were responders 1 was not. Age, weight, and height, did not affect response.

Abbreviations: BID, twice daily; NA, not applicable; QID, 4 times daily; TED, 3 times daily; yo, years old.

[a] Drug efficacy is based on definitions specific to each study (see Primary Outcomes column).

Data from Refs.[3–6,9]

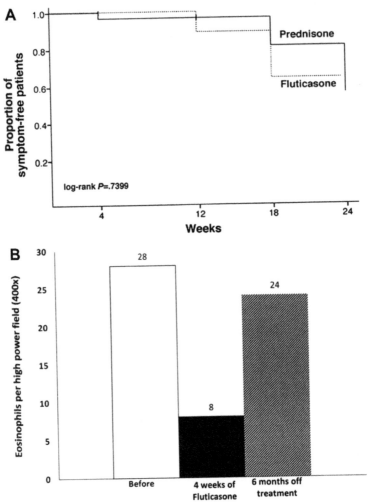

Fig. 1. (A) Proportion of symptom-free patients with prednisone and swallowed fluticasone. Patients received induction dose × 4 weeks, were weaned over 8 weeks, and were clinically monitored for next 12 weeks. (B) Recurrence of esophageal eosinophilia after withdrawal of swallowed fluticasone (220 μg twice daily). (From [A] Schaefer ET, Fitzgerald JF, Molleston JP, et al. Comparison of oral prednisone and topical fluticasone in the treatment of eosinophilic esophagitis: a randomized trial in children. Clin Gastroenterol Hepatol 2008;6:165–73, with permission; and [B] Liacouras CA, Spergel JM, Ruchelli E, et al. Eosinophilic esophagitis: a 10-year experience in 381 children. Clin Gastroenterol Hepatol 2005;3:1202, with permission.)

Budesonide

The current OVB formulation contains 10 mg sucralose per 1 mg budesonide to create an 8-mL slurry.[16] Concerns about taste, cost, and potential adverse effects of sucralose have made many patients and parents wary of OVB.[17] Some patients may use applesauce or other palatable food products that patients are not allergic to, although efficacy with these alternate vehicles has not been studied. At the authors' institution, 1 to 2 tablespoons of applesauce are allowed to be mixed with

Table 2
Dosing regimens for fluticasone propionate and oral viscous budesonide in pediatric eosinophilic esophagitis

Medication	Age (y)	Drug Formulation	Induction Dose	Weaning Dose	Instructions
FP	1–10	110 μg/puff	2 Puffs 4 times/d	2 Puffs 3 times/d × 3 wk, 2 puffs 2 times/d × 3 wk, 1 puff 2 times/d × 2 wk	1. Do not use with spacer. 2. Place inhaler in mouth, close lips around it, press down firmly on top of canister to release 1 dose of medication and swallow. Repeat as indicated. 3. No eating or drinking for 30 min after taking medication. 4. After 30 min, drink 30–60 mL of liquid to rinse medication to prevent yeast infection.
	11–18	220 μg/puff	Same as above with 220 μg/puff inhaler	Same as above with 220 μg/puff inhaler	
OVB	1–10	0.5 mg/2 mL budesonide respules	1 mg Daily		1. Open liquid budesonide respules and mix with sucralose (5g[a] per 2 mL respule). 2. Swallow mixture slowly over 5–10 min to help coat esophagus. 3. No eating or drinking for 30 min after taking medication. 4. After 30 min, drink 30–60 mL of liquid to rinse medication to prevent yeast infection.
	11–18	0.5 mg/2 mL budesonide respules	2 mg Daily		

[a] Sucralose (5 g) = 5 packets or 10 teaspoons.

2 respules (0.5 mg/2 mL) of budesonide. Hait and colleagues[18] found that 13 of 14 patients who added a hypoallergenic, amino acid–based semisolid (Neocate Nutra, Nutricia, Gaithersburg, MD) to their budesonide respules improved with post-treatment eosinophil counts less than 15 eos/hpf and continue to find results that are at least comparable to OVB with improved patient compliance (Eitan Rubinstein, personal communication, 2013).

Also in the works is a non–sucralose-based oral budesonide suspension (OBS) currently being studied in adolescents and adults. A prospective, randomized, double-blind, placebo-controlled study comparing 2 doses of OBS and placebo in children ages 2 to 18 years found panesophageal endoscopic and histologic dose-related responses.[19] Histologic response (peak $\leq$6 eos/hpf) was seen in 94% of patients in the high-dose OBS group (1.4 mg twice daily for 2–9 years old and 2 mg twice daily for 10–18 years old) versus 54% of patients in the medium-dose group (1.4 mg daily for 2–9 years old and 2 mg daily for 10–18 years old) and 5.6% in the placebo arm. This higher response in the high-dose group suggests a possible need to increase OVB dosing regimens to a higher dose of 4 mg/d in patients previously thought to fail budesonide therapy.

SYSTEMIC CORTICOSTEROIDS

Oral prednisone was the first pharmacologic agent shown effective in treating EoE[20] but can have systemic adverse effects in 40% of patients.[5] Although complete histologic resolution is more likely with prednisone compared with FP, the symptom improvement and long-term disease remissions were similar to those with FP. With the newer therapies available, systemic prednisone is now reserved for urgent situations where topical CS may not be as rapidly effective. Intravenous methylprednisolone may be considered in situations where patients are not tolerating anything by mouth.

MARKERS OF RESPONSE

The mechanism of action of topical steroids in EoE is still unknown. In randomized trials in children, 50% to 94% of children with EoE have partial to complete response to FP or OVB treatment.[4,5,9] Interpretation of published data is challenging for a variety of reasons, including varying definitions of response, type of CS, CS formulation, mode of delivery, total daily dose, number of doses per day, and adjustment of dose for clinical factors, such as age and height (discussed later). Currently, predicting who will or will not respond to CSs is not possible, but some studies have identified possible mechanisms of nonresponsiveness in these patients.

Caldwell and colleagues[21] provided evidence that topical CSs directly affect esophageal epithelial gene expression in vivo. They identified 32 transcripts altered by FP treatment in responders compared with those with untreated EoE and normal healthy controls. One of the genes, FK506 binding protein 51 (FKBP51), a known steroid-induced gene in respiratory epithelial cells and lymphocytes, was increased in FP responders and found to act as a negative regulator of FP action. In vitro, increased baseline FKBP51 levels correlated with a decreased ability of glucocorticoid to repress interleukin 13–mediated eotaxin-3 promoter activity and may suggest a mechanism for steroid nonresponsiveness.

Responders to OVB (defined as patients who had <7 eos/hpf after therapy) show a decrease in lamina propria fibrosis score, esophageal fibrosis mediators (transforming growth factor β1 [TGF-β1] and phosphorylated Smad2/3), epithelial edema, and vascular cell adhesion molecule 1–positive vessels not seen in nonresponders or untreated patients.[22] This study also suggested that genetic polymorphisms in the TGF-β1 promoter may be predictive of CS responsiveness.

Medication delivery method could affect histologic response; a recent adult study showed higher mucosal medication contact time and improved eosinophil counts with OVB versus the nebulized budesonide method.[23] Potential noninvasive markers for topical steroid therapy response include serum eosinophil cationic protein and serum eosinophil-derived neurotoxin.[24,25]

BENEFITS

A major benefit to patients of treatment with topical CS, in addition to improving their EoE, is not having to implement dietary modifications. As demonstrated in the recently validated PedsQL EoE Module, patients on restricted diets (and their parents) reported lower quality-of-life scores, with the largest gaps concerning food, eating, and food feelings.[26] Therefore, optimizing current topical CS therapy and developing other medical therapies are important in maintaining good quality of life for these patients.

Nevertheless, a variety of elimination diets are also recommended as first-line therapy for EoE; practice at the authors' institution is shown in **Fig. 2**. An adult study has shown symptomatic improvement with leukotriene antagonists but no effect on esophageal eosinophilia.[27] The authors do not note this improvement, however, in clinical practice where patients on montelukast (for their asthma management) have active EoE. In addition, cysteinyl leukotriene levels in esophageal mucosal biopsies of children with EoE were similar to those of controls.[28] A small series of children with EoE had no symptomatic or histologic response to cromolyn sodium.[13]

RISKS

As expected, 40% of children treated with prednisone for EoE exhibit systemic side effects, such as hyperphagia and weight gain.[5] Up to 15% of patients receiving FP

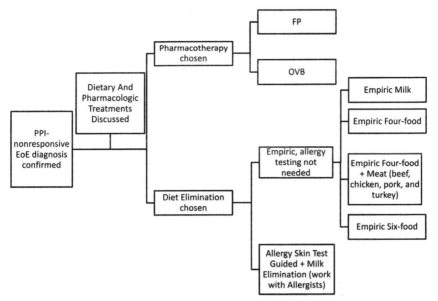

Fig. 2. Proposed algorithm for treatment of EoE.

may develop esophageal candidiasis, although this is usually found incidentally on follow-up endoscopy, is not associated with esophageal inflammation, and may not be of clinical significance.[4–6] To minimize this risk, the authors instruct patients to not eat or drink for 30 minutes after drug administration and then drink a small amount of liquid to wash the esophageal mucosa (see **Table 2** for FP and OVB dosing regimens and instructions). The incidence of esophageal candidiasis is decreasing with careful attention to drug administration.

There has been no definitive evidence of adrenal suppression with topical steroids. In the placebo-controlled trial with OVB there were no signs of adrenal suppression; serum cortisol levels were similar between pretreatment, post-treatment, and placebo-groups.[9] Long-term data regarding bone disease and/or growth rates are not yet available in patients with EoE. Asthma studies indicate that children receiving inhaled steroids grow 1 to 2 cm less than their counterparts; this height deficit does not accumulate but does persist into adulthood.[29,30] Prospective long-term studies using large EoE patient databases are needed to evaluate this.[31,32]

SUMMARY AND UNMET NEEDS

Swallowed FP and OVB are effective first-line pharmacologic therapies for EoE and an alternative to dietary restrictions. Side effects are minimal without evidence of Cushing syndrome, as seen in treatment with systemic CSs. Recent preliminary studies suggest that higher dosing and/or improved delivery may be needed to improve efficacy of these medications.[19] New studies on alternative delivery systems and different CSs (eg, ciclesonide) are encouraging. As knowledge of EoE expands, newer questions arise. Several of these are listed, recognizing that some have partial answers and others are without any answers at present. The authors hope this list will stimulate interests in the study of EoE:

1. Do the various formulations of topical CSs differ in efficacy and/or side-effect profile?
2. What are the optimal delivery mechanisms, dose strength, and dosing frequencies for topical CSs for induction and maintenance of remission?
3. What is the best length of treatment to induce remission?
4. What are long-term side effects of prolonged topical CS therapy (eg, linear growth, bone health, and adrenal suppression)? Are these adverse effects reversible or irreversible?
5. To what degree are adverse effects modified by simultaneous use of topical CSs for other conditions (eg, asthma and allergic rhinitis)?
6. Is there a benefit to cooling down the inflamed esophageal strictures with topical CSs or diet elimination prior to dilation?
7. Are CSs useful in the burnt-out esophagus without active eosinophilic inflammation but poor motility/compliance due to their effects on the fibrotic pathway?
8. Could PPI, mast cell stabilizers, or leukotriene antagonists be additive or synergistic with CS?
9. Should topical CSs be used in combination with diet and/or dilation therapy?

ACKNOWLEDGMENTS

We wish to extend our sincere appreciation to Ms Sharon McPheeters for her secretarial assistance and expert attention to this work.

REFERENCES

1. Dellon ES, Gonsalves N, Hirano I, et al. ACG clinical guideline: evidenced based approach to the diagnosis and management of esophageal eosinophilia and eosinophilic esophagitis (EoE). Am J Gastroenterol 2013;108:679–92 [quiz: 693].
2. Faubion WA Jr, Perrault J, Burgart LJ, et al. Treatment of eosinophilic esophagitis with inhaled corticosteroids. J Pediatr Gastroenterol Nutr 1998;27:90–3.
3. Teitelbaum JE, Fox VL, Twarog FJ, et al. Eosinophilic esophagitis in children: immunopathological analysis and response to fluticasone propionate. Gastroenterology 2002;122:1216–25.
4. Konikoff MR, Noel RJ, Blanchard C, et al. A randomized, double-blind, placebo-controlled trial of fluticasone propionate for pediatric eosinophilic esophagitis. Gastroenterology 2006;131:1381–91.
5. Schaefer ET, Fitzgerald JF, Molleston JP, et al. Comparison of oral prednisone and topical fluticasone in the treatment of eosinophilic esophagitis: a randomized trial in children. Clin Gastroenterol Hepatol 2008;6:165–73.
6. Boldorini R, Mercalli F, Oderda G. Eosinophilic oesophagitis in children: responders and non-responders to swallowed fluticasone. J Clin Pathol 2013;66: 399–402.
7. Ammoury RF, Rosenman MB, Roettcher D, et al. Incidental gastric eosinophils in patients with eosinophilic esophagitis: do they matter? J Pediatr Gastroenterol Nutr 2010;51:723–6.
8. Rothenberg ME, Children's Hospital Medical Center C. A double blinded, randomized trial of swallowed 1760 mcg fluticasone propionate versus placebo in the treatment of eosinophilic esophagitis. Bethesda (MD): National Library of Medicine (US); 2000 [cited 2014 Jan 10]. In: ClinicalTrials.gov [Internet]. Available at: http://clinicaltrials.gov/ct2/show/NCT00426283. NLM Identifier: NCT00426283.
9. Dohil R, Newbury R, Fox L, et al. Oral viscous budesonide is effective in children with eosinophilic esophagitis in a randomized, placebo-controlled trial. Gastroenterology 2010;139:418–29.
10. Lee JJ, Fried AJ, Hait E, et al. Topical inhaled ciclesonide for treatment of eosinophilic esophagitis. J Allergy Clin Immunol 2012;130:1011 [author reply: 1011–2].
11. Schroeder S, Fleischer DM, Masterson JC, et al. Successful treatment of eosinophilic esophagitis with ciclesonide. J Allergy Clin Immunol 2012;129:1419–21.
12. Dyer MJ, Halpin DM, Stein K. Inhaled ciclesonide versus inhaled budesonide or inhaled beclomethasone or inhaled fluticasone for chronic asthma in adults: a systematic review. BMC Fam Pract 2006;7:34.
13. Liacouras CA, Spergel JM, Ruchelli E, et al. Eosinophilic esophagitis: a 10-year experience in 381 children. Clin Gastroenterol Hepatol 2005;3:1198–206.
14. Straumann A, Conus S, Degen L, et al. Long-term budesonide maintenance treatment is partially effective for patients with eosinophilic esophagitis. Clin Gastroenterol Hepatol 2011;9:400–9.e1.
15. Aptalis Pharma. Six month safety follow-up study for PR-021 [multicenter, randomized, double-blind, placebo-controlled, safety and tolerability phase 1/2a study of two dosing regimens of EUR-1100 for oral use, in eosinophilic esophagitis subjects]. Bethesda (MD): National Library of Medicine (US); 2000 [cited 2014 Jan 10]. In: ClinicalTrials.gov [Internet]. Available at: http://clinicaltrials.gov/ct2/show/NCT01498497. NLM Identifierr: NCT 01498497.
16. Aceves SS, Bastian JF, Newbury RO, et al. Oral viscous budesonide: a potential new therapy for eosinophilic esophagitis in children. Am J Gastroenterol 2007; 102:2271–9 [quiz: 2280].

17. Schiffman SS, Rother KI. Sucralose, a synthetic organochlorine sweetener: overview of biological issues. J Toxicol Environ Health B Crit Rev 2013;16:399–451.
18. Hait E, Lee J, Fried A, et al. Neocate® Nutra is as effective as sucralose as a delivery vehicle for oral viscous budesonide to treat eosinophilic esophagitis in children [abstract]. J Pediatr Gastroenterol Nutr 2013;57:e4.
19. Gupta S, Collins M, Lewis J, et al. Efficacy and safety of oral budesonide suspension (OBS) in pediatric subjects with eosinophilic esophagitis (EoE): results from the double-blind, placebo-controlled PEER study. Gastroenterol Clin North Am 2011;140:S179.
20. Liacouras CA, Wenner WJ, Brown K, et al. Primary eosinophilic esophagitis in children: successful treatment with oral corticosteroids. J Pediatr Gastroenterol Nutr 1998;26:380–5.
21. Caldwell JM, Blanchard C, Collins MH, et al. Glucocorticoid-regulated genes in eosinophilic esophagitis: a role for FKBP51. J Allergy Clin Immunol 2010;125:879–88.e8.
22. Aceves SS, Newbury RO, Chen D, et al. Resolution of remodeling in eosinophilic esophagitis correlates with epithelial response to topical corticosteroids. Allergy 2010;65:109–16.
23. Dellon ES, Sheikh A, Speck O, et al. Viscous topical is more effective than nebulized steroid therapy for patients with eosinophilic esophagitis. Gastroenterology 2012;143:321–4.e1.
24. Schlag C, Pfefferkorn S, Brockow K, et al. Serum eosinophil cationic protein is superior to mast cell tryptase as marker for response to topical corticosteroid therapy in eosinophilic esophagitis. J Clin Gastroenterol 2013. [Epub ahead of print].
25. Subbarao G, Rosenman MB, Ohnuki L, et al. Exploring potential noninvasive biomarkers in eosinophilic esophagitis in children. J Pediatr Gastroenterol Nutr 2011;53:651–8.
26. Franciosi JP, Hommel KA, Bendo CB, et al. PedsQL eosinophilic esophagitis module: feasibility, reliability, and validity. J Pediatr Gastroenterol Nutr 2013;57:57–66.
27. Attwood SE, Lewis CJ, Bronder CS, et al. Eosinophilic oesophagitis: a novel treatment using Montelukast. Gut 2003;52:181–5.
28. Gupta SK, Peters-Golden M, Fitzgerald JF, et al. Cysteinyl leukotriene levels in esophageal mucosal biopsies of children with eosinophilic inflammation: are they all the same? Am J Gastroenterol 2006;101:1125–8.
29. Guilbert TW, Morgan WJ, Zeiger RS, et al. Long-term inhaled corticosteroids in preschool children at high risk for asthma. N Engl J Med 2006;354:1985–97.
30. Kelly HW, Sternberg AL, Lescher R, et al. Effect of inhaled glucocorticoids in childhood on adult height. N Engl J Med 2012;367:904–12.
31. Straumann A, Hruz P. What's new in the diagnosis and therapy of eosinophilic esophagitis? Curr Opin Gastroenterol 2009;25:366–71.
32. Dellon ES, Erichsen R, Pedersen L, et al. Development and validation of a registry-based definition of eosinophilic esophagitis in Denmark. World J Gastroenterol 2013;19:503–10.

Steroid Treatment of Eosinophilic Esophagitis in Adults

Jeffrey A. Alexander, MD

KEYWORDS

- Open-label trials • Placebo-controlled trials • Comparator trials • Maintenance trials
- Issues in steroid treatment of eosinophilic esophagitis

KEY POINTS

- Currently, there is no commercially available preparation designed to deliver the steroid to the esophagus. Current regimens consist of swallowing steroid preparations designed for inhalation treatment for asthma.
- When used in proper dose, steroids lead to complete histologic responses in the range of 60% to 70% of patients and at least a partial histologic response in more than 90% of patients.
- Symptom response rates appear to be somewhat less than histologic rates, with at least a partial symptomatic response of only 60% to 75%.
- Maintenance therapy seems promising in one trial, but likely needs a higher dosage than 0.25 mg budesonide twice a day.
- In the short term, steroids are associated with about a 15% to 25% incidence of asymptomatic esophageal candidiasis, but otherwise appear to be well tolerated.

OPEN-LABELED TRIALS

The first report of topical steroid therapy in adult patients with eosinophilic esophagitis (EoE) was reported by Arora and colleagues in 2003 (**Table 1**).[1] In this open-labeled study, Arora and colleagues[1] treated 21 adults with esophageal eosinophilic infiltration (EEI) and dysphagia. Patients were treated with 440 μg aerosolized swallowed fluticasone twice a day and all patients had a symptomatic response of their dysphagia to the treatment as accessed by a phone interview. Histologic follow-up was not obtained in this report.

Disclosures: The author is a consultant for Meritage Pharmacia, Aptalis Pharma. He has research funding from Meritage Pharmacia, Aptalis Pharma, and Merck Inc. He has financial interest in Meritage Pharmacia.
Division of Gastroenterology and Hepatology, Mayo Clinic School of Medicine, Mayo Clinic, 200 First Street Southwest, Rochester, MN 55905, USA
E-mail address: alexander.jeffrey14@mayo.edu

Gastroenterol Clin N Am 43 (2014) 357–373
http://dx.doi.org/10.1016/j.gtc.2014.02.001
0889-8553/14/$ – see front matter © 2014 Elsevier Inc. All rights reserved.

gastro.theclinics.com

Table 1
Open-labeled trials active treatment trials

Author	Tx	EEI/EoE	N	Duration	Symptoms Response	Definition	Histologic Response	Definition	Side Effects	Comments
Arora et al,[1] 2003	Fluticasone 440 µg twice a day	EEI	21	6 wk	90% (19/21)	Resolution of solid food dysphagia by phone interview	Not evaluated		5% (1/21) dry mouth	First report of steroid benefit in adult patients
Remedios et al,[2] 2006	Aerosolized fluticasone 500 µg twice a day	EEI	19	4 wk	5.42 pre −0.068 post (P<.001) 100% (19/19) decreased 58% (11/19) asymptomatic	Symptom score (0–18)	Proximal 25.0 pre 4.5 post (P<.0004) Distal 39.3 pre 3.8 post (P<.0001) 21% (4/19) complete response	eos/hpf	16% (3/19) asymptomatic esophageal candidiasis	53% (10/19) abnormal esophageal pH studies

Abbreviations: EEI, eosinophil esophageal infiltration; EoE, eosinophilic esophagitis; eos, eosinophils; hpf, high power field.

Data from Arora AS, Perrault J, Smyrk TC. Topical corticosteroid treatment of dysphagia due to eosinophilic esophagitis in adults. Mayo Clin Proc 2003;78:830–5; and Remedios M, Campbell C, Jones DM, et al. Eosinophilic esophagitis in adults: clinical, endoscopic, histologic findings, and response to treatment with fluticasone propionate. Gastrointest Endosc 2006;63:3–12.

A second open-labeled trial of topical steroid treatment in adult EoE was reported by Remedios and colleagues.[2] They evaluated 26 patients with symptomatic EEI and treated 19 who were accessed after treatment for histologic response, as well as symptomatic response. Pretreatment esophageal pH testing was abnormal in 53% (10/19) of the patients. All patients, regardless of pH results, were treated with topical aerosolized fluticasone 500 μg twice a day, a minimally increased dose over that used by Arora and colleagues.[1] The symptom score after treatment, as well as the histologic eosinophil levels in the proximal and distal esophagus, were markedly decreased with treatment.

In summary, both open-labeled trials showed a dramatic symptom and histologic response to aerosolized swallowed fluticasone. These studies involved patients with symptomatic EEI, and the therapeutic response was seen in those with and without gastroesophageal reflux disease (GERD) by pH testing.

PLACEBO-CONTROLLED TRIALS

There are 2 published placebo-controlled trials of topical steroid therapy in the treatment of EoE (**Table 2**). In the first trial, by Straumann and colleagues,[3] aerosolized budesonide delivered by nebulizer was used at a dosage of 1 mg twice a day for 15 days in subjects with EoE. There was a significant symptomatic response of dysphagia and histologic response in the budesonide-treated patients over the placebo treatment group. Of note, there was no symptomatic or histologic response in the placebo group. Of great interest in this trial, there were significant decreases in a semiquantitative histologic fibrosis score, markers of inflammation, and apoptosis with only 2 weeks of treatment. In histologic responders, the endoscopic findings of white exudates and furrows resolved but rings did not. Asymptomatic esophageal candidiasis was seen in 22% of patients with budesonide therapy.

The trial by Alexander and colleagues[4] studied the commonly used swallowed, aerosolized fluticasone delivered by inhaler in patients with EEI. This is currently available in the United States, requires no preparation, and is commonly used in clinical practice. In this trial, subjects were treated for 6 weeks with swallowed aerosolized fluticasone 880 μg twice a day. This is a dosage nearly double that used in the previously described open-label trials. In this trial, there, similarly, was an impressive histologic response to treatment. However, contrary to the previous uncontrolled trials of topical budesonide and fluticasone and the controlled trial of budesonide, symptoms were not improved in this trial. The per-protocol complete symptom response was 47% in the treatment group and 40% in the placebo group. Although the cause of the lack of symptomatic benefit in the treatment groups as compared with the control group is not clearly apparent, it may be due to the high symptomatic response in the placebo group, which was not seen in the Straumann and colleagues'[3] trial. Alternatively, because symptomatic response to treatment has been seen other trials of topical steroid therapy in EoE, it may be that the 2-Week Mayo Dysphagia Questionnaire failed to adequately access the patients' symptoms because the patients' symptoms were too infrequent and/or too mild to be adequately accessed with this instrument. Resolution of all endoscopic findings was uncommon in this trial and, similar to the Straumann and colleagues'[3] trial, endoscopic rings generally persisted in patients with a complete histologic response. Asymptomatic esophageal candidiasis was seen in 26% of treated patients.

In summary, placebo-controlled trials of fluticasone and budesonide confirmed the uncontrolled trials showing a strong histologic response to topical steroid treatment.[3,4] Of note, both trials showed essentially no histologic placebo response with

Table 2
Placebo-controlled trials

Author	Tx	EEI/ EoE N	Duration	Symptoms Tx Response	Symptoms Placebo Response	Symptoms Definition	Histologic Tx Response	Histologic Placebo Response	Histologic Definition	Endoscopic Tx Response	Endoscopic Placebo Response	Endoscopic Definition	Side Effects	Comments
Straumann et al,[3] 2010	Nebulized liquid suspension budesonide 1 mg twice a day	EoE 18 Tx / 18 Placebo	15 d	5.6 to 2.2 (P<.0001); 72% (13/18)	5.3 to 4.7 (ns); 22% (4/18) (P=.007)	Dysphagia scale (0–9); Pre-Post decreased >2 pts	72% (13/18); 17% (3/18)	11% (2/18) (P<.0001); 0% (0/18) (P<.0001)	Complete <5 eos/hpf; Partial 5–20 eos/hpf	White exudates 100% (10/10) to (0/10) (P=.0001); Red furrows 89% (9/9) to (P=.0036); Rings 11% (9/9) to (8/9) (ns)		Resolution of finding when present in histologic complete responders	Asymptomatic esophageal candidiasis 22% (4/18) of Tx group 0% (0/18) of placebo All mild 3 grossly, 1 histologic only	No predictors of steroid response Decrease proinflammatory markers, tissue apoptosis, fibrosis score with Tx
Alexander et al,[4] 2012	Fluticasone 440 µg twice a day	EEI 19 Tx / 15 Placebo	6 wk	Complete: ITT 43% (9/21) PP 47% (9/19) Partial: ITT: 14% (3/21) PP: 16% (3/19)	ITT 29% (6/21) (ns) PP 40% (6/15) (ns) ITT 2% (1/21) (ns) PP 7% (1/15) (ns)	Complete: No dysphagia in 2 wk by MDQ Partial: decrease in frequency/severity by MDQ	Complete: ITT 62% (13/21) PP 68% (13/19) Partial: ITT 81% (17/21) x% (4/21) PP 89% (17/19) x% (4/19)	ITT 0% (0/21) (P<.001) PP 0% (0/15) (P<.001) ITT 5% (1/21) (P<.001) PP 7% (1/15) (P<.001)	Decrease by >90% Decrease by >50%	27% (4/15) of those with complete histologic response, had 38% (3/8) endoscopic response No resolution of rings	8% (1/12) (ns)	Resolution of all endoscopic findings	Asymptomatic esophageal candidiasis 26% (5/19) of Tx group vs 0% (0/15) of placebo (ns)	Staining for eosinophil derived neurotoxin similar to histology

Abbreviations: EEI, eosinophilic esophageal infiltration; EoE, eosinophilic esophagitis; eos, eosinophils; hpf, high power field; ITT, intention to Tx; MDQ, Mayo Dysphagia Questionnaire; PP, per protocol; Tx, treatment.

Data from Straumann A, Conus S, Degen L, et al. Budesonide is effective in adolescent and adult patients with active eosinophilic esophagitis. Gastroenterology 2010;139:1526–37; and Alexander JA, Jung KW, Arora AS, et al. Swallowed fluticasone improves histologic but not symptomatic response of adults with eosinophilic esophagitis. Clin Gastroenterol Hepatol 2012;10:742–9.e1.

treatment. The placebo-controlled trials differ in the symptomatic response to therapy. In the Straumann and colleagues'[3] trial there was a robust symptomatic response and there was no symptom response in the Alexander and colleagues'[4] trial, which did have a high placebo symptom response. In both trials, about one-quarter of treated patients developed asymptomatic esophageal candidiasis.

COMPARATIVE TRIALS

Three trials compare esomeprazole and topical steroid in the treatment of EEI (**Table 3**).[5–7] In the Francis and colleagues'[6] trial, patients with GERD evidenced by an abnormal pH study were treated with esomeprazole 40 mg twice a day, whereas those without GERD were treated with oral viscous budesonide (OVB) 1 mg twice a day. The histologic response rates in both groups were similar, with a complete response rate of approximately 60% and at least a partial response rate of approximately 80%. This histologic response rate is consistent with other studies with OVB at that dosage. Of note, this study showed that EEI associated with GERD has a similarly high, but not complete, response rate to high-dose proton pump inhibitor (PPI) treatment. Symptom response in both groups was similar and modest.

In the trials by Peterson and colleagues[5] and Moawad and colleagues,[7] subjects were randomized to esomeprazole 40 mg every day or lower-dose fluticasone (440 µg twice a day) regardless of pH results. Both these studies showed lower histologic response rates with fluticasone therapy. The complete response rates were 15% and 19%, considerably lower than those seen in other controlled trials, which may be a result of the lower dose of fluticasone administered. Of note, these results are significantly lower than the response rates reported by Remedios and colleagues,[2] who used a minimally greater (500 µg twice a day) dose of fluticasone. The etiology of this discrepancy is uncertain, but could be related to sampling error, as Remedios and colleagues[2] took only 4 biopsies from the esophagus compared with 8 in the other 2 trials. Symptom response was no different between fluticasone and esomeprazole in the trial by Peterson and colleagues[5] and was better with esomeprazole in the trial by Moawad and colleagues.[7] We would conclude from these trials that (1) 440 µg twice a day aerosolized fluticasone is inadequate dosing, and (2) esomeprazole is effective in those with GERD and EEI, as well as having some effect in EEI with negative pH testing.

In a fourth comparative trial, Dellon and colleagues[8] found OVB to be more effective than the same dose of aerosolized budesonide administered by nebulizer at improving histology. Moreover, they document greater mucosal contact time by scintigraphy with the OVB preparation that may explain this finding. We would conclude from this study that viscous preparations may be preferred over swallowed aerosolized drug delivery by means of nebulizer. The generalizability of this finding to the use of drug delivery by means of an inhaler system is unknown.

MAINTENANCE STEROID TRIALS

Straumann and colleagues[3] performed the only maintenance trial of topical steroid therapy in EoE (**Table 4**).[9] This was a well-done, innovative, landmark study comparing swallowed nebulized budesonide 0.25 mg twice a day with placebo in 28 patients. This showed a modest benefit in symptoms with budesonide treatment. The symptom score from baseline to 1 year from treatment onset increased numerically, but not to a statistically significant level (0.79–2.3) in the treatment group, but increased to a statistically significant level in the placebo group (0.71–4.0). The 1-year complete remission rate was numerically, but not statistically, significantly

Table 3
Comparator-controlled trials

Author	Tx	EEI/EoE	N	Duration	Symptoms Steroid Response	Comparator Response	Definition	Histologic Steroid Response	Comparator Response	Definition	Endoscopic Tx Response	Comparator Response	Definition	Side Effects	Comments
Peterson et al,[5] 2010	Fluticasone 440 μg twice a day	EEI	12	8 wk	50% (6/12)	25% (3/12) (ns)	Dysphagia Scale (0–8)	15% (2/13)	33% (4/12) (ns)	Complete <6 eos/hpf				Not described	56% of patients with abn pH studies
	Omeprazole 40 mg qd		12				Decrease by >2 points	31% (4/13)	50% (6/12) (ns)	Partial <16 eos/hpf					
Francis et al,[6] 2012	OVB 1 mg twice a day to those with nl pH studies	EEI	28	6 wk	54% (15/28)	61% (11/18)	MDQ decrease by >1 level	57% (16/28)	61% (11/18)	Complete <5 eos/hpf	15% (3/20)	21% (3/14)	Resolution of all EoE findings	Not described	29% of pH negative pts had erosive esophagitis on fu EGD
	Omeprazole 40 mg twice a day to those with abn pH studies		18					86% (24/28)	83% (15/18)	Partial <15 eos/hpf					37% of pts with abnormal pH study

Study	Disease / n / duration	Treatment	n			MDQ score				Histology				Endoscopy	Safety	Other
Dellon et al,[8] 2012	EoE 12 8 wk	OVB 1 mg twice a day Nebulized budesonide 1 mg twice a day	13	25 to 16 (P = .04)	34 to 10 (ns) (P = .002)	Baseline to post-tx	64%	73%	27% (P = .09) 45% (P = .09)	complete <1 eos/hpf partial <15 eos/hpf	91%	Partial improvement	45% (P = .02)	Improved global assessment	14% asymptomatic esophageal candidiasis No serum budesonide detected ACTH stim test in all post-tx normal	Mucosal contact time greater for OVB by scintigraphy (P = .008) Rings resolved in 2/3 on OVB
Moawad et al,[7] 2013	EEI 21 8 wk	Fluticasone 440 µg twice a day Omeprazole 40 mg qd	21	17 to 12	19 to 1 (P<.001)	Baseline to post-tx	19%		33% (ns)	<7 eos/hpf	Partial improvement	Partial improvement (ns)		Stenosis, rings, furrows, plaques	5% (1/21) asymptomatic esophageal candidiasis	pH abnormal in 19%. GERD patients stratified to both groups. In GERD patients response to omeprazole is better (100%, 4/4) than fluticasone (0%, 0/4, P = .029)

Abbreviations: abn, abnormal; ACTH, adrenocorticotropic hormone; ct, count; EEI, eosinophilic esophageal infiltration; EGD, esophagogastroduodenoscopy; EoE, eosinophilic esophagitis; eos, eosinophils; fu, follow up; GERD, gastroesophageal reflux disease; hpf, high power field; MDQ, Mayo Dysphagia Questionnaire; nl, normal; ns, non significant; OVB, oral viscous budesonide; qd, every day; stim, stimulation; tx, treatment.
Data from Refs.[5–8]

Table 4
Placebo-controlled maintenance Tx trials

Author	Tx	EEI/EoE	N	Duration	Tx Response	Placebo Response	Definition	Tx Response	Placebo Response	Definition	Side-Effects	Comments
Straumann et al,[9] 2011	Nebulized liquid suspension budesonide 0.25 mg twice a day	EoE	14 Tx	50 wk	0.79 to 2.3 (ns)	.71 to 4.0 (P = .0004)	Dysphagia score (0-9) Pre-Post	38% (5/14)	0% (0/14) (ns)	Complete <5 eos/hpf	None	No predictors of steroid response
			14 Placebo		64% (9/14)	36% (5/14) (ns)	Clinical remission	14% (2/14) Pre 0.4 Post 32	29% (4/14) (ns) Pre 0.7 Post 65 (P = .024)	Partial 5-20 eos/hpf Eosinophil load		Decrease proinflammatory markers, tissue apoptosis, fibrosis score, mucosal thickness with Tx

Eosinophil load calculated by review of 40 hpf.

Abbreviations: EoE, eosinophilic esophagus; eos, eosiniophils; hpf, high power field; ns, nonsignificant; Tx, treatment.

Data from Straumann A, Conus S, Degen L, et al. Long-term budesonide maintenance treatment is partially effective for patients with eosinophilic esophagitis. Clin Gastroenterol Hepatol 2011;9:400–9.e1.

higher in the treatment group: 64% to 36% over placebo. Histologically there were similar results: the eosinophil density increased in both groups but this was significant in only the placebo group (treatment group: 0.4–32, placebo group: 0.7–35). The complete response rate (treatment 38%, placebo 0%) and at least partial response rate (treatment 52%, placebo 29%) were greater in the budesonide group but did not reach statistical significance. Similar to the previous steroid trials, exudates and furrows seen endoscopically tended to resolve in histologic responders, but rings persisted. Asymptomatic candida esophagitis was seen in 22% of patients, similar to previous trials. Of interest, there was no evidence of esophageal squamous epithelial thinning with steroid treatment and no clinical viral or fungal infections were seen.

Of great interest in this study, the fibrosis score, which decreased with acute EoE treatment, increased numerically less over the next year following budesonide therapy as compared with placebo. Moreover, endoscopic ultrasound was used to measure the thickness of the esophageal wall at baseline and after 1 year of therapy. The mucosal wall thickness decreased significantly at 1 year in the treatment group. There were smaller decreases in the submucosal and the muscularis propria thickness in the treatment group that did not reach statistical significance. In contrast, the values in the placebo were completely unchanged.

We feel the findings of this study strongly support the use of maintenance steroid therapy in EoE. Statistical significance was obtained with only a few of the end points, but we feel this is most likely a result of trial design, rather than a failure of steroid therapy. First, the study was small, with only 14 patients in each limb, and we strongly suspect a larger study would show these trends in symptom and histologic response to be statistically significant. Second, the steroid dose was quite low, at budesonide 0.25 mg twice a day. Of note, in a small open-label trial, Lucendo and colleagues[10] found a significant histologic benefit of liquid fluticasone 400 μg twice a day for 1 year on histology. Mean eosinophil counts at 1 year were 3.5/hpf and 7.4/hpf in the upper and lower esophagus respectively. The better histologic response in this study may reflect the relatively higher steroid dose administered in this trial compared with the Straumann and colleagues study.[3] It has been our clinical experience that maintenance doses of budesonide gel in the range of 1.5 mg/d are needed in most patients to maintain symptomatic and histologic remission.

ISSUES IN STEROID TREATMENT
Steroid Preparations

Currently, there are no drugs available specifically designed for the treatment of EoE. Furthermore, there are no medications approved by the Food and Drug Administration for the treatment of EoE. The most commonly used drugs in clinical practice are fluticasone and budesonide. Both fluticasone and budesonide are highly potent topical steroids with affinity for binding to the glucocorticoid receptor several hundred times that of dexamethasone.[11] The affinity of fluticasone is about threefold greater than budesonide. Mometasone, an even more potent steroid used for asthma, has not been studied in EoE. Ciclesonide is a similarly potent steroid that may be associated with less systemic bioavailability than fluticasone and budesonide.[12] It was effective in the treatment of EoE in a small case series.[13] Both fluticasone and budesonide have a near complete first-pass hepatic metabolism. Moreover, both of these medications have been used for some period in the treatment asthma.

Fluticasone is available as an aerosolized inhaler used to treat asthma that is commonly used to treat EoE. The aerosolized preparation is used without a spacer and swallowed. Studies to date have used dosages of 440 μg twice a day and

880 μg twice a day. The results appear less than adequate with the 440-μg twice-a-day dosing and 880 μg twice a day is the dosage of choice for this agent.[4,5,7] Whether higher doses would be of increased benefit is uncertain.

Budesonide can be nebulized and swallowed or taken in a liquid or gel form. Straumann and colleagues'[3,9] several studies have used the nebulized preparation. OVB has been used in several studies in which the commercially available liquid respules are mixed with 10 mL water and 1 to 2 teaspoons of sucralose (Splenda) to negate the bitter taste of the compound.[6,8,14,15] Budesonide has been compounded with Ricinol, a mucosal adherent preparation.[16] Budesonide is available in a generic preparation and can be compounded at centers where a compounding pharmacy is available at a considerable cost savings. Compounded budesonide tablets can be crushed in honey, maple syrup, or pancake syrup to make the preparation more palatable. Dellon and colleagues[8] compared nebulized budesonide with OVB, and found the OVB preparation to have a significantly greater mucosal contact time measured by scintigraphy and greater effect on suppressing esophageal eosinophilia than the nebulized preparation.

In studies to date, the dosage of 1 mg twice a day has been the standard for acute treatment. Similar to fluticasone, higher dosages have not been adequately evaluated. However, in an abstract, Gupta and colleagues[17] showed a histologic response that was dose dependent and was studied up to 2 mg of OVB twice a day in adolescents. Histologic response rates ($\leq$6 eos/hpf) were 16.7% with OVB 0.5 mg every day, 44.4% at 2 mg every day, and 100% at 2 mg twice a day. This suggests that studies of higher dosages of topical steroid need to be performed. In our clinic practice, we use 1.5 to 3.0 mg of budesonide every day to twice a day for treatment of active EoE. For maintenance therapy of EoE, the dosage of 0.25 mg twice a day appears to be somewhat inadequate. We use 1.5 mg qhs (once daily at bedtime) for maintenance; however, studies to determine the proper maintenance dose to adequately control inflammation and limit toxicity need desperately to be performed.

Many feel patients on fluticasone and budesonide therapy should rinse their mouths with water and expectorate after use to limit oral candidiasis, although this has never been formally studied. All studies to date have used twice-a-day dosing. Potentially, treatment might be able to be given once daily, which would improve compliance, but this has not been well evaluated. The contact time in the esophagus is extremely brief, less than 10 seconds, which might thereby favor more frequent rather than once-a-day dosing, although direct comparison studies between twice-a-day and every day dosing need to be performed.[8]

In the next few years, it is likely that a commercially available steroid medication in a delivery system designed for esophageal treatment will be available. An OVB preparation and other steroid delivery systems are currently under study.

Length of Therapy

Studies for the acute treatment of EoE have varied from 2 to 8 weeks of therapy. Straumann[3] showed a complete histologic response in 72% of patients at 2 weeks, which is similar to histologic results at 4 to 8 weeks in other trials.[1–4,6–8] In the Alexander and colleagues'[4] trial, symptom response was accessed at 2-week intervals; 89% of complete symptom responders had resolution of their dysphagia at 2 weeks, similarly suggesting a rapid response to therapy. Based on limited data, it does not appear that there is a significant delay in symptomatic response beyond that of histologic response.

Symptom relapse appears to be nearly universal following steroid therapy.[18] It is uncertain if longer treatment courses for treatment of active EoE will lead to longer disease-free interval after steroid therapy. Complete mucosal healing has been shown to lead to longer-term remission in inflammatory bowel disease.[19] This has not been directly evaluated in EoE, but indirect evidence in a study by Schaefer and colleagues[20] would not support this line of reasoning. In that study, swallowed aerosolized fluticasone was compared with oral prednisone in children and teens. The degree of histologic improvement with prednisone was greater than that with fluticasone at 4 weeks. However, the time to symptomatic relapse was similar with both treatments, thereby questioning the value of greater histologic improvement, which potentially might be obtained with longer treatment courses. Therefore, the limited data make it hard to draw firm conclusions, but currently acute treatment of EoE should be continued for 2 to 6 weeks.

Symptomatic Response

All of the budesonide and higher-dose fluticasone trials that resulted in at least 50% histologic response rates, with the exception of the Alexander and colleagues'[4] trial, which had an unusually high placebo response rate, show a symptom response to topical steroid therapy in EoE.[3,4,6,8] Multiple different dysphagia scales were used in these trials. A median score for all of the patients grouped together was used in some of the trials, and in other trials, each individual subject was classified as a responder or nonresponder. Therefore, it does make the trials somewhat difficult to compare with each other.

In general, however, the complete symptom response in these studies appears to be less than the histologic response. Complete histologic response rates tend to be in the 60% to 70% range and partial histologic response rates in the 90% range, with high-dose topical steroid therapy.[3,4,6,8] In contrast, symptom reduction, or at least partial symptom response, is reported in only about 60% to 75% of patients in these trials. One would worry about esophageal candidiasis causing symptoms that would lessen the treatment response, but that did not appear to be the case in these studies, as all infections were classified as "asymptomatic." The presence of an esophageal stricture or small-caliber esophagus is present in 50% of patients with EoE undergoing a structured esophagram, and is frequently not appreciated at esophagogastroduodenoscopy.[21,22] Moreover, esophageal loss of compliance is seen in most all patients with EoE when evaluated with the more sensitive Endoflip device (Crospon Inc, Carlsbad, CA).[23,24] Esophageal fibrosis leading to loss of compliance and esophageal narrowing will frequently cause persistent dysphagia despite resolution of EoE, and may explain the histologic response being greater than the symptom response in steroid treatment trials in EoE. This is supported by the report of Gentile and colleagues,[22] showing that those with a significantly small-caliber esophagus and complete histologic response to topical steroid therapy did not have dysphagia resolution until they underwent esophageal dilation. Steroid therapy may potentially reverse fibrosis and lead to an increase in esophageal diameter.[3,9,21,25] In the 2 maintenance steroid trials, however, the reversal of fibrosis has been mild.[9,10]

Patients with GERD

It is unclear if the response to topical steroid therapy is the same in patients with GERD and EoE versus patients with allergic EoE alone. This issue has never been directly evaluated, and studies offering any insight into this question are small. Trials using the entrance criteria of persistent eosinophilia post PPI treatment will include both patients with allergic EoE and mixed allergic EoE/GERD. More than half of the patients treated by Remedios and colleagues[2] had GERD by pH testing, all of whom had persistent symptoms on PPI; and all were described as having a "response to fluticasone treatment." The symptom response to fluticasone was similar between the patients with GERD (57% [4/7]) and without GERD (40% [2/5]) in the Peterson and colleagues' trial.[5] Francis and colleagues[6] treated only pH-negative patients and had a complete histologic response rate of 57% (16/28) and symptom response rate of 54% (15/28). This response rate is similar to response rates seen in studies including patients with allergic EoE and mixed allergic/GERD EoE (PPI nonresponders).[3,8] These data might suggest that the response to topical steroid therapy in allergic EoE and allergy/GERD EoE is similar.

Conversely, Alexander and colleagues[4] found complete histologic response to fluticasone in only 33% (3/9) of patients with erosive esophagitis compared with 100% (10/10) of patients without erosive esophagitis. Similarly, Moawad and colleagues[7] found a histologic response in 0% (0/4) of patients with GERD compared with 24% (4/17) of patients without GERD treated with low-dose fluticasone. These studies might suggest a greater response to steroid in patients without GERD. Therefore, at this point in time, this question of differential response rates to steroids of allergic EoE and allergic/GERD EoE remains unanswered.

Maintenance Therapy

The role of maintenance therapy is an area of considerable controversy. There are those who support maintenance therapy with dietary or topical steroid therapy to all patients with EoE.[26] Maintenance therapy can be indicated to prevent symptom recurrence, which is extremely common in this disease after stopping steroid therapy. Helou and colleagues[18] found symptoms to recur in 91% of patients after stopping fluticasone therapy with a mean recurrence time of 8.8 months. Schaefer and colleagues[20] found symptomatic recurrence to be nearly 50% at 24 weeks after steroid therapy. Straumann and colleagues,[9] in a placebo-controlled maintenance trial of budesonide, found after steroid-induced remission, symptomatic recurrence 64% of the time and histologic recurrence 100% of the time at 1 year in the placebo group.

Maintenance therapy also can be indicated to prevent the long-term complications of this disease. EoE is a chronic disease associated with wall fibrosis, leading to loss of compliance, esophageal stricture, and recurrent food impaction.[18,23,24,26–28] Straumann and colleagues[27] reported persistent dysphagia symptoms over 7 years in a group of 30 patients with EoE without anti-inflammatory therapy in the first natural history study of EoE. Recently Schoepfer and colleagues[26] reported on the Swiss database showing that the longer patients had symptoms without diagnosis, the greater the risk of esophageal stricture. An esophageal stricture was present in 71% of those with untreated symptoms of 20 years' duration. The Northwestern group has showed compliance abnormalities in nearly all patients with EoE leading to a nondistensible esophagus leading to dysphagia and food impaction.[23,24] These data would suggest EoE is a chronic inflammatory structuring disease, analogous to Crohn disease. EoE, therefore, should be considered a disorder that requires maintenance therapy to prevent symptoms, as well as an end-stage scarred esophagus.

There is another school of thought, however, that suggests maintenance therapy is not required for all patients with EoE. This group would argue that although symptomatic recurrence and the development of significant fibrosis is common, it is not universal in EoE. The data of Straumann and colleagues[27] and Schoepfer and colleagues,[26] mentioned previously, are retrospective looks at the Swiss practice. It is possible that patients with milder forms of disease may have had minimal long-term symptoms and did not seek medical care, and therefore may not be represented in those reports. Khanna and colleagues[29] reported the results of a structured phone interview of patients diagnosed with symptomatic EEl at 5 to 11 years after diagnosis. Nearly

70% of patients were on no EoE treatment, nearly 70% had no dysphagia in the past month, and more than 80% were eating an unlimited diet. In a similar vein, Levine and colleagues[30] found 68% of previously symptomatic patients with EEI to be asymptomatic on PPI therapy at a mean of 3 years despite 78% having persistent eosinophilia. Moreover, stricturing is not present in all patients with EoE. Lee and colleagues[21] reported a normal esophageal diameter by structured esophagram in 50% of patients with EoE, and in a meta-analysis of endoscopic findings in EoE, an esophageal stricture and/or small-caliber esophagus was reported in only 30% of patients.[31] This school of thought would suggest maintenance therapy should be reserved for patients with frequent recurrence of symptoms off therapy and those with evidence of significant fibrosis evidenced by esophageal stricture or small-caliber esophagus. Patients with infrequent symptomatic recurrence and a normal-diameter esophagus can be treated with periodic 2 to 4 weeks of on-demand treatment.

At this point in time, the question of who needs maintenance therapy remains unanswered and controversial. If we are using dietary therapy, then we would treat all patients long term. Because the long-term risks of topical steroid therapy have not been evaluated, our approach is to offer topical steroid maintenance therapy to all patients with frequent recurrent symptoms off steroid therapy, those with esophageal strictures appreciated endoscopically, and those with small-caliber esophagus determined by an esophageal maximal diameter smaller than 18 mm by structured esophagram. We find it very difficult to make a strong recommendation for lifelong therapy of an expensive medication with a relatively unstudied long-term safety profile in patients with infrequent mild symptoms and a normal-caliber esophagus. As a practical point, patients with minimal symptoms are often noncompliant with the medication long term. As mentioned previously, the budesonide 0.5-mg dose twice a day appears to be underdosed in the only performed maintenance study in EoE.[9] In our practice, for maintenance, we use budesonide 1.5 mg daily or fluticasone 440 µg to 880 µg at bedtime 4 to 7 days per week.

Cost

Cost is a significant issue with topical steroid therapy for EoE. The medications are not inexpensive and, in many cases, require potentially lifelong treatment. The purchase price (without insurance) of topical steroid therapy for EoE in our area is displayed in **Table 5**. Of note, there is dramatic cost savings in compounding budesonide over the commercially available steroid products. The cost of maintenance therapy with compounded budesonide is manageable at about $40 per month but can be potentially cost prohibitive if using brand-name commercially prepared preparations at $200 to $500 per month.

Safety

In the short term, there has been little toxicity from topical steroid therapy. Asymptomatic esophageal candidiasis has been seen in approximately 20% (0%–26%) of patients in clinical trials.[2,4,6,8] In the Straumann and colleagues[9] 1-year maintenance trial of lower-dose budesonide, no fungal or viral infections were reported or seen at the 1-year endoscopy. Whether *Candida* or viral infection, specifically herpes, which has been reported in EoE, will be an issue with higher-dose maintenance therapy is uncertain.[32,33]

Steroids have been known to cause epithelial thinning, but reassuringly, the Straumann and colleagues[9] maintenance trial found no change in epithelial thickness with 1 year of budesonide therapy.

Table 5 Costs of topical stored treatment	
Fluticasone 220 µg 4 puffs BID × 6 wk	$967[a]
Pulmicort Respules 1 mg BID × 6 wk	$1613[a]
Compounded Budesonide Ricinol 3 mg BID × 6 wk	$225[b]
Compounded Budesonide tablets 3 mg BID × 6 wk	$141[b]

Abbreviation: BID, twice a day.
[a] Average from 3 commercial pharmacies.
[b] Mayo Clinic Pharmacy.

The big concern with chronic use of a swallowed steroid is systemic absorption of steroid and steroid complications, including bone health. Fortunately, we do have an excellent long-term safety record with topical steroid therapy for asthma. Although clinical adrenal insufficiency with inhaled steroids is an extremely rare event, high-dose topical steroid therapy for asthma may have some significant effects on the hypothalamic-adrenal axis.[34–37] Of note, studies looking specifically at bone density have found it unaffected by topical inhaled steroid.[38–40] Importantly, systemic levels of steroids with a rapid first-pass hepatic metabolism appear to be significantly lower with oral than inhaled administration in healthy controls; thereby, suggesting the systemic safety profile of these medications when given orally may be even better than what has been observed with pulmonary use.[41] On the other hand, EoE is a disease with markedly dilated intracellular spaces that are associated with increased esophageal intracellular permeability. Therefore, it is not clear that data on systemic bioavailability of topical swallowed steroid therapy in healthy controls can be translated to patients with EoE. Moreover, esophageal absorption may not have the rapid first-pass clearance of these compounds that is seen with intestinal absorption. Finally, Dilger and colleagues[42] reported decreased metabolism of budesonide in EoE compared with healthy controls. The pharmokinetics and systemic toxicity of these preparations when given orally in EoE clearly need more evaluation. This information is critical to determine the role of topical steroid therapy in the long-term treatment of EoE.

SUMMARY

Topical steroid therapy has been used to treat EoE for more than 15 years. Currently, there is no commercially available preparation designed to deliver the steroid to the esophagus. Current regimens consist of swallowing steroid preparations designed for inhalation treatment for asthma. It appears a viscous liquid preparation may be more effective than a nebulized preparation. When used in proper dose, steroids lead to complete histologic responses in the range of 60% to 70% of patients and at least a partial histologic response in more than 90% of patients. Symptom response rates appear to be somewhat less than histologic rates with at least a partial symptomatic response of only 60% to 75%. Acute treatment should be for 2 to 8 weeks with fluticasone 880 μg twice a day or budesonide 1 to 2 mg twice a day in adults. Maintenance therapy seems promising in one trial, but likely needs a higher dosage than 0.25 mg budesonide twice a day. In the short term, steroids are associated with about a 15% to 25% incidence of asymptomatic esophageal candidiasis, but otherwise appear to be well tolerated.

Many unanswered questions remain regarding topical steroid therapy in EoE: What is the appropriate drug, dosage, and dosing interval for acute treatment? What is the appropriate drug and dosage for maintenance therapy? What are the systemic side effects of long-term maintenance therapy? Do all patients with EoE require long-term therapy? If not, is there a subset of patients with EoE who would benefit from maintenance treatment? Hopefully, in the second 15 years of steroid therapy in EoE, we can answer these questions and optimize therapy for this increasingly common clinical disorder.

REFERENCES

1. Arora AS, Perrault J, Smyrk TC. Topical corticosteroid treatment of dysphagia due to eosinophilic esophagitis in adults. Mayo Clin Proc 2003;78:830–5.
2. Remedios M, Campbell C, Jones DM, et al. Eosinophilic esophagitis in adults: clinical, endoscopic, histologic findings, and response to treatment with fluticasone propionate. Gastrointest Endosc 2006;63:3–12.
3. Straumann A, Conus S, Degen L, et al. Budesonide is effective in adolescent and adult patients with active eosinophilic esophagitis. Gastroenterology 2010;139: 1526–37.
4. Alexander JA, Jung KW, Arora AS, et al. Swallowed fluticasone improves histologic but not symptomatic response of adults with eosinophilic esophagitis. Clin Gastroenterol Hepatol 2012;10:742–9.e1.
5. Peterson KA, Thomas KL, Hilden K, et al. Comparison of Esomeprazole to aerosolized, swallowed fluticasone for eosinophilic esophagitis. Dig Dis Sci 2010; 55(5):1313–9.
6. Francis DL, Foxx-Orenstein A, Arora AS, et al. Results of ambulatory pH monitoring do not reliably predict response to therapy in patients with eosinophilic oesophagitis. Aliment Pharmacol Ther 2012;35:300–7.
7. Moawad FJ, Veerappan GR, Dias JA, et al. Randomized controlled trial comparing aerosolized swallowed fluticasone to esomeprazole for esophageal eosinophilia. Am J Gastroenterol 2013;108:366–72.
8. Dellon ES, Sheikh A, Speck O, et al. Viscous topical is more effective than nebulized steroid therapy for patients with eosinophilic esophagitis. Gastroenterology 2012;143:321–4.e1.
9. Straumann A, Conus S, Degen L, et al. Long-term budesonide maintenance treatment is partially effective for patients with eosinophilic esophagitis. Clin Gastroenterol Hepatol 2011;9:400–9.e1.
10. Lucendo AJ, Arias A, De Rezende LC, et al. Subepithelial collagen deposition, profibrogenic cytokine gene expression, and changes after prolonged fluticasone propionate treatment in adult eosinophilic esophagitis: a prospective study. J Allergy Clin Immunol 2011;128:1037–46.
11. Lumry WR. A review of the preclinical and clinical data of newer intranasal steroids used in the treatment of allergic rhinitis. J Allergy Clin Immunol 1999; 104:S150–8.

12. Stoeck M, Riedel R, Hochhaus G, et al. In vitro and in vivo anti-inflammatory activity of the new glucocorticoid ciclesonide. J Pharmacol Exp Ther 2004;309: 249–58.

13. Schroeder S, Fleischer DM, Masterson JC, et al. Successful treatment of eosinophilic esophagitis with ciclesonide. J Allergy Clin Immunol 2012;129:1419–21.

14. Aceves SS, Newbury RO, Dohil R, et al. Esophageal remodeling in pediatric eosinophilic esophagitis. J Allergy Clin Immunol 2007;119:206–12.

15. Dohil R, Newbury R, Fox L, et al. Oral viscous budesonide is effective in children with eosinophilic esophagitis in a randomized, placebo-controlled trial. Gastroenterology 2010;139:418–29.

16. Neumann D, Alexander G, Farrugia G, et al. A new therapy for eosinophillic esophagitis in adults: efficacy of budesonide-ricinol gel for 6 weeks in patients with dysphagia. Am J Gastroenterol 2008;103:19.

17. Gupta S, Collins MH, Lewis J, et al. Efficacy and safety of oral budesonide suspension (OBS) in pediatric subjects with eosinophilic esophagitis (EoE): results from the double-blind, placebo-controlled PEER study. Gastroenterology 2011; 140:1077 S-179.

18. Helou EF, Simonson J, Arora AS. 3-yr-follow-up of topical corticosteroid treatment for eosinophilic esophagitis in adults. Am J Gastroenterol 2008;103:2194–9.

19. Burger D, Travis S. Conventional medical management of inflammatory bowel disease. Gastroenterology 2011;140:1827–37.e2.

20. Schaefer ET, Fitzgerald JF, Molleston JP, et al. Comparison of oral prednisone and topical fluticasone in the treatment of eosinophilic esophagitis: a randomized trial in children. Clin Gastroenterol Hepatol 2008;6:165–73.

21. Lee J, Huprich J, Kujath C, et al. Esophageal diameter is decreased in some patients with eosinophilic esophagitis and might increase with topical corticosteroid therapy. Clin Gastroenterol Hepatol 2012;10:481–6.

22. Gentile N, Ravi K, Trenkner S, et al. The sensitivity and specificity of esophagogastroduodenoscopy (EGD) for the small caliber esophagus in esophageal eosinophilic infiltration (EEI). Am J Gastroenterol 2012;107:S17, 36.

23. Kwiatek MA, Hirano I, Kahrilas PJ, et al. Mechanical properties of the esophagus in eosinophilic esophagitis. Gastroenterology 2011;140:82–90.

24. Nicodeme F, Hirano I, Chen J, et al. Esophageal distensibility as a measure of disease severity in patients with eosinophilic esophagitis. Clin Gastroenterol Hepatol 2013;11:1101–7.e1.

25. Aceves SS, Newbury RO, Chen D, et al. Resolution of remodeling in eosinophilic esophagitis correlates with epithelial response to topical corticosteroids. Allergy 2010;65:109–16.

26. Schoepfer AM, Safroneeva E, Bussmann C, et al. Delay in diagnosis of eosinophilic esophagitis increases risk for stricture formation in a time-dependent manner. Gastroenterology 2013;145:1230–6.e2.

27. Straumann A, Spichtin HP, Grize L, et al. Natural history of primary eosinophilic esophagitis: a follow-up of 30 adult patients for up to 11.5 years. Gastroenterology 2003;125:1660–9.

28. Chehade M, Sampson HA, Morotti RA, et al. Esophageal subepithelial fibrosis in children with eosinophilic esophagitis. J Pediatr Gastroenterol Nutr 2007;45: 319–28.

29. Khanna S, Kujath C, Katzka D, et al. The natural history of symptomatic esophageal eosinophilia: a longitudinal follow-up over 5 years. Am J Gastroenterol 2011; 106:S19, 45.

30. Levine J, Lai J, Edelman M, et al. Conservative long-term treatment of children with eosinophilic esophagitis. Ann Allergy Asthma Immunol 2012;108:363–6.
31. Kim HP, Vance RB, Shaheen NJ, et al. The prevalence and diagnostic utility of endoscopic features of eosinophilic esophagitis: a meta-analysis. Clin Gastroenterol Hepatol 2012;10:988–96.e5.
32. Sehgal S, Darbari A, Bader A. Herpes simplex virus and eosinophilic esophagitis. J Pediatr Gastroenterol Nutr 2013;56:e1.
33. Squires KA, Cameron DJ, Oliver M, et al. Herpes simplex and eosinophilic oesophagitis: the chicken or the egg? J Pediatr Gastroenterol Nutr 2009;49:246–50.
34. Nguyen KL, Lauver D, Kim I, et al. The effect of a steroid "burst" and long-term, inhaled fluticasone propionate on adrenal reserve. Ann Allergy Asthma Immunol 2003;91:38–43.
35. Mahachoklertwattana P, Sudkronrayudh K, Direkwattanachai C, et al. Decreased cortisol response to insulin induced hypoglycaemia in asthmatics treated with inhaled fluticasone propionate. Arch Dis Child 2004;89:1055–8.
36. Adams N, Bestall JM, Lasserson TJ, et al. Inhaled fluticasone versus inhaled beclomethasone or inhaled budesonide for chronic asthma in adults and children. Cochrane Database Syst Rev 2005;(2):CD002310.
37. Casale TB, Nelson HS, Stricker WE, et al. Suppression of hypothalamic-pituitary-adrenal axis activity with inhaled flunisolide and fluticasone propionate in adult asthma patients. Ann Allergy Asthma Immunol 2001;87:379–85.
38. Kemp JP, Osur S, Shrewsbury SB, et al. Potential effects of fluticasone propionate on bone mineral density in patients with asthma: a 2-year randomized, double-blind, placebo-controlled trial. Mayo Clin Proc 2004;79:458–66.
39. Johnell O, Pauwels R, Lofdahl CG, et al. Bone mineral density in patients with chronic obstructive pulmonary disease treated with budesonide Turbuhaler. Eur Respir J 2002;19:1058–63.
40. Medici TC, Grebski E, Hacki M, et al. Effect of one year treatment with inhaled fluticasone propionate or beclomethasone dipropionate on bone density and bone metabolism: a randomised parallel group study in adult asthmatic subjects. Thorax 2000;55:375–82.
41. Mackie AE, Bye A. The relationship between systemic exposure to fluticasone propionate and cortisol reduction in healthy male volunteers. Clin Pharmacokinet 2000;39(Suppl 1):47–54.
42. Dilger K, Lopez-Lazaro L, Marx C, et al. Active eosinophilic esophagitis is associated with impaired elimination of budesonide by cytochrome P450 3A enzymes. Digestion 2013;87:110–7.

Dietary Treatment of Eosinophilic Esophagitis

Nirmala Gonsalves, MD[a], Amir F. Kagalwalla, MD[b],*

KEYWORDS

- Eosinophilic esophagitis • Treatment • Diet

KEY POINTS

- Dietary treatment offers the prospect of inducing and maintaining prolonged disease remission without the potential complications associated with pharmacologic therapy.
- Elemental diet is superior to all other therapies for the treatment of eosinophilic esophagitis.
- Empirical elimination diet offers distinct advantages over allergy test directed diets.

INTRODUCTION

Eosinophilic esophagitis (EoE) is an immune-mediated chronic inflammatory disorder of the esophagus that is triggered by food antigens in most patients.[1] Dietary therapy has been established as an effective first-line therapy in children with EoE.[2–7] However, support for the effectiveness of dietary therapy in adults is only now beginning to emerge in the literature.[8,9] The highest response rates of up to 96% are achieved with dietary treatment, and thus, dietary approach is superior to the other available therapies to treat EoE.[3,10] The natural history of EoE is progression to remodeling and subepithelial fibrosis. Dietary treatment has been shown to reverse subepithelial fibrosis and is likely to alter the natural history of EoE.[11–14]

The goals of dietary treatment in EoE include: (1) symptom resolution; (2) maintenance of sustained histologic remission and thus prevention of disease-related complications, including fibrosis and strictures; and (3) prevention of iatrogenic treatment-related adverse reactions, such as nutritional deficiencies.

Because food antigens trigger eosinophilic inflammation, the dietary approach of identification and exclusion of causative food antigens to induce and maintain both

Disclosures: Dr N. Gonsalves has no disclosures. Dr A.F. Kagalwalla serves on the speaker's bureau for Nutricia.
[a] Division of Gastroenterology & Hepatology, Northwestern University-Feinberg School of Medicine, 676 North Saint Claire, Suite 1400, Chicago, IL 60611, USA; [b] Division of Gastroenterology, Hepatology & Nutrition, Ann & Robert H. Lurie Children's Hospital of Chicago, Northwestern University-Feinberg School of Medicine, 225 East Chicago Avenue, Chicago, IL 60611, USA
* Corresponding author.
E-mail address: akagalwalla@luriechildrens.org

Gastroenterol Clin N Am 43 (2014) 375–383
http://dx.doi.org/10.1016/j.gtc.2014.02.011
0889-8553/14/$ – see front matter © 2014 Elsevier Inc. All rights reserved.

clinical and histologic remission addresses the root cause of the disease.[2] The current recommendations for treatment of EoE with diet are based on several retrospective and observational studies in children as well as prospective studies in adults.[2–10] The available dietary approaches include: (1) elemental diet with an amino acid–based complete liquid formulation,[2,3,5,10,15] (2) empirical or nondirected elimination diet with elimination of several common food antigens from the diet,[5,8,9] and (3) directed elimination diet based on the results of allergy testing.[4,6,7] The type of dietary treatment selected should be tailored to the needs of the individual patient. The treatment selection in children depends on the age of the patient, the presence of comorbid malnutrition, and feeding aversion. In adults and older children, the diet selection depends on the comfort and acceptance of the specific elimination diet. Outcomes of the different dietary approaches are summarized in **Table 1**.

ELEMENTAL DIET

Several pediatric studies have reported that ingestion of a crystalline amino acid–based elemental formula in lieu of a regular diet induced clinical and histologic remission in 88% to 96% of children.[2,3,5] Subsequent controlled reintroduction of individual specific foods resulted in recurrence of gastrointestinal symptoms, thereby establishing a clear link between food allergy and esophageal injury.[2] The likelihood of achieving mucosal healing with lower residual eosinophil counts is higher with this modality than other dietary therapy or pharmacologic treatment with corticosteroids. A recent study in a small group of adults treated with elemental diet reported histologic improvement in 70% (eosinophil count <10 per high power field) with an average decrease in the eosinophil count from 54 to 10 after the elemental diet.[15] Similar to the pediatric experience, 50% of adults had eosinophil counts less than 5 per high power field. Patients did not show symptomatic improvement; however, that may be because of limitations in the dysphagia assessment tool used in this study. The decreased efficacy in this study compared with that of pediatrics could be attributed to adherence issues on the diet in the adult population.

Although universal guidelines regarding optimal duration of dietary therapy and period of reintroduction have not been established, based on available data, we propose the following approach. After 4 to 6 weeks of exclusive elemental diet and evidence of histologic remission on repeat endoscopy with biopsy, food reintroduction is initiated, beginning with the least allergenic foods from vegetable or fruit groups; single foods may be introduced every 5 to 7 days from within these less allergenic food groups. Once all foods in a given food group are successfully introduced, endoscopy is performed to show remission before moving to the next food group. If this strategy is successful, single food reintroductions from the most allergic food group, which includes foods such as cow's milk, soy, wheat, egg, chicken, and corn, may be undertaken. The reintroductions are outlined by Markowitz and colleagues,[10] as shown in **Table 2**. In this process, if symptoms are elicited with an ingested food, then the symptom-inducing food is excluded from the diet, and the next food in that group is

Table 1				
Response with different dietary treatments				
	Elemental (%)	SFED (%)	Directed (%)	Milk Only (%)
Pediatrics	96	74	72	65
Adults	50	70	26	Not applicable

Table 2
Dietary introduction approach to food reintroduction in EoE

Start ——————————————————→ End
(Least Allergenic)   (Most Allergenic)

A	B	C	D
Vegetables (nonlegume)	Citrus fruits	Legumes	Fish/shellfish
Carrots, squash (all types),	Orange, grapefruit,	Lima beans,	Corn
sweet potato, white	lemon, lime	chickpeas,	Peas
potato, string beans,	Tropical fruits	white/black/	Peanut
broccoli, lettuce, beets,	Banana, kiwi,	red beans	Wheat
asparagus, cauliflower,	pineapple, mango,	Grains	Beef
Brussels sprouts	papaya, guava,	Oat, barley, rye,	Soy
Fruit (noncitrus, nontropical)	avocado	other grains	Egg
Apple, pear, peaches,	Melons	Meat[a]	Milk
plum, apricot, nectarine,	Honeydew,	Lamb, chicken,	
grape, raisins	cantaloupe,	turkey, pork	
Vegetables	watermelon		
Tomatoes, celery,	Berries		
cucumber, onion, garlic,	Strawberry, blueberry,		
any other vegetables	raspberry, cherry,		
	cranberry		
	Grains		
	Rice, millet, quinoa		

[a] Progress from well cooked to rarer.

Adapted from Markowitz JE, Spergel JM, Ruchelli E, et al. Elemental diet is an effective treatment for eosinophilic esophagitis in children and adolescents. Am J Gastroenterol 2003;98(4):777–82; with permission.

introduced once the symptoms have resolved. Some may wish to hold off on additional food reintroductions after that food has been removed from the diet for 4 to 6 weeks to ensure an adequate amount of time to wash out any potential histologic changes caused by the latest food reintroduction.

Although treatment with elemental formula has been shown to be highly effective in treatment of EoE, several disadvantages are worth noting, the most important one being compliance/adherence to the therapy secondary to the poor taste in both children and adults. Many children require either nasogastric or gastrostomy tubes to deliver adequate nutrients because of the palatability of the formula. Limiting a child to an exclusive elemental diet may also restrict the child's participation in social activities, because many childhood activities involve food, which can lead to impaired quality of life. Although most adults are able to drink the formula without the use of feeding tubes, quality of life is also severely affected because of the inability to participate in social eating and engagement in activities involving food intake. The elemental formulas are also expensive, and this can place significant financial and social burden on the families. There may also be additional costs related to tubes, pumps, bags, and other supplies, particularly in children who require a feeding tube to administer the formulation.

EMPIRICAL ELIMINATION DIETS

The major advantage of the empirical or nondirected elimination diet is that allergy testing is not required to determine the foods to be eliminated. One of the most recognized empirical elimination diets is the 6-food elimination diet (SFED), in which patients exclude cow's milk protein, wheat, egg, soy, peanut/tree nuts, and fish/shellfish from the diet.[5] In 74% of children, this approach has shown significant clinical and histologic improvement.[5] Two additional pediatric studies have recently validated the results of SFED, with histologic response ranging from 50% to 81%.[6,7] Subsequent food reintroduction in the SFED responders identified milk (74%) as the single most common food responsible for triggering eosinophilic esophageal inflammation, followed by wheat (26%), egg (17%), and soy (10%).[16] Other investigators have validated milk, wheat, egg, and soy as the 4 foods most likely to trigger inflammation in children with EoE.[6,7]

Empirical dietary elimination has also been shown to have comparable effectiveness in adults.[8,9] A prospective study excluding the same 6 foods as the study in children[8] reported histologic remission in 70% of the patients studied after completing the diet for 6 weeks. These results mirror the pediatric experience. In patients who responded to the diet, serial food reintroduction was undertaken and resulted in symptom recurrence within 5 days of adding the trigger food. After exposure to the trigger food, esophageal eosinophil counts also returned to pretreatment values, and endoscopic features of EoE recurred on follow-up endoscopy.[8] Common food allergens identified in this adult study were wheat (60%), milk (50%), soy (10%), nuts (10%), and egg (5%). A second adult study from Spain[9] reported similar results, with remission in 73% of adults with EoE after empirical elimination of wheat, rice, corn, legumes, peanuts, soy, egg, milk, fish, and shellfish. More than 6 foods were excluded in this study. Food reintroduction in the Spanish study identified the common triggers as milk (61%), wheat (28%), eggs (26%), and legumes (23%). These investigators also found that continued elimination of these food triggers was effective in maintaining remission.[9] Thus, in both adults and children, the 4 foods most likely to trigger esophageal inflammation include milk, wheat, egg, and soy.

In a small retrospective series of children,[17] single food elimination with milk induced clinical and histologic improvement in only 65% of patients. Validation of this approach in a prospective study of children and adults is warranted.

The primary advantage of an elimination diet over exclusive elemental diet is that it allows intake of a variety of table foods, including meats, grains, fruits, vegetables, and legumes compared with a single nutrient source taken orally or via a feeding tube. The major limitation of empirical elimination diet is the difficulty with adherence to elimination of multiple food groups, even if for a limited time. Other concerns are that because of the lack of symptom/histology correlation, multiple endoscopies are required during the food reintroduction phase to help identify food triggers until noninvasive testing becomes available.

DIRECTED ELIMINATION DIETS

In a directed elimination diet, foods are eliminated based on the results of allergy testing. Elimination diets based only on the results of a radioallergosorbent test or skin prick test (SPT) results have failed to show clinical and histologic remission in children.[18,19] However, a large retrospective study from Philadelphia using an allergy tested diet based on the results of a combination of atopic patch testing (APT) and SPT showed clinical and histologic remission in 72% of children.[4] Patients in this series were tested for a total of 23 foods in 5 food groups, which included meats (chicken, turkey, beef, and pork), vegetables (peas, string beans, squash, sweet potatoes, potatoes, and carrots), fruits (apples, pears, and peaches), grains (wheat, rice, rye, oats, barley, and corn), and the fifth group included cow's milk, soy, eggs, and peanuts. The foods most frequently identified in patients who underwent a combination of APT and SPT were milk, soy, wheat, chicken, and beef. The same investigators in a subsequent study showed a lower response of 53% on treatment based on results of SPT and APT.[6] Another study from Cincinnati showed 65% response to an allergy test directed diet.[7] Two recent communications in the literature have reported positive APT responses in the range of between 12% and 37%, which is significantly lower than 85% positive APT tests from the Philadelphia study.[6,20–22] A Cincinnati study reported that a combination of directed elimination diet based on SPT and APT results used in conjunction with SFED was 80% effective versus 82% for SFED alone.[7] In adults, SPT testing has failed to identify the causative foods.[8,9,23] The predictive value of SPT for causal foods in adults treated with empirical elimination diet and who also underwent SPT was only 13%.[8] In a recent study in Spain, a cohort of 22 adults underwent multimodal allergy testing with prick prick testing in addition to SPT and APT to identify allergens in EoE.[24] Only 26% of adults improved with this testing approach. Taken together, these results in adults and children suggest that current allergic testing methods may not be reliable to identify food triggers. Possible explanations for the inability of allergy tests to identify incriminating foods in EoE include (1) lack of validation between EoE and control population, (2) lack of standardized extracts, with both fresh or preserved food extracts used for testing, and (3) interpretation of APT results is subjective. Patch testing remains primarily a research tool.[25]

STAGES OF DIETARY THERAPY

In the interest of simplification, dietary therapy can be broadly divided into 3 stages:

1. Remission stage: during this stage multiple foods are simultaneously eliminated or elemental formula is started. Endoscopy with esophageal biopsy is typically performed after a period of dietary elimination for at least 6 weeks.
2. Reintroduction stage: this stage is typically undertaken in patients who show remission with dietary elimination. This stage is characterized by reintroduction of one of the excluded foods sequentially followed by endoscopy and biopsies. If inflammation recurs with a reintroduced food, the incriminating trigger food is excluded from the diet, and the next food is added, until all the excluded foods are reintroduced back in the diet. The reintroduction process identifies 1 or rarely 2 foods as the cause of esophageal inflammation.
3. Maintenance stage: once food trigger(s) are identified during the reintroduction stage, these are eliminated from the diet long-term to maintain continuing disease remission.

NUTRITIONAL ASSESSMENT

The success of a dietary therapy approach in EoE depends on the involvement of a registered dietitian in the process. Nutritional assessment of children and adults with EoE before initiating an elimination diet improves compliance of the prescribed nutritional therapy. It involves obtaining a detailed nutritional history; including descriptions of food and supplements being consumed (including brand names of foods), preparation methods, and eating environment. Younger children with vomiting, feeding aversion, and multiple IgE-mediated food allergies may present with malnutrition. The initial assessment may also identify preexisting nutritional deficiencies, which can be addressed concurrently when prescribing an elimination diet. Patients who are on elimination diets for a prolonged period need to have their nutritional intake monitored. In addition to anthropometric measurements, including weight, height, and body mass index, some patients, especially those who have many foods excluded, require biochemical tests, including complete blood count, prealbumin, iron, calcium, and vitamin D levels, to monitor for deficiencies.[26,27]

FOOD SUBSTITUTIONS AND CROSS-CONTAMINATION

The deleterious consequences of eliminating major foods such as milk, soy, wheat, or egg from the diet can be prevented by participation of a dietitian with understanding and expertise in food substitution. Adequate food substitution of the excluded foods ensures a nutritionally complete diet. This process requires knowledge and understanding of the nutrient deficiencies caused by elimination of specific foods, as well as the appropriate substitution for these foods, as shown in **Table 3**.

Another important aspect of eliminating foods from the diet involves understanding and preventing food cross-contamination. Cross-contamination can transform a naturally occurring antigen-free food into an antigen-containing food. Cross-contamination can occur during processing, preparing, cooking, or serving food. Many processed foods, including fast foods, may be cross-contaminated with 1 or more foods, such as milk, soy, wheat, or nuts. Cross-contamination can also occur during the process of food preparation at home and can be avoided by simple measures such as using different utensils and strict hand washing between cooking different foods.

Reading food labels is a must to ensure that those products are allowed in the diet. Food labels should be reviewed every time, because manufacturing or processing may have changed, and a food that was formerly antigen free may contain the excluded antigen.

COMPLICATIONS

Exclusion of important food elements from a growing child's diet can have disastrous consequences, including impaired growth, rickets, and vitamin deficiencies.[28–30] Kwashiorkor from protein calorie malnutrition has been reported in children with

Table 3 Potential nutritional deficiencies		
Food	**Nutrients**	**Alternative Food Sources**
Milk	Protein, calcium, vitamin D, vitamin A, vitamin B_{12}, riboflavin, phosphorus, pantothenic acid, potassium	Meats, legumes, whole grains, nuts, fortified foods/beverages (ie, enriched soy milk)
Soy	Protein, iron, zinc, magnesium, thiamin, riboflavin, pyridoxine, folate, calcium, phosphorus	Meats, allowed grains/legumes, fortified foods/beverages
Wheat	Iron, thiamin, riboflavin, niacin, folic acid	Other enriched grains (ie, oat, corn, rice, soy flour), fruits, vegetables, legumes
Egg	Protein, pantothenic acid, biotin, selenium, choline	Meat, legumes, whole grains, fish, seafood
Peanut/tree nut	Vitamin E, niacin, magnesium, manganese, chromium, folate, vitamin B_6, copper, zinc, selenium, phosphorus	Allowed legumes, whole grains, vegetable oils, fish, seafood
Fish/shellfish	Protein, omega 3 fatty acids, phosphorus, zinc, selenium, vitamin B_{12}	Whole grains, meats, milk, nuts, soy, flaxseed, nuts, oils

only milk protein exclusion from the diet of toddlers suspected of milk protein allergy.[30] Frequently, it is not only the exclusion of 1 specific food that results in nutritional deficiency; it is also the concurrent exclusion of processed foods, which may contain that particular food antigen.

Elimination diets with the emphasis on excluding milk, wheat, soy, and nuts among other foods also can be challenging for children and adults on a vegan diet. Participation of a registered dietitian ensures a calorically adequate diet for growth, provides education on appropriate food substitutions, prevents contamination with excluded food antigens, and is an ongoing resource for families as they learn to adapt to the diet modification.

SUMMARY

Dietary treatment is a logical and effective approach to treating EoE. Identification and exclusion of specific food triggers leads to resolution of symptoms and esophageal mucosal healing. Implementation of the various dietary treatments can often be challenging and is contingent on the involvement of a nutritional support team and available local resources. Elemental diet with complete elimination of all intact food antigens offers the best outcome results as well as most complete healing; however, the major drawback is excluding all solid foods and the long food reintroduction process, which are often frustrating for patients. An empirical elimination diet requiring the elimination of a limited number of foods is more readily acceptable by patients and allows for food trigger identification more quickly. Although responses to directed and empirical elimination diets are similar in children, the directed elimination diet has not been shown to be effective in adults. Also, allergy testing has been shown to have limitations in identifying food triggers in EoE, and therefore, we currently do not recommend allergy testing to guide dietary intervention in children and adults. The future availability of a minimally or noninvasive test would alleviate the current difficulties with administering dietary management. The overall success of implementing dietary therapy is contingent on a multidisciplinary approach, involving nutritional support, in addition to tailoring the specific treatment to the individualized needs of each patient.

REFERENCES

1. Liacouras CA, Furuta GT, Hirano I, et al. Eosinophilic esophagitis: updated consensus recommendations for children and adults. J Allergy Clin Immunol 2011;128(1):3–20.e6 [quiz: 21–2].
2. Kelly KJ, Lazenby AJ, Rowe PC, et al. Eosinophilic esophagitis attributed to gastroesophageal reflux: improvement with an amino acid-based formula. Gastroenterology 1995;109(5):1503–12.
3. Liacouras CA, Spergel JM, Ruchelli E, et al. Eosinophilic esophagitis: a 10-year experience in 381 children. Clin Gastroenterol Hepatol 2005;3(12):1198–206.
4. Spergel JM, Andrews T, Brown-Whitehorn TF, et al. Treatment of eosinophilic esophagitis with specific food elimination diet directed by a combination of skin prick and patch tests. Ann Allergy Asthma Immunol 2005;95(4):336–43.
5. Kagalwalla AF, Sentongo TA, Ritz S, et al. Effect of six-food elimination diet on clinical and histologic outcomes in eosinophilic esophagitis. Clin Gastroenterol Hepatol 2006;4(9):1097–102.
6. Spergel JM, Brown-Whitehorn TF, Cianferoni A, et al. Identification of causative foods in children with eosinophilic esophagitis treated with an elimination diet. J Allergy Clin Immunol 2012;130(2):461–7.e5.

7. Henderson CJ, Abonia JP, King EC, et al. Comparative dietary therapy effectiveness in remission of pediatric eosinophilic esophagitis. J Allergy Clin Immunol 2012;129(6):1570–8.

8. Gonsalves N, Yang GY, Doerfler B, et al. Elimination diet effectively treats eosinophilic esophagitis in adults; food reintroduction identifies causative factors. Gastroenterology 2012;142(7):1451–9.e1 [quiz: e14–5].

9. Lucendo AJ, Arias A, Gonzalez-Cervera J, et al. Empiric 6-food elimination diet induced and maintained prolonged remission in patients with adult eosinophilic esophagitis: a prospective study on the food cause of the disease. J Allergy Clin Immunol 2013;131(3):797–804.

10. Markowitz JE, Spergel JM, Ruchelli E, et al. Elemental diet is an effective treatment for eosinophilic esophagitis in children and adolescents. Am J Gastroenterol 2003;98(4):777–82.

11. Chehade M, Sampson HA, Morotti RA, et al. Esophageal subepithelial fibrosis in children with eosinophilic esophagitis. J Pediatr Gastroenterol Nutr 2007;45(3): 319–28.

12. Aceves SS, Newbury RO, Dohil R, et al. Esophageal remodeling in pediatric eosinophilic esophagitis. J Allergy Clin Immunol 2007;119(1):206–12.

13. Rea B, Akhtar N, Jacques K, et al. Epithelial mesenchymal transition induced esophageal remodeling in eosinophilic esophagitis reverses with treatment. Gastroenterology 2011;140(5, Suppl 1). S-180.

14. Kagalwalla AF, Akhtar N, Woodruff SA, et al. Eosinophilic esophagitis: epithelial mesenchymal transition contributes to esophageal remodeling and reverses with treatment. J Allergy Clin Immunol 2012;129(5):1387–96.e7.

15. Peterson KA, Byrne KR, Vinson LA, et al. Elemental diet induces histologic response in adult eosinophilic esophagitis. Am J Gastroenterol 2013;108(5): 759–66.

16. Kagalwalla AF, Shah A, Li BU, et al. Identification of specific foods responsible for inflammation in children with eosinophilic esophagitis successfully treated with empiric elimination diet. J Pediatr Gastroenterol Nutr 2011; 53(2):145–9.

17. Kagalwalla AF, Shah A, Ritz S, et al. Cow's milk protein-induced eosinophilic esophagitis in a child with gluten-sensitive enteropathy. J Pediatr Gastroenterol Nutr 2007;44(3):386–8.

18. Noel RJ, Putnam PE, Collins MH, et al. Clinical and immunopathologic effects of swallowed fluticasone for eosinophilic esophagitis. Clin Gastroenterol Hepatol 2004;2(7):568–75.

19. Teitelbaum JE, Fox VL, Twarog FJ, et al. Eosinophilic esophagitis in children: immunopathological analysis and response to fluticasone propionate. Gastroenterology 2002;122(5):1216–25.

20. Assa'ad AH, Putnam PE, Collins MH, et al. Pediatric patients with eosinophilic esophagitis: an 8-year follow-up. J Allergy Clin Immunol 2007;119(3):731–8.

21. Rizo Pascual JM, De La Hoz Caballer B, Redondo Verge C, et al. Allergy assessment in children with eosinophilic esophagitis. J Investig Allergol Clin Immunol 2011;21(1):59–65.

22. Paquet B, Begin P, Paradis L, et al. Variable yield of allergy patch testing in children with eosinophilic esophagitis. J Allergy Clin Immunol 2013;131(2):613.

23. Simon D, Straumann A, Wenk A, et al. Eosinophilic esophagitis in adults–no clinical relevance of wheat and rye sensitizations. Allergy 2006;61(12):1480–3.

24. Molina-Infante J, Martin-Noguerol E, Alvarado-Arenas M, et al. Reply: to PMID 22867695. J Allergy Clin Immunol 2013;131(2):613–4.

25. Assa'ad A. Detection of causative foods by skin prick and atopy patch tests in patients with eosinophilic esophagitis: things are not what they seem. Ann Allergy Asthma Immunol 2005;95(4):309–11.
26. Salman S, Christie L, Burks W, et al. Dietary intakes of children with food allergies: comparison of the food guide pyramid and the recommended dietary allowances 10th ed. J Allergy Clin Immunol 2002;109:S214.
27. Mofidi S. Nutritional management of pediatric food hypersensitivity. Pediatrics 2003;111(6 Pt 3):1645–53.
28. Carvalho NF, Kenney RD, Carrington PH, et al. Severe nutritional deficiencies in toddlers resulting from health food milk alternatives. Pediatrics 2001;107(4):E46.
29. Noimark L, Cox HE. Nutritional problems related to food allergy in childhood. Pediatr Allergy Immunol 2008;19(2):188–95.
30. Liu T, Howard RM, Mancini AJ, et al. Kwashiorkor in the United States: fad diets, perceived and true milk allergy, and nutritional ignorance. Arch Dermatol 2001; 137(5):630–6.

Eosinophilic Esophagitis
Emerging Therapies and Future Perspectives

Alex Straumann, MD

KEYWORDS

- CRTH2 antagonists • Disease monitoring • Eosinophilic esophagitis
- Esophageal distensibility • Esophageal string test • IL-4 antagonist
- IL-13 antagonist

KEY POINTS

- Twenty years have passed since eosinophilic esophagitis was first recognized as a new and distinct entity; this time span has been long enough for research to ascertain several fundamental principles, and also long enough to pose certain critical questions regarding the diagnosis, therapy, and long-term management of this disease.
- In eosinophilic esophagitis, several therapeutic modalities are available but all have important limitations; there is thus an urgent need for alternative treatment options.
- With respect to medications, second-generation CRTH2 antagonists and biologicals targeting IL-13 and/or IL-4 are promising candidates.
- As for dietary treatment, there is hope that a simplified induction regimen, more accurate allergy tests to identify causative food antigens, as well as an individualized maintenance diet will increase the utilization of the dietary approach.

INTRODUCTION

Somewhat more than 20 years have passed since eosinophilic esophagitis (EoE) was first recognized as a new and distinct entity.[1,2] In the early days, the discussion was often dictated by the question, "Do you believe in eosinophilic esophagitis?" This question illustrates the broadly held skepticism that occurs when a disturbing factor invades an established concept which, at that time, was that EoE indicates gastro-esophageal reflux. Twenty years later, this question and the initial skepticism have clearly disappeared and gastroenterologists are informed about, and are familiar with, this immune-mediated esophageal disease. Huge educational efforts, including establishing well-defined diagnostic criteria and therapeutic algorithms,[3–5] combined with personal clinical experience coming from their own EoE patients, have led to this

Conflict of Interest: The author has no conflicts to declare regarding this article.
Swiss EoE Clinic and Swiss EoE Research Network, Roemerstrasse 7, Olten 4600, Switzerland
E-mail address: alex.straumann@hin.ch

change among practitioners. Nevertheless, EoE is still a relatively new disease and one may ask the question, quo vadis? In this article, the focus is on promising therapeutic developments and subsequently on more general perspectives.

EMERGING TREATMENT MODALITIES FOR EoE

EoE is defined as a chronic, mainly Th2-type inflammatory disorder of the esophagus, characterized clinically by symptoms reflecting esophageal dysfunction and, histologically, by an eosinophil-predominant infiltration of the esophageal mucosa.[3–5] Adults and adolescents with EoE usually cope for years with their swallowing disturbances until a food impaction forces them to seek medical attention.[5] This behavior by those affected raised the question of whether EoE patients should continue with their coping strategy or be actively encouraged to seek treatment. Today, the results of several natural history studies suggest that there are at least 3 reasons to treat patients suffering from active EoE: First, dysphagia has a markedly negative impact on the quality of life and this handicap can be precluded by proper treatment.[3–5] Second, untreated EoE patients are at risk for experiencing long-lasting food impactions with the danger of suffering severe esophageal injury.[5] Third, treatment should be sought to prevent esophageal damage caused by tissue remodeling due to uncontrolled eosinophilic inflammation.[4,5] All of the above-mentioned reasons for treatment are valid for both children and adults.[5] Physicians caring for EoE patients are therefore encouraged to inform their patients comprehensively and to offer effective treatment options.

LIMITATIONS OF ESTABLISHED TREATMENT MODALITIES

Currently, the treatment modalities for EoE include the 3 Ds: drugs, allergen avoidance by elimination or elemental diets and, finally, esophageal dilation.[3–5] Furthermore, each of these 3 modalities encompasses several particular options: for instance, at least 10 different drugs are recommended for medical treatment; 3 different dietary regimens are available for allergen avoidance strategy; and 2 types of dilation are currently used. With respect to the long list of available therapeutic modalities, one could ask the question of whether there is actually a need for developing further therapies.

Drugs have the limitation that only corticosteroids have a proven efficacy; indeed, most other compounds have shown only limited or even no effect.[3–5] Swallowed topical corticosteroids (TCS) have undergone the most investigation; they achieve successful remission in up to 80% of patients with active EoE symptoms and inflammation.[6–11] Some 10% of EoE patients require higher doses of TCS to achieve this goal and, with the higher dose, there is an increased risk of systemic side effects.[5] In another 10% of patients, symptoms and inflammation are refractory to TCS treatment.[6–11] Moreover, swallowed TCS have only a limited efficacy in sustaining EoE in clinical and histologic remission over a longer period of time.[12] Systemically administered corticosteroids or immunosuppressants are alternatives,[6] but according to the literature, not superior to TCS[8] and, in addition, their efficacy has not yet been adequately evaluated.[3–5] In several controlled, randomized clinical trials, specific eosinophil-targeted drugs, such as the 2 anti-IL-5 antibodies, mepolizumab and reslizumab, have demonstrated rather disappointing results with persistence of symptoms and endoscopic abnormalities, despite a significant reduction in eosinophils in esophageal tissue and peripheral blood.[13–15] A new approach using the prostaglandin pathway to treat Th2-type inflammations was recently evaluated in EoE: an 8-week blockade of the so-called CRTH2 receptor with the orally available small molecule, OC000459, led to a significant reduction in the eosinophilic inflammation in esophageal tissue, and to a moderate resolution of symptoms and endoscopic abnormalities.

Although the drug was well tolerated, this first-generation CRTH2 antagonist was less effective than swallowed TCS.[16]

Allergen avoidance by dietary measures, the second D, was one of the first modalities attempted to treat EoE.[17] Since the initial endeavors, 3 different dietary approaches that reduce the exposure of the esophagus to allergens have been established.[3–5] All 3 approaches have demonstrated efficacy in bringing active EoE into remission, with complete elimination of food proteins by amino acid formulae proving to be the most successful.[18] Of note, these dietary restrictions likely need to be maintained indefinitely because symptoms and inflammation reappear rapidly after the reintroduction of the causative food.[19,20] Unfortunately, each of these dietary restrictions interferes markedly with the patient's quality of life, either through restricting daily eating habits with amino acid formulae or by elimination of several staple foods, such as milk, wheat, and eggs.[3–5] In addition, severe dietary restrictions entail a risk of malnutrition.

The third D, dilation, has been used to treat EoE since the disease was first recognized[1,2] and provides a rapid and unexpected long-lasting relief of symptoms. Nevertheless, because it does not modulate the underlying inflammation,[21] dilation cannot be considered a first-line treatment of EoE.

In summary, the list of potential therapeutic modalities is, in theory, long, but in reality, rather short. Furthermore, each of the available treatments has severe limitations and none is currently approved. Indeed, even today, in a substantial number of EoE patients, the disease cannot be controlled, and the search continues for successful alternative therapeutic options.[3–5]

THE SEARCH FOR NEW TARGETS

The first step in the discovery and development of any new and novel anti-inflammatory drug consists of the identification of targets that are critically involved in the pathway of the particular inflammation.[22] Identification of relevant pro-inflammatory mediators and their corresponding receptors requires a profound understanding of the disease-specific inflammatory properties.[22] Of note, one difficulty in this procedure is the redundancy of almost all relevant signaling mechanisms. This harbors the risk that blockade of an assumed key signaling pathway does not necessarily lead to the expected effect. Before addressing several candidate drugs, some key properties of the eosinophilic inflammation characterizing EoE are discussed.

EoE presents many features of a Th2-type inflammation.[23] Eosinophils, mast cells, and T cells are involved in this type of inflammatory response, but eosinophils are visually predominant and likely the key effectors. After maturation in the bone marrow, eosinophils relocate to the peripheral circulation and, finally, traffic to specific tissues, primarily the gastrointestinal tract, where they reside for at least 1 week.[24] Although a multitude of cytokines and growth factors are vital in enhancing eosinophil development, it is important to point out that the proliferation and terminal differentiation of eosinophils from precursor myeloblasts depend critically on the presence of interleukin-5 (IL-5).[25] IL-5 is a major eosinophil-specific regulator that is not only responsible for the proliferation and maturation of eosinophils in the bone marrow and release into the circulation, but also for promoting eosinophil survival and activation. In addition, IL-5 primes the response to chemoattractants, such as eotaxin-1, also known as CC-chemokine ligand 11 (CCL11). Expressed by gastrointestinal epithelial and other cells, eotaxin-1 is important for trafficking and accumulation of eosinophils in the gastrointestinal tract in both the steady state and inflammatory conditions. In addition to eotaxin-1, 2 other members of eosinophil-specific chemokines, eotaxin-2 (CCL24) and eotaxin-3 (CCL26), have been identified in humans. Eotaxin-1, eotaxin-2, and eotaxin-3 act through CC-chemokine receptor 3 (CCR3), which is expressed in high levels on eosinophils.[26–28] Among these eosinophil-specific chemokines, eotaxin-3 appears to play a key role in the pathogenesis of EoE, as it has been demonstrated that the level of expression of the eotaxin-3 gene is increased by 53-fold in EoE patients when compared with control subjects.[29] This RNA response has been confirmed at the protein level by immunohistochemistry showing that, in biopsies of EoE patients, the levels of eotaxin-3 correlated with the density of the eosinophils in the esophageal tissue.[29] Allergen exposure in patients with EoE results in an influx of activated Th2 lymphocytes to the site of inflammation and an increase in the tissue levels of Th2 cytokines, thereby leading to eosinophil recruitment and activation at the site of exposure.

The process of eosinophil activation is regulated by a multitude of cytokines, such as IL-5, IL-13, IL-4, and tumor necrosis factor α, which are produced by activated Th2 and mast cells.[3–5,23] On activation, eosinophils produce IgE, up-regulate production of numerous cytokines and chemokines, and then degranulate, thereby releasing preformed granules containing at least 4 major cationic and cytotoxic proteins: eosinophil peroxidase, eosinophil cationic protein, eosinophil-derived neurotoxin, and major basic protein. In the presence of an antigen, the complex interplay between the esophageal epithelium and many of the immune cells, including antigen-presenting cells, Th2, mast cells, and eosinophils, eventually leads to chronic esophageal inflammation.[23] The effect of IL-5 blockade with mepolizumab and reslizumab on EoE has been evaluated in 3 controlled trials.[13–15] This highly selective IL-5 blockade was well tolerated but, unfortunately, neither in children nor in adults, did it fulfill expectations. The significant but isolated eosinophil reduction in esophageal tissue and blood did not lead to a substantial resolution of EoE symptoms,[13–15] thereby indicating that this approach might be too selective. Based on these results, IL-4, IL-13, and the eotaxin-receptor, CCR3, might prove more promising targets.

In addition to this eosinophil-centered pathway, it has been demonstrated that several cells centrally involved in Th2-type inflammation express a common receptor on their surface.[30] This so-called CRTH2 (chemoattractant receptor expressed on Th2 cells) is a G protein-coupled receptor expressed, in particular, by Th2 lymphocytes, eosinophils, and basophils. It mediates chemotaxis of these cells in response to prostaglandin D_2, a key prostanoid in allergic responses produced by mast cells.[30] It can therefore be expected that a blockade of the CRTH2 receptor abolishes the ability of prostaglandin D_2 to cause chemotaxis and activation of Th2 lymphocytes and eosinophils, resulting finally in a suppression of the eosinophilic tissue inflammation associated with EoE.

In summary, based on the above-outlined understanding of EoE's immunopathogenic mechanisms, as well as on the results of in vitro studies, animal models, and clinical trials, the Th2 cytokines, IL-13 and IL-4, the CRTH2 receptor, and the eosinophil-specific chemokine, eotaxin-3, are currently the most promising targets for discovering new antieosinophil drugs.

EMERGING THERAPEUTIC OPTIONS

This section presents promising treatment modalities that are currently under evaluation, but not yet ready for use in clinical practice.

CRTH2 Antagonism

The effect of a selective CRTH2 receptor blockade on EoE has been evaluated using OC000459, the first orally bioavailable CRTH2 antagonist.[31] In a randomized, double-blind, placebo-controlled trial, adult patients with active, severe EoE, dependent on or refractory to corticosteroids, were treated either with OC000459 or with placebo.[16] The primary endpoint was the reduction of eosinophil infiltration in the esophageal tissue. After an 8-week treatment with OC000459, the esophageal eosinophilic load decreased significantly by 36%, whereas no reduction was observed with placebo. In addition, the physician's global assessment of disease activity decreased significantly with OC000459. Summarizing, the first trial evaluating the principle of a CRTH2 blockade in adult patients with severe, active, corticosteroid-refractory EoE has shown a moderate, but significant, anti-eosinophil effect and a beneficial clinical outcome; furthermore, the drug was well tolerated.[16] Based on the results of this first trial and the excellent safety profile, this pathway merits further evaluation, and since the initial study, CRTH2 blockers with a much higher in vitro activity have been developed.

IL-13 Antagonism

A first proof of mechanism study using a fully human anti-IL-13 monoclonal antibody (mAb) in adult patients with active EoE has shown an impressive normalization of the altered genetic pattern, a remarkable (approximately 60%) reduction in the eosinophil load in the esophageal tissue, and a trend toward resolving EoE-related symptoms. Data from this initial study underscore the optimistic perspective of this therapeutic approach, although further investigation is needed.

Empiric 4-Food and Individually Restricted Elimination Diet

To limit the disadvantages of the established dietary allergen avoidance, 2 steps have been proposed: first, several reports indicate that an empiric 4-food elimination regimen might be just as efficient as the established 6-food elimination diet. Unfortunately, the 2 staple foods, "milk" and "wheat," are still excluded in the diet.[32,33] Second, it has been demonstrated that identification of the causative food categories by a controlled reintroduction procedure, followed by an individually restricted elimination of the identified causative food, is sufficient to maintain EoE in remission over a 1-year time period.[20] In one-third of patients, only one food category is implicated; in one-third, 2 food categories, and in the last third, 3 food categories are affected. There is hope that the modified induction diet schedule as well as the individualized maintenance diet will make the dietary approach easier to follow.

In conclusion, simplified diet regimens should soon be standardized and able to replace complex established diets. As for medical treatment, second-generation CRTH2 antagonists as well as biologicals interfering with the IL-13 pathway are under evaluation and should shortly be available, at least in the setting of clinical trials, for patients suffering from severe EoE.

FUTURE THERAPEUTIC OPTIONS

This section discusses novel therapeutic concepts that have the potential to expand the future spectrum of pharmacologic EoE treatments.

IL-4/IL-13 Antagonism

IL-4 and IL-13 signal through 2 different, but overlapping, receptors, both of which contain an identical type II, α-subunit receptor.[34] Blocking this α-subunit could thus potentially inhibit the downstream pathways of both cytokines. A 12-week treatment with dupilumab, a fully human mAb targeting the α-subunit of the IL-4 receptor, improved lung function and reduced Th2-associated inflammatory markers in

52 patients with moderate to severe asthma.[35] Asthma and EoE are both Th2-type inflammations and share several other similarities. The impressive results from basic research and from translational studies performed in asthma encourage the evaluation of the efficacy of similarly blocking the α-subunit of the IL-4 receptor in EoE.

CCR3 Receptor Antagonism

Expanding the idea of receptor blockade, findings from basic research and translational studies again compel an assessment of the efficacy of blocking the CCR3 receptor in EoE.[26–29] CCR3 receptor blockers, oral, small molecules, are currently under development and awaiting evaluation for this application.

As illustrated by this catalog of emerging and future therapeutic options, there is justifiable hope that the near future holds even more therapeutic options for treating EoE patients, especially those suffering from an aggressive form or nonresponders to traditional modalities.

FUTURE PERSPECTIVES FOR EoE

In the 20 years since EoE was first recognized as a distinct entity, much has been learned and some patient suffering has been alleviated. Whether a 20-year period can be considered a long time depends very much on one's perspective. For EoE patients still suffering from dysphagia, 20 years is indeed a long time. However, for researchers assiduously studying this "new" disease, the same period seems rather short. Their progress can be summarized as identification of disease-specific features and development of future-directed perspectives that are discussed below.

NECESSITY OF A PROPER MONITORING STRATEGY

First of all, 20 years has been long enough to learn that EoE is a *chronic disease.*[3–5] Inherent to chronic disease is the fact that proper diagnosis is only the first step in management; establishing long-term medical care is equally important. For EoE, the question is, what does "long-term medical care" entail? Which markers should be surveyed? Can we rely on symptoms or do we need to monitor endoscopic and histologic features on a regular schedule? Which follow-up intervals are reasonable?

In these 2 decades, it has been recognized that, in EoE, symptoms and inflammatory activity are, surprisingly, not closely linked,[11] and that the risk of impending food impaction cannot be reliably assessed based on symptoms alone.[36] Current standard recommendations that will likely remain valid for the near future entail regular annual follow-up examinations with invasive and costly endoscopic and histologic evaluation. Promising alternatives that loom on the horizon include a minimally invasive 1-hour esophageal string test[37] and the noninvasive determination of eosinophil-derived specific markers in the feces.

NECESSITY OF A RELIABLE ASSESSMENT OF ESOPHAGEAL FUNCTION

In these 20 years, it has been recognized that *ongoing eosinophilic inflammation leads to so-called remodeling of the esophagus.*[3–5] This process has been proven and characterized on the molecular, cellular, and tissue levels. Mural thickening, stiffness, increased fragility, and friability with an ensuing loss of function are the clinical results of this process. Indeed, symptoms reflecting esophageal dysfunction are even included in the conceptual definition of EoE.[4] This EoE-inherent feature raises the question, "How can one assess esophageal function in EoE?" This question is of particular interest as, so far, the established functional esophageal tests (eg, high-resolution manometry, impedance/pH-monitoring, or the barostat) have shown uncharacteristic or even conflicting results.[3,4]

First studies measuring the esophageal wall distensibility using the EndoFlip (endo-luminal functional lumen imaging probe) imaging system (Crospon, Carlsbad, CA, USA), a tool that determines the relationship between esophageal cross-sectional area and pressure, have delivered promising results.[38] This method thus has the potential to be of use both at diagnosis and during the follow-up of EoE patients; it demonstrates both inflammatory activity and the stage of remodeling.

NECESSITY OF EARLY AND CONSISTENT CONTROL OF EOSINOPHILIC INFLAMMATION

Moreover, 20 years have been long enough to learn that *stricture formation is a serious concern in EoE.* "Narrow esophagus," "small-caliber esophagus," "ringed esophagus," and "esophageal strictures" are only some of the terms used in association with EoE. They all illustrate that EoE can lead to a shrinking of the esophageal lumen. Indeed, a recently published long-term study has shown that the longer EoE goes untreated, the higher the risk of developing strictures.[39] Of note, currently in North America and in Europe, EoE is, on average, not diagnosed before 5 to 6 years after onset of symptoms.[3–5] This long period of untreated inflammation poses the question of what could be done to shorten the time that the esophagus is exposed to an ongoing, untreated eosinophilic inflammation in EoE patients.

Attempts should be undertaken to promote the information that "dysphagia for solids" is a red flag symptom and should be taken just as seriously as, for instance, a positive test for occult blood in the feces. In addition, after establishing the diagnosis, a consistent long-term treatment should be started to control the inflammation as much as possible.

NECESSITY OF AN INDIVIDUALIZED THERAPEUTIC APPROACH

Twenty years have also been long enough to learn that *EoE is not at all a uniform disease, but that different EoE phenotypes* exist. Clinicians are confronted with a broad spectrum of EoE types, ranging from mild, almost asymptomatic forms with only few eosinophils in the tissue, up to severely diseased patients. Thus, it is not yet clear whether patients suffering from an aggressive form have an overall poorer prognosis than do those with a milder variant, then posing the question of whether all these different phenotypes should be managed according to the same principles.

There is evidence that more long-term natural history studies are required to understand and to manage appropriately all these different forms of the same underlying disease.

NECESSITY OF A NEW DISEASE CONCEPT

Finally, 20 years have also been long enough to learn that a sizable subgroup of patients suffer from symptoms of esophageal dysfunction, often leading to bolus impaction, and have endoscopically typical EoE signs, but show only few or even no eosinophils in the esophageal tissue, briefly, *"EoE without eosinophils"* or *"noneosinophilic esophagitis."* This curious observation raises the question of the actual role of the eosinophil in the immunopathogenesis of this disease. Attempts are underway to improve the understanding of this intriguing phenomenon. As more information is collected, it will surely improve the understanding of EoE's immunopathogenesis and, in turn, even open new paths for effective therapeutic concepts.

As highlighted by this discussion of emerging concepts, EoE is still a relatively new and enigmatic disease. These perspectives will certainly stimulate further research; it is hoped to result in improved care and treatment of EoE patients.

SUMMARY

- Most patients suffering from active EoE can be treated adequately with the currently available therapeutic modalities. However, up to one-third of patients do not achieve clinical and histologic remission despite medication or diet therapies.
- EoE is a chronic inflammatory disease requiring long-term treatment; nevertheless, with currently available options, as many as one-half of patients experience a relapse within 1 year, despite proper adherence to treatment.
- Biologicals targeting IL-13 and/or IL-4 have the potential to improve response rates in patients suffering from severe or refractory EoE.
- Second-generation CRTH2 antagonists and, empirically, limited elimination diets, afford the possibility of reducing the relapse rate on a long-term basis.
- EoE is a chronic disease presenting with a variety of clinical and histologic phenotypes; a more profound understanding of these different forms including their long-term risks is urgently needed.

ACKNOWLEDGMENTS

We are grateful to Kathleen Bucher for editorial assistance and to all our EoE patients for their committed collaboration.

REFERENCES

1. Attwood SE, Smyrk TC, Demeester TR, et al. Esophageal eosinophilia with dysphagia. A distinct clinicopathologic syndrome. Dig Dis Sci 1993;38: 109–16.
2. Straumann A, Spichtin HP, Bernoulli R, et al. Idiopathic eosinophilic esophagitis: a frequently overlooked disease with typical clinical aspects and discrete endoscopic findings. Schweiz Med Wochenschr 1994;124:1419–29 [in German with English abstract].
3. Furuta GT, Liacouras C, Collins MH, et al. Eosinophilic esophagitis in children and adults: a systematic review and consensus recommendations for diagnosis and treatment. Gastroenterology 2007;133:1342–63.
4. Liacouras CA, Furuta GT, Hirano I, et al. Eosinophilic esophagitis: updated consensus recommendations for children and adults. J Allergy Clin Immunol 2011;128:3–20.
5. Straumann A, Aceves SS, Blanchard C, et al. Pediatric and adult eosinophilic esophagitis: similarities and differences. Allergy 2012;67:477–90.
6. Liacouras CA, Wenner WJ, Brown K, et al. Primary eosinophilic esophagitis in children: successful treatment with oral corticosteroids. J Pediatr Gastroenterol Nutr 1998;26:380–5.
7. Konikoff MR, Noel RJ, Blanchard C, et al. A randomized, double-blind, placebo-controlled trial of fluticasone propionate for pediatric eosinophilic esophagitis. Gastroenterology 2006;131:1381–91.
8. Schaefer ET, Fitzgerald JF, Molleston JP, et al. Comparison of oral prednisone and topical fluticasone in the treatment of eosinophilic esophagitis: a randomized trial in children. Clin Gastroenterol Hepatol 2008;6:165–73.

9. Dohil R, Newbury R, Fox L, et al. Oral viscous budesonide is effective in children with eosinophilic esophagitis in a randomized, placebo-controlled trial. Gastroenterology 2010;139:418–29.

10. Straumann A, Conus S, Degen L, et al. Budesonide is effective in adolescent and adult patients with active eosinophilic esophagitis. Gastroenterology 2010;139:1526–37.

11. Alexander JA, Jung KW, Arora AS, et al. Swallowed fluticasone improves histologic but not symptomatic response of adults with eosinophilic esophagitis. Clin Gastroenterol Hepatol 2012;10:742–9.

12. Straumann A, Conus S, Degen L, et al. Long-term budesonide maintenance treatment is partially effective for patients with eosinophilic esophagitis. Clin Gastroenterol Hepatol 2011;9:400–9.

13. Straumann A, Conus S, Grzonka P, et al. Anti-interleukin-5 antibody treatment (mepolizumab) in active eosinophilic esophagitis: a randomised, placebo-controlled, double-blind trial. GUT 2010;59:21–30.

14. Assa'ad AH, Gupta SK, Collins MH, et al. An antibody against IL-5 reduces numbers of esophageal intraepithelial eosinophils in children with eosinophilic esophagitis. Gastroenterology 2011;141:1593–604.

15. Spergel JM, Rothenberg ME, Collins MH, et al. Reslizumab in children and adolescents with eosinophilic esophagitis: results of a double-blind, randomized, placebo-controlled trial. J Allergy Clin Immunol 2012;129:456–63.

16. Straumann A, Hoesli S, Bussmann Ch, et al. Anti-eosinophil activity and clinical efficacy of the CRTH2 antagonist OC000459 in eosinophilic esophagitis. Allergy 2013;68:375–85.

17. Kelly KJ, Lazenby AJ, Rowe PC, et al. Eosinophilic esophagitis attributed to gastroesophageal reflux: improvement with an amino acid-based formula. Gastroenterology 1995;109:1503–12.

18. Henderson CJ, Abonia JP, King EC, et al. Comparative dietary therapy effectiveness in remission of pediatric eosinophilic esophagitis. J Allergy Clin Immunol 2012;129:1570–8.

19. Gonsalves N, Yang GY, Doerfler B, et al. Elimination diet effectively treats eosinophilic esophagitis in adults; food reintroduction identifies causative factors. Gastroenterology 2012;142:1451–9.

20. Lucendo AJ, Arias Á, González-Cervera J, et al. Empiric 6-food elimination diet induced and maintained prolonged remission in patients with adult eosinophilic esophagitis: a prospective study on the food cause of the disease. J Allergy Clin Immunol 2013;131:797–804.

21. Schoepfer AM, Gonsalves N, Bussmann C, et al. Esophageal dilation in eosinophilic esophagitis: effectiveness, safety and impact on the underlying inflammation. Am J Gastroenterol 2010;105:1062–70.

22. Levin JI, Laufer S, editors. Anti-inflammatory drug discovery in. London: RSC Drug Discovery; 2012. p. 1–4 Series, No 26.

23. Straumann A, Bauer M, Fischer B, et al. Idiopathic eosinophilic esophagitis is associated with a $T_{(H)}2$-type allergic inflammatory response. J Allergy Clin Immunol 2001;108:954–61.

24. Rothenberg ME, Mishra A, Brandt EB, et al. Gastrointestinal eosinophils in health and disease. Adv Immunol 2001;78:291–328.

25. Yamaguchi Y, Suda T, Suda J, et al. Purified interleukin 5 supports the terminal differentiation and proliferation of murine eosinophilic precursors. J Exp Med 1988;167:43–56.

26. Mishra A, Hogan SP, Lee JJ, et al. Fundamental signals that regulate eosinophil homing to the gastrointestinal tract. J Clin Invest 1999;103:1719–27.

27. Garcia-Zepeda EA, Rothenberg ME, Ownbey RT, et al. Human eotaxin is a specific chemoattractant for eosinophil cells and provides a new mechanism to explain tissue eosinophilia. Nat Med 1996;2:449–56.
28. Forssmann U, Uguccioni M, Loetscher P, et al. Eotaxin-2, a novel CC chemokine that is selective for the chemokine receptor CCR3, and acts like eotaxin on human eosinophil and basophil leukocytes. J Exp Med 1997;185:2171–6.
29. Blanchard C, Wang N, Stringer KF, et al. Eotaxin-3 and a unique conserved gene-expression profile in eosinophilic esophagitis. J Clin Invest 2006;116:536–47.
30. Pettipher R, Hansel TT, Armer R. Antagonism of the prostaglandin D2 receptors DP1 and CRTH2 as an approach to treat allergic diseases. Nat Rev Drug Discov 2007;6:313–25.
31. Pettipher R, Vinall SL, Xue L, et al. Pharmacologic profile of OC000459, a potent, selective, and orally active D prostanoid receptor 2 antagonist that inhibits mast cell-dependent activation of T helper 2 lymphocytes and eosinophils. J Pharmacol Exp Ther 2012;340:473–82.
32. Gonsalves N, Doerfler B, Hirano I. Long term maintenance therapy with dietary restriction in adults with eosinophilic esophagitis [abstract]. Gastroenterology 2011;140. S-180-S-181.
33. Kagalwalla AF, Amsden K, Shah A, et al. Cow's milk elimination: a novel dietary approach to treat eosinophilic esophagitis. J Pediatr Gastroenterol Nutr 2012;55:711–6.
34. Wills-Karp M, Finkelman FD. Untangling the complex web of IL-4- and IL-13-mediated signaling pathways. Sci Signal 2008;1(51):pe55.
35. Wenzel S, Ford L, Pearlman D, et al. Dupilumab in persistent asthma with elevated eosinophil levels. N Engl J Med 2013;368:2455–66.
36. Nicodème F, Hirano I, Chen J, et al. Esophageal distensibility as a measure of disease severity in patients with eosinophilic esophagitis. Clin Gastroenterol Hepatol 2013;11:1101–7.
37. Furuta GT, Kagalwalla AF, Lee JJ, et al. The oesophageal string test: a novel, minimally invasive method measures mucosal inflammation in eosinophilic oesophagitis. Gut 2013;62:1395–405.
38. Kwiatek MA, Hirano I, Kahrilas PJ, et al. Mechanical properties of the esophagus in eosinophilic esophagitis. Gastroenterology 2011;140:82–90.
39. Schoepfer AM, Safroneeva E, Bussmann C, et al. Delay in diagnosis of eosinophilic esophagitis increases risk for stricture formation in a time-dependent manner. Gastroenterology 2013;145:1230–6.

Index

Note: Page numbers of article titles are in **boldface** type.

Gastroenterol Clin N Am 43 (2014) 395–403
http://dx.doi.org/10.1016/S0889-8553(14)00046-6
0889-8553/14/$ – see front matter © 2014 Elsevier Inc. All rights reserved.

gastro.theclinics.com

Moving?

Make sure your subscription moves with you!

To notify us of your new address, find your **Clinics Account Number** (located on your mailing label above your name), and contact customer service at:

Email: journalscustomerservice-usa@elsevier.com

800-654-2452 (subscribers in the U.S. & Canada)
314-447-8871 (subscribers outside of the U.S. & Canada)

Fax number: 314-447-8029

Elsevier Health Sciences Division
Subscription Customer Service
3251 Riverport Lane
Maryland Heights, MO 63043

*To ensure uninterrupted delivery of your subscription, please notify us at least 4 weeks in advance of move.